Psychiatric Institutions and Society

The book probes how the serious and sometimes fatal decision was made to admit individuals to asylums during Germany's age of extremes. The book shows that—even during the Nazi killing of the sick—relatives played an even more important role in most admissions than doctors and the authorities.

In light of admission practices, this study traces how ideas about illness, safety, and normality changed when the Nazi regime collapsed in 1945 and illuminates how closely power configurations in the psychiatric sector were linked to political and social circumstances.

Stefanie Coché is a historian at the Justus-Liebig-University, Giessen. Her research interests are history of psychiatry, religious history, German history, and American history.

Routledge Studies in Modern European History

The Laboratory of Progress
Switzerland in the Nineteenth Century, Volume 2
Joseph Jung

The Brandt Commission and the Multinationals
Planetary Perspectives
Bo Stråth

Obscene Traffic
Prostitution and global migrations from the Italian perspective (1890–1940)
Laura Schettini

Mussolini and the Rise of Populism
The Man Who Made Fascism
Spencer M. Di Scala

Britain, France and the Battle for the Leadership of Europe, 1957–2007
Richard Davis

A British Education Control Officer in Occupied Germany, 1945–1949
The Letters of Edward Aitken-Davies
David Phillips

Print and the Celtic Languages
Publishing and Reading in Irish, Welsh, Gaelic and Breton, 1700–1900
Niall Ó Ciosáin

Psychiatric Institutions and Society
The Practice of Psychiatric Committal in the "Third Reich," the Democratic Republic of Germany, and the Federal Republic of Germany, 1941–1963
Stefanie Coché

For more information about this series, please visit: https://www.routledge.com/Routledge-Studies-in-Modern-European-History/book-series/SE0246

Psychiatric Institutions and Society

The Practice of Psychiatric Committal
in the "Third Reich,"
the Democratic Republic of Germany,
and the Federal Republic of Germany,
1941–1963

Stefanie Coché
Translated by Alex Skinner

The translation of this work was funded by the Hamburger Stiftung zur Förderung von Wissenschaft und Kultur, the Deutsche Gesellschaft für Geschichte der Nervenheilkunde (DGGN) e.V. (German Society for the History of Neurosciences), and the Justus Liebig University Giessen.

Routledge
Taylor & Francis Group

LONDON AND NEW YORK

First published in English 2024
by Routledge
4 Park Square, Milton Park, Abingdon, Oxon OX14 4RN

and by Routledge
605 Third Avenue, New York, NY 10158

Routledge is an imprint of the Taylor & Francis Group, an informa business

© 2024 Stefanie Coché

Translated by Alex Skinner

© Brill Deutschland GmbH, Vandenhoeck & Ruprecht, Psychiatrie
und Gesellschaft. Psychiatrische Einweisungspraxis im Dritten Reich,
in der DDR und der Bundesrepublik 1941–1963, Stefanie Coché
(Göttingen, 2017)

British Library Cataloguing-in-Publication Data
A catalogue record for this book is available from the British Library

ISBN: 978-1-032-71617-6 (hbk)
ISBN: 978-1-032-71622-0 (pbk)
ISBN: 978-1-032-71623-7 (ebk)

DOI: 10.4324/9781032716237

Typeset in Times New Roman
by MPS Limited, Dehradun

Contents

Acknowledgments

This book is a slightly revised version of my PhD dissertation, originally written in German, which was accepted by the Faculty of Arts and Humanities at the University of Cologne in December 2014. The English edition of my book would not have been possible without the generous support of the Hamburg Foundation for the Promotion of Science and Culture (Hamburger Stiftung zur Förderung von Wissenschaft und Kultur), the German Society for the History of Neurosciences (Deutsche Gesellschaft für Geschichte der Nervenheilkunde e.V. or DGGN), and the head of my department at Justus Liebig University Giessen, Friedrich Lenger. Working with Alex Skinner, who did an outstanding job translating the German manuscript into English, was a pleasure: I am deeply impressed by his accuracy and speed and the interest he showed in my book beyond mere questions of translation.

At Routledge, Robert Langham supported my proposal from the outset and guided me through the editorial and production process. This was a wonderful experience from start to finish.

It is a great pleasure to express my gratitude to my doctoral advisor Ralph Jessen, who played a major role in making my doctoral studies a carefree, enjoyable time replete with stimulating discussions. I thank him for the many conversations, his unwavering support, and his keen interest in and enthusiasm for my doctorate. I also extend my gratitude to Ulrike Lindner for acting as second examiner and to Margit Szöllösi-Janze for her all-round support and extremely helpful comments on my manuscript as the third examiner. My thanks to Mitchell Ash for welcoming me to speak at the "Natural Sciences in Historical Context" ("Naturwissenschaften im Historischen Kontext") colloquium in Vienna in the fall of 2013 and for the opportunity to discuss my project in that circle and with him. I am thankful to Sybille Steinbacher for facilitating my participation in her colloquium and for providing valuable feedback on my dissertation during the initial stages of its composition in Vienna. Klaus-Michael Mallmann deserves thanks for his in-depth assessment of my dissertation idea at the very beginning of the project. To Thomas Stamm-Kuhlmann I owe a debt of gratitude for the opportunity to take part in his colloquium during my archival trip to Greifswald. I would also like to thank Hedwig Richter and Frank Möller for a pleasant and intellectually stimulating time there.

My research was supported by generous scholarships from the a.r.t.e.s. Graduate School for the Humanities and the German Academic Exchange Service (Deutscher Akademischer Austauschdienst or DAAD). The a.r.t.e.s. Graduate School for the Humanities not only provided secure funding for my entire doctoral period but also financed my numerous and extensive archival trips without red tape. Above all, though, it gave me the opportunity to work on its premises while continuously exchanging ideas with other researchers, including several from different disciplines. Thanks to this ongoing dialogue and the friendship with Corinna Kühn, Jule Schaffer, Cornelia Kratz, and Britta Tewordt, I look back on my time at a.r.t.e.s with great fondness. In addition, I would like to thank Stefan Grohé, who led the a.r.t.e.s. class together with Ralph Jessen, for his strong support of the "Erste Generation Promotion" (EGP) project as Dean of the Faculty of Arts and Humanities. My thanks also go to Manuela Günther for the positive and helpful discussions and her support during the final phase of my doctorate as an EGP mentor. I owe a debt of gratitude to my colleagues Frauke Scheffler, Sandra Vacca, Verena Limper, and Ann-Kristin Kolwes for the enjoyable and successful collaboration within the EGP initiative. Over the years, many friends have helped me by discussing ideas and texts with me. As prime examples, I would like to thank Maximilian Ruland, Barbara Manthe, Robert Fuchs, Brian K. Feltman, Frauke Scheffler, Sascha Penshorn, Jens Gründler, and Susanne Schregel.

My heartfelt thanks also go to the staff at the numerous archives I visited. The provision of almost 1,500 psychiatric case files was highly time-consuming and, in some cases, legally complicated. My special thanks to Christina Vanja and Dieter Ingold at the Archive of the Hesse Land Welfare Association (Landeswohlfahrtsverband Hessen), Nikolaus Braun at the Archive of the District of Upper Bavaria (Archiv des Bezirk Oberbayern), Tobias Crabus at the Chemnitz State Archive (Staatsarchiv Chemnitz), Dirk Alvermann at the Greifswald University Archive (Universitätsarchiv Greifswald), and Kerstin Stockhecke at the Main Archive of the von Bodelschwingh Foundations Bethel (Hauptarchiv der von Bodelschwinghschen Stiftungen Bethel).

I would also like to express my gratitude for the awards I received for my dissertation manuscript from the German Society for the History of Neurosciences (Deutsche Gesellschaft für Geschichte der Nervenheilkunde), the German Society for the History of Hospitals (Deutsche Gesellschaft für Krankenhausgeschichte e. V.), the Academy of Useful Science, Erfurt (Akademie gemeinnütziger Wissenschaften zu Erfurt), the Documentation Center of Austrian Resistance (Dokumentationsarchiv des Österreichischen Widerstands or DÖW), and the University of Cologne (Offermann Hergarten Preis).

I owe a special debt of gratitude to my family. I thank Daniel Brewing not only for numerous conversations about my dissertation, but also for a wonderful time outside of work. I also thank my siblings, Svenja, Moritz, and Joel. It is a pleasure to dedicate this book to my parents, Michael and Annette Coché. Annette taught me in the most spontaneous and natural ways to look at things from many different perspectives and to relate these points of view to each other. Without her influence, the present book would likely never have seen the light of day.

Introduction

Topic and period of investigation

The 36-year-old Martina R.[1] crossed the institutional threshold in March 1946, presenting herself for admission to the Marburg Land Sanatorium (Landesheilanstalt or LHA) accompanied by her mother-in-law. The mother of four thus became a psychiatric patient. "Patient has been suffering from depressive moods for several days,"[2] was the GP's finding on which the referral for "immediate treatment and specialist medical assessment" was based.[3] Her mother-in-law was quoted as stating that the "patient has been severely depressed for about eight weeks. Yesterday she flew into a kind of rage at her child."[4] Yet this committal was no automatic medical process. Martina R. signed a declaration of voluntariness when she was admitted, making this a civil committal. Her mother-in-law was cited as follows: "She brought her daughter-in-law here because the [female] doctor had stated that [her family] could no longer bear responsibility for her. It takes some time, [her mother-in-law remarked], to admit that a member of your own family is no longer mentally normal, because you are unwilling to believe it yourself."[5] Her mother-in-law provided a psychologizing explanation for the need for treatment that referred directly to specific contemporary conditions: "The blows of fate she has suffered in the last few years were too much for this delicate little woman. Her husband is still in a political camp as a member of the SS. He lost his job at the outset, his property has been confiscated, and the patient's parents have also lost everything. [...]"[6] In this respect, the case of Martina R. is exemplary: psychiatric committals are complex negotiation processes involving a variety of institutional and non-institutional actors whose reasoning varies. The constellation of actors in a particular case, how these processes unfolded, and the rationales put forward by different actors make psychiatric committals a high-yield object of historical study. Who was committed and why—and who was involved in this? What does this tell us about ideas of "normality," security (the terms "security" and "safety" are used in this book to convey the German *Sicherheit* depending on context), illness, and health in a society? The core interest of the present study is in the practice of psychiatric committals between 1941 and 1963 in three specific

DOI: 10.4324/9781032716237-1

time periods: I probe continuities and ruptures—in terms of the history of both everyday life and science—in the "Third Reich" and in the two German successor states. How and why did people end up in an asylum or psychiatric clinic during World War II, and in the early German Democratic Republic (GDR or East Germany) and Federal Republic of Germany (FRG or West Germany)? What does this say about these societies?

The period under investigation begins in wartime, which is particularly informative when it comes to analyzing exclusionary mechanisms under National Socialism: the war accelerated the "radicalization of hierarchizing, selective and exclusionary ways of dealing with patients."[7] The year 1941 makes sense as a starting point for this study for two reasons. At least after the public speeches by Bishop von Galen, we can assume that knowledge of the Nazi murder of the sick was widespread among the German population,[8] a policy that was carried out in a decentralized manner after the regime brought a halt to the T4 campaign.[9] Decisions on committal subsequent to the cessation of T4 must be interpreted against the background of this substantial degree of public knowledge.[10] Moreover, the year 1941 represents a turning point in the war in several respects,[11] one that altered the situation on the "home front." Well aware of the war-weariness of the German public during World War I, the Nazi regime initially strove to achieve the greatest possible degree of normality. When the fortunes of war shifted in 1941, however, the government pivoted to a more pragmatic approach. Against this backdrop, both asylums and the conditions of committal practices underwent major change as beds were increasingly appropriated for injured soldiers. We also have to consider the numerous transfers between asylums that occurred within the framework of the Brandt Campaign, which began in 1942.[12] The period under investigation ended before demands for psychiatric reforms gained traction in East and West Germany. The so-called "Rodewisch Propositions" (*Rodewischer Thesen*), a list of demands for the reform of psychiatry in the GDR composed in 1963, mark the end of the period considered in this book. For the Federal Republic of Germany, no phenomenon comparable to the Rodewisch Propositions can be identified prior to the Psychiatry Inquiry of 1975, though this was the outcome of lengthy public and professional debates. Against this background, the Rodewisch Propositions are an apt means of marking off an era because psychiatrists from West Germany also took part in the conference at which they were formulated.[13]

Martina R.'s committal is symptomatic of German society in the immediate postwar period, one of upheaval and "collapse."[14] Her medical history features the impressions and evaluations of her relatives, which convey the ways in which the patient's behavior clashed with what was considered desirable. One of them remarked, for example, that Martina R. had failed to adapt to her new situation after the loss of her house and property by "pitching in." Her (female) cousin claimed that the patient had "white hands from doing nothing."[15] This case demonstrates that a range of different criteria and their potentially gender- or class-specific definitions overlapped in committal practices. Doctors considered these statements and referred to the family in their own reasoning. The (female) family doctor in this instance referred to the family and its social status as well as to a telephone conversation with another institution, the Marburg University Psychiatric Clinic (Universitäts- und Nervenklinik Marburg), which preceded the admission. The patient's mother-in-law cited the family doctor's expert opinion to legitimize her daughter-in-law's impending stay in the asylum. Her mother-in-law's statements precede those of the patient herself in her medical file. In this case, all the medical laypersons who made statements were family members, but individuals from the patient's work environment or neighbors could also be involved. As Martina R.'s committal was of a civil character, she signed a declaration of voluntariness when she was admitted. In the course of compulsory committals, meanwhile, police officers and lawyers could also be involved in the committal process.

Committals did not depend on "clear" or "objective" criteria but on the interaction of different actors under circumstances specific to the time and context. The special relevance of the relationship between different rationales lies in the fact that committals are one of the most consequential "negotiations" in modern societies. The removal—for a more or less limited period of time—of people from their ordinary lives through admission to a psychiatric institution emerges as a litmus test not only of individual freedom, autonomy, and life chances, but also of the social understanding of health, normality, security and decency.

In line with this, the present study not only provides examinations of committal processes during World War II, and in the early FRG and GDR, but also proceeds on an integrative basis, asking what this tells us about these societies and whether we can identify continuities and ruptures.[16] Using a combination of approaches from the history of science, the history of the justice system, and the history of everyday life, it makes a contribution to German social history that addresses conditions in both "totalitarian" dictatorships and in the West German postwar democracy in relation to one another. In the present work, my core interest is in practice, the analysis of which often allows more profound conclusions to be drawn about the mechanisms of a society than the mere examination of rules, concepts, and intentions.[17]

Committal practices took place at the *threshold* of the institution. Here I adhere to Cornelia Brink's definition of the threshold as a "zone [belonging to] the inside and outside"[18] of the asylum.[19] This liminal zone was co-constituted and reconstituted in each individual case by actors inside the asylum, in other words, psychiatrists, neurologists, and in the case of religious establishments also clergy, as well as by actors outside of them, including patients, their families, family doctors and medical specialists, and police and the courts. While just a few articles on the German-speaking countries take account of the patient's social environment, research on the English-speaking world shows how crucial decisions outside the asylum were in the institutional run-up to committals.[20] When it comes to the National Socialist era, the GDR, and the

FRG, changes in societal ideas about what psychiatric establishments were for and whom they ought to serve, and in the associated processes of inclusion and exclusion, have as yet only been investigated in relation to regulatory systems and with respect to the history of scandals.[21] Almost no studies, especially for the twentieth century, take into account the patients' families and social environment.[22] Cornelia Brink's work deals primarily with regulations on compulsory committal and discourses on this topic. The same applies to the comparative study on the FRG and the GDR by Sabine Hanrath. In neither case are patient files used as a source.[23] As a result of the public interest in the political abuse of psychiatric institutions, which was ignited as early as 1990 by a series in *Stern* magazine on the Waldheim Clinic, it was this topic that was initially foregrounded in post-1989 research on psychiatry in East Germany. The seminal study by Sonja Süß, however, concludes that, in contrast to the Soviet Union, there was no systematic political abuse of psychiatry in the GDR.[24] Studies that go beyond topics of this kind can be found mainly in the English-speaking world and are mostly oriented toward the history of psychology rather than psychiatry.[25]

For the first time, then, the present study scrutinizes the nature of power relations between different groups of actors—institutional as well as non-institutional—in relation to psychiatric committals in specific, mid-twentieth-century contexts, while seeking to reveal the room for maneuver available in each case.[26] *Power* is understood in relational terms, in other words as a social relationship. As such, power is not static, but a "dynamic phenomenon" in which "the relationship between individuals, groups and institutions is constantly changing due to their asymmetrical and reciprocal relations."[27] I thus work with a broad concept of power to comprehend the actors involved in the practice of committal in the light of their relations to each other. This also allows me to emphasize the varying degrees of openness of the committal situation even in cases of compulsory committals formally subject to clear regulations. My approach thus enables me to investigate the various groups involved in a nuanced way. The key figures here are psychiatrists in asylums and university psychiatric clinics, public health officers in the health offices, hospital doctors, and independent physicians. This approach also facilitates examination of the relationship between medical institutions and the police,[28] as well as the purposeful (*eigensinnig*) behavior of the patient's relatives within committal practices. Following Alf Lüdtke, I deploy the concept of purposefulness (*Eigensinn*) to analyze the actions of patients and their families. I show that they displayed this purposeful conduct in many ways, by initiating committals and seizing opportunities for committal, as well as by adopting certain rationales, which they often transformed or articulated in a nuanced manner.[29]

The present study thus differs from a strongly discourse-oriented, Foucauldian tradition of psychiatric historiography, but also from interpretations informed by the work of Erving Goffman, which analyze patients as actors but always place them in a reactive position.[30] This book, in contrast, seeks to examine in an open-ended way the power relations among all the actors involved in committals to six psychiatric institutions under the specific conditions of World War II and the early GDR and FRG, taking emphatic account of the committed persons themselves and their social milieu. This conceptual framework furnishes us with a rare opportunity to shine a light on the inclusionary and exclusionary processes characteristic of non-institutional actors during the war and in the postwar period.[31]

The present study works on the assumption that the relationship between institutions and lay people can be best described through the push-and-pull model that is an established feature of English-language research. In line with this template, I assume that committals cannot be explained without considering the involvement of doctors and police on the one hand and families and the social environment on the other. So far, studies on periods after World War I have not used the push-and-pull model.[32] The present book thus offers an alternative interpretation of the role of psychiatric establishments in the mid-twentieth century. A praxeological perspective unsettles established attributions of relevance and agency: while state coercion remains significant, as do regulatory and scientific knowledge, they take a back seat to everyday knowledge and power relations in social microcosms. This allows us to question established narratives and research foci vis-à-vis all three societies. In the course of this book, I will show that the practice of committing patients to psychiatric institutions took on more radical forms during World War II, with significant participation of the general public despite knowledge of the regime's murder of the sick. As yet, very little attention has been paid to non-institutional actors in research on the history of psychiatry during the Nazi era.[33] The scholarly focus on rules and public debates, especially with regard to the Federal Republic of Germany, risks portraying the history of psychiatry as a grand narrative in which locking people up was superseded by de-hospitalization from the 1970s onwards. The praxeological perspective, in contrast, reveals that even in the 1950s and 1960s, asylums were used for a wide variety of reasons and also for very short stays. The buzzwords "coercion" and "locking up" in themselves create a distorted picture of how psychiatry was embedded in society. Other important factors included individuals' hopes of gaining medical help and restoring their ability to work. Examination of the practice of committals, meanwhile, shows that in the GDR, those carried out against the patient's will did not usually involve any form of state intervention. Here, the findings of a praxeological study call into question entrenched interpretations of the relationship between state power and society.[34]

Object of inquiry

This study focuses on the committal of "adult" patients. Rather than foregrounding the legal age of majority in this regard,[35] I examine individuals committed to adult wards, a group that often included adolescents of around sixteen and above.

The process of inpatient committal to a psychiatric institution can be divided analytically into three successive steps. A committal decision was followed by the formal initiation of admission and finally the patient's entry into the asylum. The decision to commit concluded with the official instigation of committal, which could be undertaken by medical, police, or judicial personnel in the period under investigation here. At the same time, this official move was already part of the formal initiation of the committal. Admission itself describes the physical entry into the clinic or asylum; during World War II and in the FRG this almost always came after the committal decision. Only in the GDR could the decision to commit and admission itself coincide in time and place. Entry into an establishment is discussed here only if it coincided with the committal decision, since the institution as a place is not the subject of this study.[36] The core focus of my analysis is the decision to commit. I pay little attention to the formal initiation of admission, as this was essentially an inter-institutional process not influenced by those committed or their milieu. Moreover, there was usually no discussion between institutions as to whether the person to be committed did in fact require institutionalization.[37] The formal initiation of admission does become relevant, however, when it plays a role in concrete committal decisions or when—as a prerequisite for committal practices—it helps us understand psychiatric institutions in a given society.

Committal practices are examined with reference to six psychiatric institutions: the Eglfing-Haar Sanatorium-Nursing Home (*Heil- und Pflegeanstalt*) in Munich, the Marburg an der Lahn Land Sanatorium (*Landesheilanstalt* or LHA), the von Bodelschwingh Asylums Bethel (von Bodelschwinghsche Anstalten Bethel) in Bielefeld, the Saxony Land Sanatorium-Nursing Home for the Mentally Ill (Sächsische Landes-Heil- und Pflegeanstalt für Geisteskranke) in Untergöltzsch (later Rodewisch) in the district of Karl-Marx-Stadt,[38] the Großschweidnitz Sanatorium-Nursing Home near Görlitz, and the Greifswald University Psychiatric Clinic (Psychiatrische und Nervenklinik der Universitätsklinik Greifswald).[39] These facilities were located in different West German federal states or East German districts, which allows me to bring out regional differences and similarities. The same applies to the religious dimension. Some of these institutions were located in predominantly Catholic areas, such as Eglfing-Haar, others in mainly Protestant ones, such as Untergöltzsch. The establishments also differed in terms of their participation in the Nazi murder of the sick, though death rates were high in all of them.[40] A huge number of patients were transferred to Saxony, which was a regional stronghold of murder by medication.[41] Eglfing-Haar, under its director Hermann Pfannmüller (1886–1961), was also directly involved in the decentralized murder of the sick. In early 1943, two so-called "hunger houses" (*Hungerhäuser*) were set up especially for this purpose, with patients being deliberately and systematically neglected. Residents there were also killed through overdose of medication. In the LHA Marburg, mortality due to malnutrition was already rising before the war. As far as is known, however, this establishment was not a site of selective murder through the targeted administration of a "starvation diet" (*Hungerkost*) or overdose of medication.[42] The same applies to the von Bodelschwingh Asylums and the Greifswald University Psychiatric Clinic.

All these facilities admitted both men and women and served urban and rural areas.[43] In making my selection, I also considered different types of clinics and asylums. Eglfing-Haar and Untergöltzsch/Rodewisch were sanatorium-nursing homes. In contrast to this institutional model, the Greifswald University Psychiatric Clinic and the Marburg Land Sanatorium were not oriented toward nursing care and quartering people (*Verwahrung*; in other words, providing accommodation for people who may or may not have had mental problems) but admitted patients for diagnosis and treatment for shorter periods,[44] referring those requiring longer stays to sanatorium-nursing homes. In line with this, after 1949 there was one type of institution in both the FRG and the GDR that catered to long-term patients and another that was intended for shorter stays. I also examine the von Bodelschwingh Asylums as a Protestant institution, for which there was no equivalent in East Germany during the period under study.[45] My selection allows conclusions to be drawn about committal mechanisms in certain types of institutions and regions, without making sweeping claims about the entire national territory of the "Third Reich," the FRG, or the GDR.

Hospitals and asylums had both psychiatric and neurological departments during the period studied here. I consider both in this book. Although my focus is on psychiatric illnesses, a strict division makes no sense in this context, as very few disorders were viewed exclusively from a psychiatric or neurological perspective.[46] This applies in particular to the process of committal and admission, in which there was often disagreement about which illness was involved. In the hospital or asylum, neurological and psychiatric examinations were carried out upon admission. Psychiatrists and neurologists published in the same journals in all three societies (Nazi Germany, the GDR, and the FRG) and the same textbooks served both medical sub-disciplines. For the medical layperson too, there was no clear separation between neurology and psychiatry. Patients were subject to the same admission regulations. Nor was the stigmatization of diseases that are nowadays typically classified as neurological, such as epilepsy, any less severe. This condition was thus subject to the Nazi Law for the Prevention of Hereditarily Diseased Offspring (*Gesetz zur Verhütung erbkranken Nachwuchses* or GzVeN). Neurological diseases were in fact one of the main targets of Nazi propaganda, and it was a neurological condition that was highlighted in the most famous Nazi propaganda film propagating "euthanasia," *Ich klage an* ("I accuse"),[47] namely, multiple sclerosis (MS).[48] Despite this shared approach to neurological and psychiatric diseases in the public sphere and in the same medical institutions, however, the division between neurology and psychiatry as two sub-disciplines was real and shaped physicians' self-image. This engendered a field of tension involving close cooperation and to some extent shared clientele on the one hand and both competition and attempts at demarcation on the other.

Methodology, complexes of theory and research, and the book's structure

Operationalizing comparison

The present study undertakes a diachronic comparison of the "Third Reich" and its two successor states while also providing a synchronic analysis of the GDR and FRG. As in virtually every comparative work, elements of transfer also play a role.[49] A comparative approach not only helps bring out commonalities and differences, but also makes it possible, first, to probe continuities and ruptures between the "Third Reich" and East and West Germany, second, to shed light on trends toward mutual demarcation and convergence between the two successor states, and third, by expanding our perspective to include transfer history, to analyze possible processes of "Westernization" (in West Germany) and "Sovietization" (in East Germany). The comparative units are the three states or, as the case may be, the occupation zones. The practice of committal is analyzed for the different states at four interlocking levels of investigation: patients, their social milieu, regulations and scientific discourses, and medical practice. Hence, this is a case of inter-societal comparison rather than the comparison of nation-states.[50] All four levels of investigation are not always accessible or meaningful with respect to every question, but each topic is examined from at least two perspectives.[51] The object of comparison is psychiatric committal practice, which I consider in light of four *tertia comparationes* in specific chapters: scope of power and action in committal practices, disease and diagnostics, security and danger, and work and performance. While these four categories also inform the arrangement of the chapters, the classical analytical categories of class,[52] race, and gender, as well as the less prominent category of age, are understood as cross-cutting conceptions and they appear in every chapter. The category of "race" plays an essentially subordinate role in this book: Jewish citizens were no longer committed in the period under investigation, beginning in 1941. The category of "race" is thus significant chiefly in the context of "internal racism."[53]

The key advantage of the chapter-dividing categories of disease and diagnostics, security and danger, and work and performance is that they enable us to link the four levels of investigation directly. We can thus connect individual cases and societal ideas, plus rules and scientific discourses. The themes of illness, danger, work, gender, class, and age crop up explicitly in case histories and psychiatric evaluations. At the same time, they constituted topics of discussion in all three societies, and thus function as key categories for understanding the practice of committal. The concept of scope of power and action, which cuts across the above categories, allows us to analyze different perspectives on committals as they relate to one another, namely, those of patients, their milieu, and physicians, as well as those embedded in rules and psychiatric knowledge.

One-to-one comparison, it should be noted, is not always possible or desirable. Different investigative foci reflect shifts in relevance and power.

For the wartime period, for example, it makes sense to delve into the process of negotiation between the police and the patient's social environment. In the postwar period, on the other hand, there were far fewer police committals, so this phenomenon is of considerably less salience. Here, we can learn more by examining the role of the social environment in light of the now prevailing mode of committal and by scrutinizing changes in the actor constellations associated with compulsory committals. The themes foregrounded in the present book thus reflect the varying significance of the above-mentioned analytical categories in the three societies, as well as changes in their semantic content. This approach leaves no gaps and allows us to consider the object of study in line with its relevance and function in a given society, thus throwing changes into relief. I argue that practices of psychiatric committal were attuned directly to social conditions, which means that psychiatric facilities were multifunctional. I include the altered function and variable embedding of psychiatry in society in my narrative, and these variations also find expression in the chapters' differing focal points. The practice of committal and the function of psychiatry were always bound up with the realities of a particular state, medical developments, and the needs of society. Ultimately, due to the influence of the social microcosm on committal decisions, which can hardly be overstated, inclusion and exclusion at the threshold of the institution could—I argue—only be steered to a very limited extent by the state and by scientific expertise. Psychiatry thus emerges as an institution that eluded the logic of knowledge-based planning.[54] Sanatorium-nursing homes were not limited to a clearly defined clientele or subject matter. I work on the assumption that it was this multifunctionality that underpinned the persistent (and generally rising) demand for places in psychiatric establishments. Psychiatric clinics and asylums, then, were about more than discipline and quartering, healing and recovery, or reintegration into the world of work. They served all these ends to differing degrees, depending on whose perspective we spotlight.[55]

Complexes of theory and research: state and psychiatry

Before I delve into this functional diversity and seek to determine its precise form within the practice of committals between 1941 and 1963, Chapter 1, "Historical Parameters of Committal Practice," discusses in highly condensed form the relationship between psychiatry and society from the nineteenth century to 1941, providing a foundation for the empirical chapters. Chapter 2, "The State and Psychiatric Institutions," grapples mainly with civil committals between 1941 and 1963. For the wartime period, the focus is on the way doctors and families approached the sick at a time when the Nazi regime was seeking to kill many of them; I also explore how patients dealt with referrals for inpatient stays. The polarized use of the asylum as a site of "healing and extermination" (*Heilen und Vernichten*) and the murders of the sick have been widely researched.[56] In particular, a vast array of studies have appeared on the latter topic,[57] with those that embed these killings broadly within society being especially useful for the purposes of the present book— though they are few and far between.[58] Here, illuminating the practice of committal, a key process that often preceded the murder of the sick, can help us understand the connections between psychiatric institutions—as sites of these killings—and society. In this context, exploring committal practices can help shed light on German wartime society and contribute to the debate on the *Volksgemeinschaft* (National Community), though I do not use this term as a category of analysis in the present book. Ever more research on the *Volksgemeinschaft* has been conducted in recent years and has come to en- compass so many specific aspects as well as overarching interpretations that it has reasonably been suggested that we should really refer to research on the "social history of National Socialism."[59] I follow this proposal here: the present work's conception as a comparative study that goes beyond the Nazi period rules out the foregrounding of a term so deeply embedded in research on Nazism.[60] Given my goal of unpacking practices of inclusion and exclusion, I build on research on the *Volksgemeinschaft* as a social practice, a body of work strongly oriented toward Alf Lüdtke's concept of domination (*Herrschaft*) as social practice when it comes to the topic of inclusion and toward Detlef Peukert's research with respect to exclusion.[61] Analyzing inclusionary and exclusionary strategies through the prism of committal practices enables us to probe the deep structures of Nazi society and thus to extend our knowledge of that social formation during the war in several respects, while also testing empirically some of the assumptions that typify the *Volksgemeinschaft* debate. Most studies on the *Volksgemeinschaft* have focused either on inclusionary or exclusionary practices[62] or have looked only at actors engaged in the margin- alization of others, but not those affected by exclusion.[63] An analysis of committal practices makes it possible to examine inclusionary and exclusionary conduct within a single study and allows us to probe, at least to some extent, patients' reasoning strategies with the aid of ego-documents.[64] Drawing on the findings of research on denunciation under National Socialism, I argue[65] that the demarcating of borders in everyday contexts took place to a significant extent through the participation of non-institutional and non-organized ac- tors.[66] This raises the question of whether differences associated with the pa- tient's social status played a role in interactions between doctors and lay people. In the nineteenth century, the bourgeoisie, in contrast to the "lower class" and the rural population, was typified by trust in doctors and hopes of recovering one's health through a stay at an institution.[67] I explore whether, in view of the murder of the sick, the "middle class" maintained this more positive attitude toward psychiatrists during and after World War II. In addition, I seek to show that there was no static boundary within the practice of committal: a variety of actors negotiated the threshold between inclusion and exclusion.[68] The wartime health system has been analyzed by Winfried Süß with particular emphasis on its internal competition and radicalization.[69] However, very little research has been conducted on physicians' practices outside of large medical institutions, such as asylums and hospitals, nor has much attention been paid to the perspective of medical laypersons, whether patients or their relatives. In terms of the existing body of research, the present work can merely draw on the small number of studies that have touched hypothetically on the relationship between doctors and patients in the Nazi era.[70] What I show in the present book, meanwhile, is that people continued to use asylums as a place to "quarter" their relatives, though to some degree they tried to avoid state institutions, assuming—often incorrectly—that private ones were safer.[71] Hence, many of them sought to find a place for their family members in the von Bodelschwingh Asylums examined here, often by making unofficial enquiries there.

When it comes to the immediate postwar period, I seek to illuminate changes on a number of different levels. I consider material shortages and their consequences for the keeping of medical records and scrutinize the effects of the "collapse" of German society (*Zusammenbruchgesellschaft*) on committal practices. Crucial here are the disrupted family relationships characteristic of displaced persons and the function of psychiatric assessment. As we will see, psychiatry geared itself primarily toward the requirements of society. I then examine whether and if so how committal pathways changed due to the founding of the new German states. When it comes to the structure of the health and welfare systems in the FRG and GDR, the key sources are the *Geschichte der Sozialpolitik in Deutschland seit 1945* ("History of Social Policy in Germany since 1945") as well as publications by Hans Günter Hockerts, Udo Schagen, Sabine Schleiermacher, Dagmar Ellerbrock and Ulrike Lindner.[72] On the East German health system, another key text is the seminal study by Anna Sabine Ernst on doctors and medical school teachers.[73] Neither the Allies nor either of the two German states had much interest in psychiatry in the 1950s; the asylum itself was not subject to any particular innovations or reforms following the founding of the new states. But did this apply to the routes of committal and the function of the asylum? Who inpatient places, which of course always required funding, were meant for[74] was discussed in both the FRG and the GDR and this permits certain conclusions about the place of psychiatry within the newly founded states. The chapter concludes with a diachronic overview of the patients' perspective and an attempt to shed light on their position within the committal process. In this context, a distinction can be made between compulsory and civil committals. But to what extent does this help us grasp the patient's position? What emerges is that even in the case of civil committals, patients found themselves in a field of tension between voluntariness and coercion. This leads us to the topic of compulsory committals, to which the next chapter, "Danger and Security," is dedicated.

Complexes of theory and research: danger and security

Since involuntary committals—unless they were instances of forensic detention—did not necessarily take place after a hazard had arisen, the question of the relationship between security (or safety) and freedom is particularly salient in this context. Who could be deprived of their freedom, when, by whom, and for what reasons because of a potential security risk? Here, we can turn to the rationales given for initiating compulsory committals, which provide a clear indication of how security was understood and what was accepted as constituting a threat to it. Equally important is the question of who could express their views on this with any chance of getting their way. I do not, therefore, give the terms security and danger a specific definition at this point, which allows me to examine how different actors endowed them with variable meanings.[75] I will merely provide some structural pointers: following Franz-Xaver Kaufmann, security is understood here as a utopian concept. Kaufmann underlines that the appeal of the concept lies in the fact that it is "unattainable and yet points to a desirable state."[76] He underscores that security is usually a fuzzy concept at the political level while being easily understood in everyday life.[77] The value ascribed to security, in combination with the fact that it is never completely attainable, means that the concept of danger exhibits the same sort of openness. The notion of the "threat to public safety" as grounds for committal neatly conveys the interdependence of the two terms. In individual cases of committal, however, specific reasons were given as to why various actors perceived a "safety risk." Arguments used to justify compulsory committals thus entailed an attempt to approach the notion of security, which ultimately remained utopian but had very real consequences for those committed. The extent to which the concept of security was de facto expanded within a given rationale for committal and who was responsible for defining danger—doctors, police officers, courts, and/or families—tells us a great deal about the relationship between security and freedom, one of crucial import in modern societies.[78]

Involuntary committals took different forms in the "Third Reich," the GDR, and the FRG. The wartime regulations were identical to those introduced in the early 1930s. When we consider the war, then, what matters is not the establishing of new rules but how the existing rules were applied. In the case of compulsory committals, one of the key issues, especially in light of the murder of the sick, is how people first came to the attention of the police and health offices. Here, following on from the previous chapter, the question arises as to what extent the familial and social environment, but also medical institutions, were involved in decisions on forcible committals that preceded admission. For the wartime period, I examine three groups of people who were regularly subject to compulsory committals. First, I provide a fairly brief discussion of soldiers as patients.[79] I then go on to analyze the files of elderly patients before finally turning to the role of sexuality[80] in the committal of women.[81]

For the postwar period, the question arises as to the impact of new legal regulations in West Germany. Article 104 of the Basic Law (*Grundgesetz* or GG) introduced compulsory judicial committal. Did this result in a changed dynamic between patients, their relatives, and physicians? In a similar vein, given West Germany's federal system, we might ask whether there were regional differences in practices and in responses to the new regulations. The present book scrutinizes continuities and ruptures in inclusionary and exclusionary practices and arguments over a period extending from the war into both German successor states. In this respect, the social microcosm has barely been researched for the postwar period. It is true that numerous studies have appeared in recent times that seek to determine the effects of National Socialism on postwar society. These, however, focus almost exclusively on public discourse[82] and continuities of personnel,[83] but pay almost no attention to the societal micro-level. An exception for East Germany is the study by Sven Korzilius, which provides insights into the exclusion of "asocials."[84] In addition, we can draw on studies of the history of everyday life in the GDR, a profoundly neglected field when it comes to the early FRG.[85]

One key question about the GDR is how the vacuum of rules that existed until 1968[86] was filled in practice. Was committal still carried out mainly by police through health offices, as in the Nazi period, or did a new *modus operandi* emerge here? I illuminate the enduring lack of rules and the question of how actors proceeded in their absence by considering differing interpretations of the relationship between state power and society. To what extent was the state present within the practice of committal? At what levels can we identify state guidelines and state interests in the first place, with which relatives, for example, were potentially confronted during the committal process? The present book argues that established interpretations, such as the notion of the GDR as a *durchherrscht* society—one governed to the point of saturation—and the idea of a "dictatorship of the borders,"[87] offer us little analytical purchase here.

Questions about the relationship between state power and society also arise when it comes to the wartime period and West Germany. Tatjana Tönsmeyer and Annette Vowinckel point out that with respect to the twentieth century, it is particularly important to analyze concepts of security directly in the context of a given structure of power and authority.[88] The topic of security touches on two overarching, interrelated research complexes. The first is centered on social security. This figures in the present study, for example, in discussions about who places in inpatient facilities were intended for and who was expected to pay for them.[89] Second, and crucial to Chapter 3, a number of studies have explored the executive security organs, namely, the police, and for World War II, the Secret State Police (Geheime Staatspolizei or Gestapo). As research on the Gestapo so strikingly shows, the production of "security" required constant interaction between the police and the general population. In recent years, Gestapo research has identified an endemic willingness among German citizens to denounce neighbors for a variety of reasons.[90] One of the key insights of this research is that, from the Gestapo's perspective, this practice of denunciation was more than a supplement to its work and more than a matter of citizens relieving it of a certain amount of effort: as Gisela Diewald-Kerkmann underlines, "in many cases, the Gestapo was not itself active, but merely reactive, as work colleagues, neighbors, acquaintances, former friends, and even family members informed the persecuting authorities about potential or real opponents of the Nazi regime."[91] The work of the Gestapo would have been quite inconceivable without the large number of denunciations.[92] The same goes for health offices in the context of committals. Without the willing participation of family members, official compulsory committals by public health officers (*Amtsärzte*) would in most cases have been impossible.

Complexes of theory and research: disease and diagnosis

While Chapters 2 and 3 often focus on non-medical actors, Chapter 4, "Disease and Diagnostics," is devoted to psychiatrists and the relationship between physicians and medical laypersons. Ultimately, the threshold to the asylum was in part a medical one. *Medicine* is conceptualized in what follows as "a form of social and cultural practice that observes, codifies, and understands certain phenomena regarded as ailments in a historically contingent manner."[93] One key assumption of the present study is that *psychiatric illness* is both a historically given object and a socially constructed ascription.[94] The illness itself and the correctness of the diagnosis are not the object of my analysis; I explore only the social and scientific-professional construction, attribution, and legitimization of illness. Entry into an asylum was tied to the attribution of a (mental) illness by a physician, while all other possible grounds for institutionalization were necessarily linked to the ascription of a psychiatric or neurological illness to those committed.[95] Conversely, the belief that an individual had a psychiatric illness or was "mentally ill" was by no means automatically taken as grounds for committal.

Expanding on a research perspective highlighted by Margit Szöllösi-Janze, analysis of the multilayered attributions of illness within the committal context in the three different states enables us to get at the connections between the nature of the state, the social system, and psychiatric discourse, as well as between rationalization and the definition of "deviance" in social microcosms. Szöllösi-Janze underscores the importance of examining "interdependencies between the character of the state, social system, the organization of science, research programs, and intellectual dispositions,"[96] especially when it comes to twentieth-century German history. As she emphasizes, her approach provides a particularly fruitful perspective on the history of Germany during that era as it eschews an exclusive focus on the major political ruptures. Even the Nazi period, as she argues, was integrated into the overall flow of German history through processes of scientification, and these processes played a key role in both postwar German states.[97] The view "from below," which I adopt here by foregrounding the social microcosm, opens up this panorama to questions about the relationship between formalized knowledge and its "quotidian" counterpart.[98]

Chapter 4 begins by addressing the self-image of psychiatrists in the context of diagnosis and committal. I analyze these phenomena with reference to discussions of diagnostic classifications in general and by looking at a specific disorder, namely, schizophrenia. Here I elaborate psychiatrists' professional self-image as it was marked off from psychiatry's sister discipline of neurology. Furthermore, I examine the circulation of practical knowledge between local institutions and the national context as well as its embedding in the Cold War order, while also exploring the preservation of tradition and scrutinizing mechanisms of epistemic appropriation. When it comes to the FRG, with regard to psychiatric knowledge and its practical application I assume continuity in basic attitudes, but this does not exclude the possibility of changes. New practices and theoretical tropes may have been integrated into the prevailing doctrine while its core theoretical premises were retained. With respect to the GDR, one key question is how broad-based psychiatric discussions were. Was it legitimate to hold and articulate Western positions or traditional viewpoints that contradicted the Soviet view? The chapter then turns to medical laypersons' conceptions of illness and health, while exploring the position of patients and their relatives vis-à-vis physicians. Chapters 2 and 3 demonstrate that during the war, due to knowledge of the Nazi murder of the sick as well as the general wartime circumstances, rationales for committal primarily revolved around pragmatic considerations or were justified in pragmatic terms. Central to the reasons identified for committal were scenarios of threat and patients' and their families' eagerness to avoid (state) asylums. In comparison, medical aspects clearly took a back seat, before becoming more important again in the postwar period. After the war, scientific publications in East and West Germany increasingly focused on diagnostic problems and diagnostic classifications, which had not played a comparable role in wartime. Chapter 4 thus focuses on the postwar period. Here, the thematic disparity reflects the new parameters, actor constellations, and prevailing interests.

Complexes of theory and research: work and performance

The example of Martina R.'s committal, outlined at the start of this introduction, has already shown that medical histories, in addition to the aspects of illness and danger, reveal everyday expectations of behavior at a deeper level. This culminates figuratively in the reference to the patient's hands as white from doing nothing. The themes of work and performance and their counterparts of unwillingness or inability to work were not only present in Martina R.'s committal. Work, the ability to work, and the will to work were not official reasons for psychiatric committals—unlike threats to self or others and illness—but they were frequently cited as factors justifying committals.[99] Moreover, during the Nazi era physicians increasingly referred to *Leistungsfähigkeit* ("performance") to ascribe illness and health.[100] The category of work thus constitutes a potent means of illuminating key issues in the history of psychiatry and social history as they relate to one another. Work undoubtedly played an important role in the asylum in the context of occupational therapy.[101] But work and performance were also key to the self-image of state and society in the "Third Reich," the GDR, and the FRG, in different ways in each case. In Nazi Germany, the focus on work and performance constituted a component of "internal racism,"[102] which was directed against those declared "asocial." In East Germany, the privileging of work played a profound role in the self-image of the "workers' state," while both the GDR and the FRG saw themselves as *Leistungsgesellschaften*, that is, performance- or achievement-oriented societies. By looking through the prism of psychiatric committal practices we can scrutinize both social exclusion and inclusion as informed by the criteria of work and performance, while also shedding light on the role of work and performance in everyday self-perceptions under National Socialism, in the GDR, and in the Federal Republic. Only a few studies here and there have explored the extent to which work and notions of performance or achievement shaped social relations and everyday life.[103] Studies of work in the mid-twentieth century under National Socialism, meanwhile, have, for good reason, mostly adopted a "top-down" perspective on the persecution and systematic exclusion of so-called "asocials."[104]

In the context of committal practices, I interpret evaluations and self-descriptions relating to the topic of work against the background of previous research in the history of medicine, the history of everyday life, and social history. Key texts here are Alf Lüdtke's studies on the significance of "quality German work" to the self-image of workers in the German Empire, under National Socialism, and in the GDR and FRG.[105] When it comes to East Germany, a large number of studies have explored everyday working life.[106] In the history of medicine, meanwhile, Nicole Schweig highlights the importance of "ability to work" (*Arbeitsfähigkeit*) to male attributions of health during the first half of the twentieth century, while Susanne Hoffmann makes similar points in her study of gender-specific health discourses in the twentieth century.[107] However, very little research has been conducted on possible continuities with the Nazi period in the treatment of so-called "asocials" in the case of the GDR[108] and especially that of the FRG.[109] Conversely, with reference to early West Germany, a lively debate was conducted on the "de-browned," in other words de-Nazified, ethic of achievement among West German elites postulated by Hans-Ulrich Wehler, which, he contended, had contributed to the young state's economic success.[110] Only a very small number of recent studies have examined the relationship between individuals and their work in the postwar period.[111] Eschewing a focus on the "elite," in contrast to the debate initiated by Wehler, these foreground blue- and white-collar workers.

In what follows, work includes not only all forms of gainful employment but also domestic work.[112] I consciously avoid positing a narrower definition of work here as this allows me to approach the topic from different angles and then draw a more nuanced picture in light of the sources. I examine work and health within the inclusionary and exclusionary rationales put forward by relatives and patients, in the ideas held by those committed about a healthy self, and in psychiatric conceptions of illness at the level of both theory and practice. I probe the extent to which notions of work and a healthy self were gender-, class-, or state-specific, which in some cases prompts me to revise or add nuance to prevailing interpretations. Did men, unlike women, define their health chiefly in terms of the capacity for work? Is the characterization of a healthy self as a hard-working self a basic feature of states that saw themselves as centered on work and performance, as did Nazi Germany, the GDR, and the FRG in their different ways? When it comes to psychiatrists, I examine to what extent the assessments and explanatory models they deployed in dealing with patients who saw themselves as "overworked" were specific to the society involved. Another important question is whether new theoretical approaches were followed by changes in practice. For the GDR, as in Chapter 4, I will explore whether the dominant assumption among researchers that the Pavlov campaign did not change medical practice[113] holds true for such practice in the wake of psychiatric committals, or whether a more differentiated view is appropriate here.

Sources

Source materials and their evaluation: a qualitative study with quantitative underpinnings

I draw on three different types of sources in the present book. The first comprises records in the Federal Archives in Koblenz and Lichterfelde, and in the state and Land archives[114] of the territories in which the clinics or asylums under consideration were located. These archival records relate to compliance with rules on committal and discussions of committal practices. Second, I consult psychiatric writings, including various editions of psychiatric textbooks and two psychiatric journals, namely, the 1941–1963 issues of *Der Nervenarzt* ("The Neurologist"), which was first published in 1928 and continued to appear in the Federal Republic of Germany, and the journal *Psychiatrie, Neurologie und medizinische Psychologie* ("Psychiatry, Neurology, and Medical Psychology"), first published in the Soviet occupation zone in 1949 and subsequently in the GDR. Third, a total of 1,424 patient files from the 6 psychiatric institutions examined here constitute the main corpus of source material. In the latter case, I draw on a pool of sources that is subject to strict legal limitations on access and which I was able to examine for the first time in such breadth for the period after World War II. Due to access restrictions, I could evaluate the medical records of the Eglfing-Haar Sanatorium-Nursing Home only for the period from 1941 to 1949. From the second half of the 1950s, the medical records at Rodewisch were archived on a selective basis. As a result, I consulted only the files up to 1955, while examining the records of the Großschweidnitz Sanatorium-Nursing Home for the period 1956–1963.[115] In most cases, doctors' personnel files were either not accessible or unavailable. A fair number of files cannot be clearly assigned to the physician who conducted the admission interview. Abbreviations were often used for signatures—and sometimes these were lacking entirely. The size of the asylums and clinics, along with the rotation of physicians, thus makes it extremely difficult to keep track of the staff involved.[116]

I carry out a mostly qualitative analysis of committal practices, but I provide quantitative insights as well, especially in Chapter 2.[117] I selected files covering four time periods, namely, from 1941 to the end of the war, from the end of that conflict to the founding of the FRG and GDR in 1949, from 1950 to 1955, and from 1956 to 1963. Where possible, I selected the individual case files at random, and I strove to take account of the gender ratio within the asylum or clinic.[118] However, since this was not always feasible because, for example, the total quantity of medical records was not known or the holdings had not yet been registered, I make no claim to representativeness in the social scientific sense. In addition, in some cases—especially for the years 1945–1949—committal forms were filled out incompletely, making the data set patchy. I do not aim to provide exact figures and thus make no attempt to interpret minor changes.[119] Figures are cited in an attempt to trace the pathways of committal and identify major changes with reference to them.

A social history of medicine that takes account of Science Studies: journals and textbooks as complementary sources for interpreting medical records

This book aims to analyze in context the perspective of patients, their milieu, and physicians, in other words, I seek to write a social history of committal practices that takes account of Science Studies. Within this framework, the aim of qualitative source analysis is to examine the (self-)descriptions of patients and members of their milieu. I neither attempt to reconstruct an entire world of experience nor do I claim that these descriptions perfectly convey the thoughts and feelings of patients and their relatives. A hermeneutic analysis of medical records is facilitated here by the fact that my goal is to reconstruct rationales for committal, not the inner world of the clinic or asylum. This is significant to the evaluation of the source material. The oft-lamented disappearance of patients' voices from medical records, which is a key argument against relying on such records to construct our interpretations, applies to stays in hospitals, not entry to them.[120] Furthermore, the relationship between laypersons and physicians was subject to a greater power imbalance in the clinic than in the case of decisions on inpatient stays. I also assume, and seek to demonstrate in this book, that the rationales for committal were, at least from the point of view of those involved, meaningful pieces of reasoning that lay within the realm of the sayable in a given political-social context and did not fundamentally defy all logic and comprehensibility. In particular, I consult letters and so-called "subjective" and "objective" anamneses. The "subjective" anamnesis is data provided by the patient, while the "objective" anamnesis is information provided by the family or another person from the social environment of the person committed. Although admissions in the 1940s–1960s certainly entailed highly formalized aspects,[121] medical histories do not provide strictly formalized information about the course of an illness or the reasons for committal.[122]

In addition to the perspective of the patients and their relatives, I scrutinize the relationship between scientific knowledge and practice. My goal here is not to endorse the frequently made and unsurprising observation that practice deviates to some degree from the theoretical knowledge of the prevailing doctrine. Especially in psychiatry, in which scientific knowledge and lay knowledge are traditionally closely interwoven,[123] a perfect fit with theory seems unlikely. Instead, I set out to elucidate in detail, with respect to small fields of action, what was or was not practiced, where, when, and why, while seeking to determine what this tells us about relationships between science and politics and between science and the social microcosm.[124] I thus pursue a social and cultural approach to the history of science.[125] In addition, I analyze the explanations given by contemporary psychiatry itself for these divergences between theory and practice, a topic it certainly reflected upon. It is important to emphasize here that such an investigation can only be carried out with regard to narrowly defined areas of knowledge that were directly related to the practice of committal. An example of such a small area is "work within the psychiatric committal": I seek neither to survey interdisciplinary research on the topic of work as a whole nor to examine every facet of work-related diagnoses that often went far beyond this topic. Again and again, then, I address psychiatric knowledge as scientific knowledge. For these specific fields, I examine legitimation, enforcement, change, and discussion on the basis of psychiatric textbooks and two psychiatric journals, as these allow us to trace[126] scholarly *discourse*.[127] This in turn enables me to examine the limited areas of knowledge illuminated by psychiatric committal practice within a double field of tension: first, that situated between theory and practice and, second, that lying between local, national, and/or larger epistemic spaces, such as the European, Western, or Soviet.

Notes

1 All names of patients and relatives have been anonymized. The names of doctors who worked in the various institutions are abbreviated when parts of the patients' files are reproduced. Doctors' names that appear in publications are given. When individual patients and their families are cited several times and in detail in the book, place names have been anonymized as well.
2 LHA Marburg, Patient file sign. 16K10740F, certificate, 15.3.1946, LWV Hessen, 16.
3 Ibid.
4 Ibid, statement by mother-in-law, 15.3.1946. All the statements by the mother-in-law were recorded in the file; she did not write them herself.
5 Ibid.
6 Ibid.

7 Süß, Winfried, "Medizin im Krieg," in Robert Jütte, *Medizin im Nationalsozialismus. Bilanz und Perspektiven der Forschung* (Göttingen 2011), 190–200, here 191.

8 On knowledge of the murder of the sick, see for example the summary in Brink, Cornelia, *Grenzen der Anstalt. Psychiatrie und Gesellschaft in Deutschland 1860–1980* (Göttingen 2010), 327ff; Aly, Götz (ed.), *Die Belasteten. "Euthanasie" 1939–1945. Eine Gesellschaftsgeschichte* (Frankfurt/M. 2013), 266 ff.

9 *Aktion T4*, the state-organized murder of physically and mentally "handicapped" people, began toward the end of 1939 and was officially terminated on August 23, 1941, probably due in part to public protests by Catholic clergy. From August 1942 onward, however, the murders were resumed, this time pursued not by the central government but on a decentralized basis that varied by region and institution. See for example Pohl, Dieter, *Verfolgung und Massenmord in der NS-Zeit 1933–1945* (Darmstadt 2003), 30 f.; Schmuhl, Hans-Walter, "Die Patientenmorde," in Angelika Ebbinghaus and Klaus Dörner (eds.), *Vernichten und Heilen. Der Nürnberger Ärzteprozeß und seine Folge* (Berlin 2001), 295–331.

10 The history of psychiatry under National Socialism can be divided into three phases, the third of which began in 1941 with the end of the T4 campaign. On this division, see ibid., 315.

11 In the wake of the German invasion of the Soviet Union, the failure of the "Blitzkrieg" concept and finally the United States' entry into the war, the entire dynamic of the conflict changed and, as it dragged on, the situation on the "home front" changed as well. Hospital care for the civilian population was no longer guaranteed from around 1941–42. See Süß, Winfried, *Der "Volkskörper" im Krieg. Gesundheitspolitik, Gesundheitsverhältnisse und Krankenmord im natio- nalsozialistischen Deutschland, 1939–1945* (Munich 2003), 210.

12 The main purpose of *Aktion Brandt* was to create special hospitals for the treatment of injured soldiers and *Volksgenossen* ("national comrades"), for example, by requiring old people's homes and psychiatric institutions to make some of their beds available. On *Aktion Brandt*, see for example Süß, *"Volkskörper,"* 76ff.

13 On the Rodewisch Propositions, see Schulz, Jörg, "Die *Rodewischer Thesen* von 1963. Ein Versuch zur Reform der DDR-Psychiatrie," in Franz-Werner Kersting (ed.), *Psychiatriereform als Gesellschaftsreform. Die Hypothek des Nationalsozialismus und der Aufbruch der sechziger Jahre* (Paderborn 2003), 87–100.

14 The term *Zusammenbruchgesellschaft* or "society in a state of collapse" was coined in Kleßmann, Christoph, *Die doppelte Staatsgründung: Deutsche Geschichte 1945–1955* (Bonn 1991), 37–63.

15 LHA Marburg, Patient file sign. 16K10740F, entry, 15.3.1946, LWV Hessen, 16.

16 Given this interest in examining a medical institution in terms of its use within society, the present book interfaces with classical questions in the social history of medicine. For detailed information on that field, see Labisch, Alfons and Reinhard Spree, "Neuere Entwicklungen und aktuelle Trends in der Sozialgeschichte der Medizin in Deutschland—Rückschau und Ausblick," VSWG, vol. 3, 1997, 305–321.

17 A praxeological approach assumes the existence of several competing strands of actional knowledge that are not merely antecedent to action in the sense of norms and mentalities, but that generate, maintain, and transform these through action. In line with this, regulatory knowledge is only one of several important factors. See Reichhardt, Sven, "Praxeologische Geschichtswissenschaft. Eine Diskussionsanregung," *Sozial.Geschichte*, vol. 3, 2007, 43–65. A seminal work in praxeologically oriented research is Bourdieu, Pierre, *Sozialer Sinn. Kritik der theoretischen Vernunft* (Frankfurt/M. 1987).

18 Brink, *Psychiatrie*, 20. On the significance of liminal spaces in the context of psychiatry and modernity, see also the following anthology: Hess, Volker and

Heinz-Peter Schmiedebach (eds.), *Am Rande des Wahnsinns. Schwellenräume einer urbanen Moderne* (Vienna 2012).

19 The choice of research object here thus dovetails with the insight, viewed as Foucault's fundamental presupposition within one subset of his reception, according to which "society's way of dealing [with the excluded] takes shape and form" on the basis of the demarcation of boundaries, as performed at the *threshold of the institution.* On this view, this demarcation process itself—and not chiefly the institution—is a particularly revealing object of investigation for the history of society and psychiatry, which converge here. See Raffnsøe, Sverre et al., *Foucault. Studienhandbuch* (Munich 2011), 105. For a summary of other readings of *Histoire de la folie,* see ibid., 88ff. It should be noted that I merely draw on the epistemological potential of boundary-drawing, first foregrounded by Foucault, as a starting point. I do not unquestioningly presuppose the Foucauldian understanding of the asylum or "madness." Instead, I analyze mechanisms of committal, constellations of action, and ideas about illness, normality, and security in an open-ended way with reference to six specific psychiatric institutions in the period 1941 to 1963.

20 On the English-speaking world, see for example Suzuki, Akihito, *Madness at Home. The Psychiatrists, the Patient, and the Family in England 1820–1860* (Berkeley 2006); Gründler, Jens, *Armut und Wahnsinn. "Arme Irre" und ihre Familien im Spannungsfeld von Psychiatrie und Armenfürsorge in Glasgow 1875–1921* (Munich 2013). On the German-speaking countries, see Nellen, Stefan and Robert Suter, "Unfälle, Vorfälle, Fälle: Eine Archäologie des polizeilichen Blicks," in Sybille Brändli et al. (ed.), *Zum Fall machen, zum Fall werden. Wissensproduktion und Patientenerfahrung in Medizin und Psychiatrie des 19. und 20. Jahrhunderts* (Frankfurt/M. 2009), 159–181.

21 Brink, *Psychiatrie*; Hanrath, Sabine, *Zwischen Euthanasie und Psychiatriereform. Anstaltspsychiatrie in Westfalen und Brandenburg: Ein deutsch-deutscher Vergleich (1945–1964)* (Paderborn 2004).

22 A quite different situation pertains outside Germany. See for example Suzuki, *Madness*; Gründler, *Armut und Wahnsinn*; Vijselaar, Joost, "Out and In. The Family and the Asylum. Patterns of Admission and Discharge in Three Dutch Psychiatric Hospitals 1890–1950," in Marijke Gijswijt-Hofstra (ed.), *Psychiatric Cultures Compared. Psychiatry and Mental Health Care in the Twentieth Century. Comparisons and Approaches* (Amsterdam 2005), 277–294. Of the many texts on Germany, see for example Lutz, Petra, et al., "NS-Gesellschaft und 'Euthanasie.' Die Reaktionen der Eltern ermordeter Kinder," in Christoph Mundt et al. (eds.), *Psychiatrische Forschung und NS-"Euthanasie." Beiträge zu einer Gedenkveranstaltung an der Psychiatrischen Universitätsklinik Heidelberg* (Heidelberg 2001), 97–113; and in rudimentary form: Aly, *Belasteten*.

23 Cornelia Brink examines public debates ("expert disputes, media interest, and lay critique"), using them to locate psychiatry in society. Sabine Hanrath was denied access to the patient files of the two institutions she studied. See Brink, *Psychiatrie*, 29; Hanrath, *Euthanasie und Psychiatriereform*, preface. The same does not apply to Svenja Goltermann's work on war returnees in the early Federal Republic of Germany, which was written with the help of patient files. Goltermann writes the history of "traumatized" war returnees—on the basis of patient files, among other things—as a history of patients, their families, medical models of diagnosis and illness, and popularization through films. Goltermann, Svenja, *Die Gesellschaft der Überlebenden. Deutsche Kriegsheimkehrer und ihre Gewalterfahrungen im Zweiten Weltkrieg* (Munich 2009).

24 Süß Sonja, *Politisch mißbraucht? Psychiatrie und Staatssicherheit in der DDR* (Berlin 1999).

22   *Introduction*

25 See esp. Ash, Mitchell G., "Kurt Gottschaldt and Psychological Research in Nazi and Socialist Germany," in Kristie Macrakis and Dieter Hoffmann (eds.), *Science under Socialism. East Germany in Comparative Perspective* (Cambridge 1999), 286–301; Eghigian, Greg, "The Psychologization of the Socialist Self. East German Forensic Psychology and its Deviants, 1945–1975," *German History*, vol. 2, 2004, 181–205; Leuenberger, Christine, "Socialist Psychotherapy and its Dissidents," *Journal of the History of the Behavioral Sciences*, vol. 37, 2001, 261–273; see also Grashoff, Udo, *"In einem Anfall von Depression ..." Selbsttötung in der DDR* (Berlin 2006).

26 On the call to pay serious attention to power relations in the history of psychiatry, see also Engstrom, Eric J., et al., "Preface," in Engstrom, Eric J., et al., (eds.), *Knowledge and Power. Perspectives in the History of Psychiatry* (Berlin 1999), 9–10, here 10.

27 Imbusch, Peter, "Macht und Herrschaft in der wissenschaftlichen Kontroverse," in Peter Imbusch (ed.), *Macht und Herrschaft. Sozialwissenschaftliche Theorien und Konzeptionen* (Wiesbaden 2013), 10. I deliberately refrain from referring to Foucault here. It is true that Foucault's concept of power is also relational. But I do not take Foucault's interpretation of power relations in modernity as read in the present work. This means that I do not assume from the outset that power in the twentieth century has generally been concentrated in the hands of welfare states or health experts to such an extent that the Foucauldian notions of "governmentality" or "biopower" can function as the key concepts guiding my analysis. On the power of the welfare-based society and related security regimes and on the regulating power of biopolitics, see Foucault, Michel, *Sicherheit, Territorium, Bevölkerung. Geschichte der Gouvernementalität I. Vorlesungen am Collège de France (1977–1978)* (Frankfurt/M. 2004); Foucault, Michel, *Die Geburt der Biopolitik. Geschichte der Gouvernementalität II. Vorlesungen am Collège de France (1978–79)* (Frankfurt/M. 2004).

28 On police responsibility beyond "public safety," see the anthology by Lüdtke, Alf, *"Sicherheit" und "Wohlfahrt." Polizei, Gesellschaft und Herrschaft im 19. und 20. Jahrhundert* (Frankfurt/M. 1992).

29 Lüdtke, Alf, *Eigen-Sinn. Fabrikalltag, Arbeitererfahrungen und Politik vom Kaiserreich bis in den Faschismus* (Hamburg 1993), 25.

30 Goffman, Erving, *Asyle. Über die soziale Situation von Patienten und anderer Insassen* (Berlin 1973). On the debate on Goffman, see also the following anthology: Bretschneider, Falk et al. (eds.), *Personal und Insassen von "Totalen Institutionen"—zwischen Konfrontation und Verflechtung* (Leipzig 2011). A detailed picture of the state of research on patients and their families as actors is provided by Gründler, *Armut und Wahnsinn*, 6ff.

31 On the social microcosm in the postwar period, see Seegers, Lu, "Being Fatherless. Memories of War Children in Germany, England and Poland," *The International Journal of Evacuee and War Child Studies*, vol. 4, 2006, 87–90; as a point of interface between privacy and institution in the Nazi era, the Gestapo in particular has been researched in some depth. See for example the following two anthologies: Paul, Gerhard and Klaus-Michael Mallmann (eds.), *Die Gestapo. Mythos und Realität* (Darmstadt 1995); Paul, Gerhard and Klaus-Michael Mallmann, *Die Gestapo im Zweiten Weltkrieg. "Heimatfront" und besetztes Europa* (Darmstadt 2000). At the Institute of Contemporary History, Munich, this interface is being investigated in the project "Private Life and Privacy in Nazi Germany": http://www.ifz-muenchen. de/aktuelles/themen/das-private-im-nationalsozialismus/. On West Germany, see Hähner-Rombach, Sylvelyn, *Gesundheit und Krankheit im Spiegel von Petitionen an den Landtag von Baden-Württemberg 1946 bis 1980* (Stuttgart 2011).

32 Cf. studies covering the period up to World War I: Finnane, Mark, *Insanity and the Insane in Post-Famine Ireland* (London 1981); Walton, John L., "Lunacy in the Industrial Revolution. A Study of Asylum Admissions in Lancashire, 1845–50," *Journal of Social History*, vol. 13, 1979, 1–21; Wright, David, "Getting Out of the Asylum. Understanding the Confinement of the Insane in the Nineteenth Century," *Social History of Medicine*, vol. 10, 1997, 137–155; Suzuki, *Madness*; Gründler, *Armut und Wahnsinn*.

33 For detailed information on the state of research, see point 3 in this introduction.

34 For detailed information on the state of research, see ibid.

35 Under National Socialism and in the early Federal Republic, the age of majority was twenty-one. In the GDR it had been lowered to eighteen by May 1950. http://www.verfassungen.de/de/ddr/volljaehrigkeitsgesetz50.htm (retrieved 16.12.2013).

36 In line with this, I will not be discussing whether or to what extent the psychiatric institutions studied in this book are "total institutions." For a discussion of the usefulness of Goffman's concept, see Watzka, Carlos, "Zur Interdependenz von Personal und Insassen in 'Totalen Institutionen.' Probleme und Potentiale von Erving Goffmans 'Asyle,'" in Falk Bretschneider et al. (eds.), *Personal und Insassen von "Totalen Institutionen"—zwischen Konfrontation und Verflechtung* (Leipzig 2011), 25–56.

37 The formal initiation of committal to state institutions took place in a similar way in all three systems: an application for coverage of costs had to be submitted, the health offices were informed, then the responsible *Kreis*, *Bezirk*, or provincial association (*Provinzialverband*)/Land welfare association (*Landeswohlfahrtsverband*) officially set the committal in motion. The formal initiation of committals to university clinics was much less complicated than to psychiatric institutions. Often, neither the municipal nor supra-municipal administrative level (*Kreise*, *Regierungsbezirke*, provincial associations) nor welfare associations were involved.

38 I use the names of cities at the time of committal. I thus refer either to Chemnitz or Karl-Marx-Stadt depending on the period in question.

39 Literature exists on all the asylums and clinics, though some of it deals exclusively with the Nazi period. Only the Greifswald Psychiatric Clinic and the LHA Marburg have been researched for the postwar period. Committal practice is not studied in any of the relevant publications—except in the specific case of committals to the LHA Marburg carried out by military doctors during World War II. On the individual institutions, see Stockdreher, Petra, "Heil- und Pflegeanstalt Eglfing-Haar," in Michael von Cranach and Hans-Ludwig Siemen (eds.), *Psychiatrie im Nationalsozialismus. Die Bayerischen Heil- und Pflegeanstalten zwischen 1933 und 1945* (Munich 1999), 327–363; Fischer, Wolfgang and Hans-Peter Schmiedebach (eds.), *Die Greifswalder Universitäts- und Nervenklinik unter dem Direktorat von Hanns Schwarz 1946 bis 1965* (Greifswald 1999); Sandner, Peter et al., *Heilbar und nützlich. Ziele und Wege der Psychiatrie in Marburg an der Lahn* (Marburg 2001); Krumpolt, Holm, "Die Landesanstalt Großschweidnitz als 'T4' Zwischenanstalt und als Tötungsansanstalt (1939–1945)," in Stiftung Sächsische Gedenkstätten (ed.), *Nationalsozialistische Euthanasieverbrechen. Beiträge zur Aufarbeitung ihrer Geschichte in Sachsen* (Dresden 2004), 137–147; Wagner, Christina, *Psychiatrie und Nationalsozialismus in der Sächsischen Landesheil- und Pflegeanstalt Untergöltzsch* (Dresden 2002); Degen, Barbara, *Bethel in der NS-Zeit. Die verschwiegene Geschichte* (Bad Homburg von der Höhe 2014). The medical records can be found in the following archives: Greifswald University Archive, Saxony Land Archive Chemnitz, Saxony Main Land Archive Dresden, Archive of the Upper Bavarian District, Main Archive of the von Bodelschwingh Foundations, and the Archive of the Hesse Land Welfare Association.

40 In Saxony, the "starvation diet" affected almost half of all patients; this also applies to the Untergöltzsch asylum studied here. See Faulstich, Heinz, *Hungersterben in der Psychiatrie* (Freiburg 1993), 481.

41 Ibid., 500.

42 Faulstich, *Hungersterben*, 540.

43 Eglfing-Haar was originally intended to cater to the city of Munich, while the Gabersee Sanatorium-Nursing Home served its rural hinterland. However, Gabersee was closed in January 1941. I consciously opted not to analyze an institution in Berlin, as this would have meant studying a mainly metropolitan clientele. On the Gabersee Sanatorium-Nursing Home, see Bischof, Hans-Ludwig, "Heil- und Pflegeanstalt Gabersee," in Michael von Cranach and Hans-Ludwig Siemen (eds.), *Psychiatrie im Nationalsozialismus. Die Bayerischen Heil- und Pflegeanstalten zwischen 1933 und 1945* (Munich 1999), 363–379.

44 The original plan was to analyze the patient files of the Cologne University and Psychiatric Clinic in order to examine one university clinic in the GDR and one in the Federal Republic. However, access to the Cologne medical records was denied. The Marburg Land Sanatorium is a good alternative as it represents a functional equivalent with regard to committals. On Marburg's specific orientation toward "curable" patients, see the anthology: Sandner et al., *Heilbar*.

45 In the GDR, religious facilities did take on care tasks on a large scale. However, their focus was on people with physical "disabilities" and children. On religious nursing care, see Thiekötter, Andrea, *Pflegeausbildung in der Deutschen Demokratischen Republik* (Frankfurt/M. 2006), 142ff.

46 Age-related diseases and epilepsy, for example, stood at the threshold between psychiatry and neurology. But "classic" psychiatric disorders, such as schizophrenia, were also examined with a view to possible neurological peculiarities.

47 Roth, Karl Heinz, "'Ich klage an'—Aus der Entstehungsgeschichte eines Propaganda-Films," in Götz Aly (ed.), *Aktion T4. 1939–1945. Die "Euthanasie"-Zentrale in der Tiergartenstrasse 4* (Berlin 1989), 93–116.

48 Multiple sclerosis is a condition that can lead to neurological problems of many different kinds due to inflammation of the brain and spinal cord. These may include paralysis, dizziness, and stomach or kidney problems. Due to the wide range of symptoms, the disease often went undetected for years; the cause of the inflammation was unknown and there was no cure. See Murray, T. Jock, *Multiple Sclerosis. The History of a Disease* (New York 2005), 2.

49 For a summary of the debate on comparison and transfer, see for example, Kaelble, Hartmut, "Die Debatte über Vergleich und Transfer und was jetzt?," *H-Soz-u-Kult*, 8.2.2005, URL: http://hsozkult.geschichte.hu-berlin.de/forum/id= 574&type=artikel (retrieved 7.6.2014); Arndt, Agnes et al., *Vergleichen, verflechten, verwirren? Europäische Geschichtsschreibung zwischen Theorie und Praxis* (Göttingen 2011).

50 On the critique of comparisons between nation-states, see for example Welskopp, Thomas, "Stolpersteine auf dem Königsweg. Methodische Anmerkungen zum internationalen Vergleich in der Gesellschaftsgeschichte," *AfS*, vol. 35, 1995, 339–367.

51 On the need to adopt at least two different perspectives on an object of study, see Werner, Michael, and Bénédicte Zimmermann, "Vergleich, Transfer, Verflechtung," *GG*, vol. 4, 2002, 618.

52 A distinction between the lower and middle classes is made in the present book on the basis of two criteria. Rather than a differentiated sociological classification into lower, middle, and upper middle class, I work with a rough, expedient subdivision. First, I use occupational data as an indicator. The self-employed, mid-level and senior staff, and mid-level and senior civil servants are counted as

middle class. To classify wives and children in education, I use the occupation of the husband or father. Second, the class of accommodation in the clinic or asylum serves as a point of reference. The families of patients admitted to class I or II—in contrast to those in the large class III—were not dependent on support from welfare associations. On the demarcation of the lower and middle classes in light of the criterion that the "lower class" is dependent on the support of third parties (poor and welfare associations), see Pfister, Ulrich, "Unterschicht," in Friedrich Jaeger (ed.), *Enzyklopädie der Neuzeit*, vol. 13 (Stuttgart 2011), 1090.

53 The term was coined by Herbert, Ulrich, "Traditionen des Rassismus," in Ulrich Herbert, *Arbeit, Volkstum, Weltanschauung. Über Fremde und deutsche im 20. Jahrhundert* (Frankfurt/M. 1995), 11–29.

54 It is considered typical of the governance of modern societies that they adhere to a logic of knowledge-based planning. The associated assumption is that inclusionary and exclusionary mechanisms in "modernity" are regulated by state-recognized experts. See Dipper, Christof, "Moderne, Version: 1.0," *Docupedia-Zeitgeschichte*, URL: http://docupedia.de/zg/Moderne?oldid=84639 (retrieved 9.4.2014).

55 Thus, in his overview of the research on the history of psychiatry, Eric Engstrom challenges monocausal explanatory approaches and asks "whether the historical dynamics of psychiatric care were driven more by professional concerns or by humanitarian imperatives, more by medical interests and corrective technologies or by emotional and psychological needs." Engstrom, Eric J., "Beyond Dogma and Discipline. New Directions in the History of Psychiatry," *Current Opinion in Psychiatry*, vol. 19, 2006, 596.

56 For more detail, see Jütte, Robert, *Medizin im Nationalsozialismus. Bilanz und Perspektiven der Forschung* (Göttingen 2011).

57 See for example Burleigh, Michael, *Tod und Erlösung. Euthanasie in Deutschland 1900–1945* (Zürich 2002); Faulstich, *Hungersterben*; Friedländer, Henry, *Der Weg zum NS-Genozid. Von der Euthanasie zur Endlösung* (Berlin 1997); Klee, Ernst, *"Euthanasie" im NS-Staat. Die Vernichtung lebensunwerten Lebens* (Frankfurt/M. 1983); Ebbinghaus, Angelika and Klaus Dörner, *Vernichten und Heilen. Der Nürnberger Ärzteprozeß und seine Folgen* (Berlin 2002); for a comprehensive account of the state of research, see Jütte, *Medizin*.

58 Lutz, Petra, "Herz und Vernunft. Angehörige von 'Euthanasie'-Opfern im Schriftwechsel mit den Anstalten," in Heiner Fangerau and Karen Nolte (eds.), *"Moderne" Anstaltspsychiatrie im 19. und 20. Jahrhundert—Legitimation und Kritik* (Stuttgart 2006), 143–168; Fuchs, Petra et al. (eds.), *"Das Vergessen ist Teil der Vernichtung selbst." Lebensgeschichten von Opfern der nationalsozialistischen "Euthanasie"* (Göttingen 2007); Aly, *Belasteten*.

59 This term is not intended to reduce the diversity of research to a common denominator, but rather to do justice to its diversity. See Steuwer, Janosch, "Was meint und nützt das Sprechen von der 'Volksgemeinschaft'? Neue Literatur zur Gesellschaftsgeschichte des Nationalsozialismus," AfS, vol. 53, 2013, 533; Wildt, Michael, "'Volksgemeinschaft'. Eine Antwort auf Ian Kershaw," *Zeithistorische Forschungen*, vol. 8, 2011, 369.

60 In addition to the conceptual vagueness of the term *Volksgemeinschaft*, which is rarely made explicit when it is deployed, and the period under investigation in this book, there is another substantive reason to refrain from using it. At the level of content, the present study shows that, at least in the wartime period under consideration here, rational self-interest of various kinds was of considerable importance to committal decisions. Here, to use sociological terminology, we find a process of "sociation" (*Vergesellschaftung*) rather than "communalization" (*Vergemeinschaftung*). Janosch Steuwer points out that it is far from uncommon

for mechanisms that were cases of "sociation" in this sense to be subsumed under the term *Volksgemeinschaft* and that this tends not to enhance conceptual clarity. See Steuwer, "Volksgemeinschaft," 516. On the sociological terminology, see Weber, Max, *Wirtschaft und Gesellschaft. Grundriss der verstehenden Soziologie* (Tübingen 2013), 21–23.

61　Lüdtke, Alf, "Einleitung. Herrschaft als soziale Praxis," in Alf Lüdtke (ed.), *Herrschaft als soziale Praxis. Historische und sozialanthropologische Studien* (Göttingen 1991), 9–63; Peukert, Detlef, *Volksgenossen und Gemeinschaftsfremde. Anpassung, Ausmerze und Aufbegehren unter dem Nationalsozialismus* (Cologne 1982); on the field of research on the *Volksgemeinschaft* that goes beyond these topics, see the summary in Steuwer, "Volksgemeinschaft."

62　Nevertheless, some of these studies draw conclusions, sometimes quite far-reaching ones, about the supposed counterparts of these practices that have not been empirically examined. For example, Kathrin Kollmeier looks at the disciplinary policy of the Hitler Youth, and thus exclusionary processes, and comes to the conclusion that these were essential to integration into the *Volksgemeinschaft*: Kollmeier, Kathrin, *Ordnung und Ausgrenzung. Die Disziplinarpolitik der Hitler-Jugend* (Göttingen 2007), 277.

63　On the lack of knowledge about the perspective of the excluded, see Wildt, "Volksgemeinschaft," 105. This perspective is considered in Meyer, Beate, "Erfühlte und erdachte 'Volksgemeinschaft.' Erfahrungen 'jüdischer Mischlinge' zwischen Integration und Ausgrenzung," in Frank Bajohr and Michael Wildt (eds.), *Volksgemeinschaft. Neue Forschungen zur Gesellschaft des Nationalsozialismus* (Frankfurt/M. 2009), 144–164.

64　The ego-documents are mostly letters written by patients and relatives. In the context of committal, these are chiefly missives composed by subsequently committed persons prior to their admission or those sent by relatives to the institution. The question of how to deal with letter censorship, then, does not arise.

65　One of the reasons why the Gestapo operated so effectively was that about half of those it persecuted had been denounced. See Mallmann, Klaus-Michael, "Die V-Leute der Gestapo. Umrisse einer kollektiven Biographie," in Gerhard Paul and Klaus-Michael Mallmann (eds.), *Die Gestapo. Mythos und Realität* (Darmstadt 1995), 268–288; Diewald-Kerkmann, Gisela, "Denunziantentum und Gestapo. Die freiwilligen 'Helfer' aus der Bevölkerung," in Gerhard Paul and Klaus-Michael Mallmann (eds.), *Die Gestapo. Mythos und Realität* (Darmstadt 1995), 288–305; for a summary see Mallmann, Klaus-Michael and Gerhard Paul, "Die Gestapo. Weltanschauungsexekutive mit gesellschaftlichem Rückhalt," in Klaus-Michael Mallmann and Gerhard Paul (eds.), *Die Gestapo im Zweiten Weltkrieg. "Heimatfront" und besetztes Europa* (Darmstadt 2000), 599–650.

66　Many of the most recently published works on the *Volksgemeinschaft* examine organized actors in some way, such as the HJ, the NSDAP district leaderships, and shooting clubs: Kollmeier, *Disziplinarpolitik der Hitler-Jugend*; Borggräfe, Henning, *Schützenvereine im Nationalsozialismus. Pflege der "Volksgemeinschaft" und Vorbereitung auf den Krieg (1933–1945)* (Münster 2011); Thieler, Kerstin, "Volksgenossen unter Vorbehalt. Die Herrschaftspraxis der NSDAP-Kreisleitungen und die Zugehörigkeit zur 'Volksgemeinschaft,'" in Detlef Schmiechen-Ackermann (ed.), *"Volksgemeinschaft." Mythos, wirkungsmächtige soziale Verheißung oder soziale Realität im "Dritten Reich"? Propaganda und Selbstmobilisierung im NS-Staat* (Paderborn 2011), 211–225. The same applies to the other contributions in this anthology.

67　Goldberg, Ann, "Conventions of Madness. Bürgerlichkeit and the Asylum in the Vormärz," *Central European History*, vol. 2, 2000, 178.

68 One of the few studies that looks at the construction of inclusion and exclusion is by Birthe Kundrus. She brings out this negotiation process with reference to the "definition" of people living in the Warthegau as Polish or German. See Kundrus, Birthe, "Regime der Differenz. Volkstumspolitische Inklusion und Exklusion im Warthegau und im Generalgouverment, 1939–1945," in Frank Bajohr and Michael Wildt (eds.), *Volksgemeinschaft. Neue Forschungen zur Gesellschaft des Nationalsozialismus* (Frankfurt/M. 2009), 105–123.

69 Süß, *Volkskörper.*

70 Thus, Winfried Süß assumes that trust in doctors was probably not particularly high. At the same time, he has mulled whether a long-term bond between doctor and GP might have prevented National Socialist ideology from being implemented in medical practice. Ibid., 373 and 378.

71 On the religious institution of Schönbrunn—one relevant to and discussed in the present book—see for example Christians, Annemone, *Amtsgewalt und Volksgesundheit. Das öffentliche Gesundheitswesen im nationalsozialistischen München* (Göttingen 2013).

72 Particularly relevant in the context of this book are Hockerts, Hans Günter, *Sozialpolitische Entscheidungen im Nachkriegsdeutschland. Alliierte und deutsche Sozialversicherungspolitik* (Stuttgart 1980); Schagen, Udo and Sabine Schleiermacher, "Gesundheitswesen und Sicherung bei Krankheit," in *1949–1961 Deutsche Demokratische Republik. Im Zeichen des Aufbaus des Sozialismus (Geschichte der Sozialpolitik in Deutschland seit 1945*, vol. 8, Berlin 2004), 390–435; Helwig, Gisela and Barbara Hille, "Familie-, Jugend- und Altenpolitik," in ibid., 495–553; Gitter, Wolfgang, "Soziale Sicherung bei Unfall und Berufskrankheit," in ibid., 437–452; Hoffmann, Dierk and Michael Schwartz, "Gesellschaftliche Strukturen und sozialpolitische Handlungsfelder," in ibid., 75–158; Hoffmann, Dierk and Michael Schwartz, "Politische Rahmenbedingungen," in ibid., 1–73; Schwartz, Michael and Constantin Goschler, "Ausgleich von Kriegs- und Diktaturfolgen, soziales Entschädigungsrecht," in ibid., 589–654; Conrad, Christoph, "Alterssicherung," in Hans Günter Hockerts (ed.), *Drei Wege deutscher Sozialstaatlichkeit. NS-Diktatur, Bundesrepublik und DDR im Vergleich* (Munich 1998), 101–116; Schulz, "Soziale Sicherung von Frauen und Familien," in ibid., 117–150; Hockerts, Hans Günter, "Einführung," in ibid., 7–27; Hachtmann, Rüdiger, "Arbeitsverfassung," in ibid., 27–55; also helping elucidate this thematic complex are Ellerbrock, Dagmar, *"Healing Democracy"—Demokratie als Heilmittel. Gesundheit, Krankheit und Politik in der amerikanischen Besatzungszone, 1945–1949* (Bonn 2004); Lindner, Ulrike, *Gesundheitspolitik in der Nachkriegszeit. Großbritannien und die Bundesregierung Deutschland im Vergleich* (Munich 2004).

73 Ernst, Anne Sabine, *"Die beste Prophylaxe ist der Sozialismus." Ärzte und medizinische Hochschullehrer in der SBZ/DDR 1945–1961* (Münster 1997).

74 A debate on the costs of asylums had already flared up in the Weimar Republic. Among other things, sterilization was discussed as a cost-effective alternative to institutionalization. During the Nazi era, the idea that money was flowing into psychiatric institutions that could be better spent elsewhere on "valuable," healthy "national comrades" (*Volksgenossen*) finally prevailed. See Brink, *Psychiatrie,* 208ff. and 239.

75 Various definitions of coercion, security, and freedom in light of "everyday understanding," the "legal definition," a "social and cultural-historical perspective," the "inherent medical standpoint" and the "institutional standpoint" are presented in Meier, Marietta et al., *Zwang zur Ordnung. Psychiatrie im Kanton Zürich, 1870–1970* (Zürich 2007), 31ff. The authors conclude that it is unhelpful to presuppose a "correct" definition; ibid, 32.

76 He comes to the same conclusion about the counter-concept of "freedom." Kaufmann, Franz-Xaver, "Sicherheit. Das Leitbild beherrschbarer Komplexität," in Stephan Lessenich (ed.), *Wohlfahrtstaatliche Grundbegriffe. Historische und aktuelle Diskurse* (Frankfurt/M. 2003), 74.

77 Ibid.

78 On the importance of security in understanding the Federal Republic, see Conze, Eckart, "Sicherheit als Kultur. Überlegungen zu einer 'modernen Politikgeschichte' der Bundesrepublik Deutschland," VfZ, vol. 3, 2005, 357–380.

79 Military committals were always compulsory in nature, but only a few committed soldiers feature in the sample collated for this book.

80 Ulrike Lindner has examined the health policy of the early West Germany and, among other things, highlighted continuities in the approach to women with STDs. See for example Lindner, *Gesundheitspolitik*, 304ff. STDs, sexuality, gender-specific behavioral expectations, and attributions of illness are also of great relevance to committal practices and represent an important set of topics in the history of psychiatry as a whole. See for example Goldberg, "Conventions of Madness," 173–193; Andrews, Jonathan, and Anne Digby, "Introduction. Gender and Class in the Historiography of British and Irish Psychiatry," in Jonathan Andrews and Anne Digby (eds.), *Sex and Seclusion, Class and Custody. Perspectives on Gender and Class in the History of British and Irish Psychiatry* (Amsterdam 2004), 7–44; Showalter, Elaine, *The Female Malady. Women, Madness and English Culture 1830–1980* (New York 1985); Kaufmann, Doris, "Nervenschwäche, Neurasthenie und 'sexuelle Frage' im deutschen Kaiserreich," in Christine Wolters et al. (eds.), *Abweichung und Normalität. Psychiatrie in Deutschland vom Kaiserreich bis zur Deutschen Einheit* (Bielefeld 2013), 197–209.

81 Women were subject to compulsory committal disproportionately often during the war, while the forcible committal of the elderly often featured direct reference to the war.

82 This applies to both German- and English-language publications. See for example Moeller, Robert, *War Stories. The Search for a Usable Past in the Federal Republic of Germany* (Berkeley 2001); Cornelia Brink's book on psychiatry is also based on print media and parliamentary debates.

83 Mallmann, Klaus-Michael and Andrej Angrick, *Die Gestapo nach 1945. Konflikte, Karrieren, Konstruktionen* (Darmstadt 2009); Mallmann, Klaus-Michael and Gerhard Paul, *Karrieren der Gewalt. Nationalsozialistische Täterbiographien* (Darmstadt 2004); in light of a single case: Herbert, Ulrich, *Best. Biographische Studien über Radikalismus, Weltanschauung und Vernunft 1903–1989* (Bonn 1996).

84 Korzilius, Sven, *"Asoziale" und "Parasiten" im Recht der SBZ/DDR* (Cologne 2005).

85 Fulbrook, Mary, *Ein ganz normales Leben. Alltag und Gesellschaft in der DDR* (Darmstadt 2008); Fulbrook, Mary, *Dissonant Lives. Generations and Violence through German Dictatorships* (Oxford 2011); Hürtgen, Renate, *Ausreise per Antrag: der lange Weg nach drüben. Eine Studie über Herrschaft und Alltag in der DDR-Provinz* (Göttingen 2014); on aspects of everyday history in East and West, see Sachse, Carola, *Der Hausarbeitstag. Gerechtigkeit und Gleichberechtigung in Ost und West 1939–1994* (Göttingen 2002).

86 Hanrath, *Euthanasie und Psychiatriereform*, 263ff. and 351ff.

87 Lindenberger, Thomas, "Die Diktatur der Grenzen. Zur Einleitung," in Thomas Lindenberger (ed.), *Herrschaft und Eigen-Sinn in der Diktatur. Studien zur Gesellschaftsgeschichte der DDR* (Cologne) 1999, 13–44; Kocka, Jürgen, "Eine durchherrschte Gesellschaft," in Hartmut Kaelble et al. (eds.), *Sozialgeschichte der DDR* (Stuttgart 1994), 547–553.

88 Tönsmeyer, Tatjana and Annette Vowinckel, "Sicherheit und Sicherheitsempfinden als Thema der Zeitgeschichte: Eine Einleitung," *Zeithistorische Forschungen/Studies in Contemporary History*, online edition, vol. 2, 2010, URL: http://www.zeithistorische-forschungen.de/16126041-Inhalt-2-2010 (retrieved 1.4.2014).
89 On police jurisdiction over both areas, "public security" and welfare, see the following anthology: Lüdtke, *"Sicherheit."*
90 See esp. Diewald-Kerkmann, Gisela, "Denunziantentum und Gestapo. Die freiwilligen 'Helfer' aus der Bevölkerung," in Gerhard Paul and Klaus-Michael Mallmann (eds.), *Die Gestapo. Mythos und Realität* (Darmstadt 1995), 288–305.
91 Quoted in ibid, 290.
92 Paul and Mallmann, *Gestapo*; Paul and Mallmann, *Gestapo im Zweiten Weltkrieg*. For this research perspective beyond the Gestapo, see also Peter Fritzsche's conception of the "Third Reich" as a "consensus dictatorship," in Fritzsche, Peter, *Life and Death in the Third Reich* (Harvard 2008).
93 Schlich, Thomas, "Wissenschaftliche Fakten als Thema der Geschichtsforschung," in Norbert Paul and Schlich, Thomas (eds.), *Medizingeschichte. Aufgaben, Probleme, Perspektiven* (Frankfurt/M. 1997), 125. On this conception, see also Eckart, Wolfgang, and Robert Jütte, *Medizingeschichte. Eine Einführung* (Cologne 2007).
94 See Schlich, "Fakten," 123.
95 This opened up the possibility, for example, of placing offenders in a forensic psychiatry department rather than prison, and of prescribing institutionalization rather than a course of treatment for overburdened mothers.
96 Szöllösi-Janze, Margit, "Wissensgesellschaft—ein neues Konzept zur Erschließung der deutsch-deutschen Zeitgeschichte?," in Hans Günter Hockerts (ed.), *Koordinaten deutscher Geschichte in der Epoche des Ost-West-Konflikts* (Munich, 2004), 277–307, here 280.
97 Ibid., 282. A similar position from a history-of-psychiatry perspective is adopted by Hess, Volker, and Benoit Majerus, "Writing the History of Psychiatry in the 20th century," *History of Psychiatry*, vol. 22, 2011, 142.
98 Szöllösi-Janze notes that her reflections on the knowledge society provide room for the integration of "actional and orientational knowledge" and also highlights psychiatry as an object of investigation. Szöllösi-Janze, "Wissensgesellschaft," 280 and 284.
99 Arguments related to work were certainly important before World War II, and they were not purely German phenomena. In a long-term study on the Netherlands, Joost Vijselaar highlights the great importance of economic circumstances and labor relations within the family: Vijselaar, "Out and In"; on the aspect of work, and the ability to work, in the context of both committal practices and everyday practice in asylums around 1900, see Ankele, Monika, *Alltag und Aneignung in Psychiatrien um 1900. Selbstzeugnisse von Frauen aus der Sammlung Prinzhorn* (Vienna 2009).
100 Bruns, Florian, *Medizinethik im Nationalsozialismus. Entwicklungen und Protagonisten in Berlin (1939–1945)* (Stuttgart 2009).
101 On the issue of work within everyday practice in asylums around 1900, see Ankele, *Alltag und Aneignung.*
102 Herbert, "Traditionen."
103 Research on other aspects of "labor history," on the other hand, is much more common, including: Kleßmann, Christoph, *Arbeiter im "Arbeiterstaat" DDR. Deutsche Traditionen, sowjetisches Modell, westdeutsches Magnetfeld (1945–1971)* (Bonn 2007); Rupieper, Hermann-J. et al. (eds.), *Die mitteldeutsche Chemieindustrie und ihre Arbeiter im 20. Jahrhundert* (Halle 2005); Hübner, Peter, *Arbeiter in der SBZ-DDR* (Essen 1999); Hübner, Peter, *Arbeit, Arbeiter und Technik in der DDR*

1971 bis 1989. Zwischen Fordismus und digitaler Revolution (Bonn 2014); in addition, studies have been published on various academically trained professions,
including physicians and professors: Ernst, "Sozialismus"; Jessen, Ralph,
*Akademische Elite und kommunistische Diktatur. Die ostdeutsche Hochs-
chullehrerschaft in der Ulbricht-Ära* (Göttingen 1999); incorporating a cultural
studies perspective: Wagner-Kyora, Georg, *Vom "nationalen" zum "sozialistischen"
Selbst. Zur Erfahrungsgeschichte deutscher Chemiker und Ingenieure im 20.
Jahrhundert* (Stuttgart 2009).

104 On persecution under Nazism, see esp. Ayaß, Wolfgang, *"Asoziale" im
Nationalsozialismus* (Stuttgart 1995). On exclusion in the GDR, see
Lindenberger, Thomas, "'Asociality' and Modernity. The GDR as a Welfare
Dictatorship," in Katherine Pence and Paul Betts (eds.), *Socialist Modern.
East German Everyday Culture and Politics* (Ann Arbor 2011), 211–233; Korzilius,
"Asoziale"; when it comes to the Federal Republic, continuities have so far been
established only with respect to the approach to "asocial" female prisoners at
Ravensbrück and to women with STDs who were declared "asocial." See the
chapter "Geschlechtskrankheiten als medizinisches und soziales Phänomen," in
Lindner, *Gesundheitspolitik*, 283ff. and Schikorra, Christa, *Kontinuitäten der
Ausgrenzung. "Asoziale" Häftlinge im Frauen-Konzentrationslager Ravensbrück*
(Berlin 2001).

105 Lüdtke, Alf, "'Helden der Arbeit'—Mühen beim Arbeiten," in Hartmut Kaelble
et al. (eds.), *Sozialgeschichte der DDR* (Stuttgart 1994), 189–213; Lüdtke, Alf,
"People Working. Everyday Life and German Fascism," *History Workshop
Journal*, vol. 50, 2000, 76–92; Lüdtke, Alf, "The World of Men's Work, East and
West," in Katherine Pence and Paul Betts (eds), *Socialist Modern. East German
Everyday Culture and Politics* (Ann Arbor 2011), 234–249.

106 See for example Port, Andrew I., *Die rätselhafte Stabilität der DDR. Arbeit und
Alltag im sozialistischen Deutschland* (Berlin 2010); Wagner-Kyora, *Selbst*; Kohli,
Martin, "Die DDR als Arbeitsgesellschaft? Arbeit, Lebenslauf und soziale
Differenzierung," in Hartmut Kaelble et al. (eds.), *Sozialgeschichte der DDR*
(Stuttgart 1994), 31–61; Roesler, Jörg, "Die Produktionsbrigaden in der Industrie
der DDR. Zentrum der Arbeitswelt?" in Hartmut Kaelble et al. (eds.),
Sozialgeschichte der DDR (Stuttgart 1994), 144–170; Hübner, Peter, "Die Zukunft
war gestern. Soziale und mentale Trends in der DDR-Industriearbeiterschaft," in
Hartmut Kaelble et al. (eds.), *Sozialgeschichte der DDR* (Stuttgart 1994), 171–187.

107 Schweig, Nicole, *Gesundheitsverhalten von Männern. Gesundheit und Krankheit in
Briefen 1800–1950* (Stuttgart 2008), 117; Hoffmann, Susanne, *Gesunder Alltag im
20. Jahrhundert? Geschlechterspezifische Diskurse und gesundheitsrelevante
Verhaltensstile in deutschsprachigen Ländern* (Stuttgart 2010).

108 On exclusion in the GDR, see Lindenberger, "Asociality"; Korzilius, "Asoziale."

109 Lindner, *Gesundheitspolitik*, 283ff; Schikorra, "Asoziale."

110 Wehler, Hans-Ulrich, *Deutsche Gesellschaftsgeschichte*, vol. 5: *Bundesrepublik
und DDR 1949–1990* (Munich 2008); on the debate, see Bahners, Patrick and
Alexander Cammann (eds.), *Bundesrepublik und DDR. Die Debatte um Hans-
Ulrich Wehlers "Deutsche Gesellschaftsgeschichte"* (Munich 2009), 107–124.

111 Bänzinger, Peter-Paul, "Der betriebsame Mensch: ein Bericht (nicht nur) aus der
Werkstatt," *Österreichische Zeitschrift für Geschichtswissenschaften*, vol. 2, 2012,
222–236; Bernet, Brigitta and David Gugerli, "Sputniks Resonanzen. Der Aufstieg
der Humankapitaltheorie im Kalten Krieg—eine Argumentationsskizze,"
Historische Anthropologie, vol. 3, 2011, 433–446.

112 In this chapter, I work with the conceptual pair of domestic work and gainful
employment, since in this context it is unrealistic to hope for deeper insights
through the use of newer concepts. On the terminological debate, see Uta

Gerhard, who argues for the term "care work." Gerhard, Uta, "Editorial," *L'Homme. Europäische Zeitschrift für feministische Geschichtswissenschaft*, vol. 19, 2008, 7.

113 Anna Sabine Ernst assesses the Pavlov campaign as unsuccessful, concluding that Pavlovian research in the 1950s was carried out alongside other research and had no impact. See Ernst, *Sozialismus*, 335ff.

114 Main State Archive Munich, State Archive Munich, City Archive Munich, Hesse State Archive Marburg, Land Archive Greifswald/Branch Office of the Mecklenburg State Archive Schwerin. In the Saxony Main State Archive Dresden, circulars to the "sanatoria" (call numbers 2007, 2008, 2009, 2010, 2011, and 2013) from the Landesregierung Sachsen, Ministerium für Arbeit und Sozialfürsorge, 1945–52 fonds were not accessible during the entire period of investigation.

115 Großschweidnitz, however, functioned less well than Rodewisch during the occupation. Both located in Saxony, they were subject to the same regional traditions and regulations, but Großschweidnitz was larger than Rodewisch.

116 In the Greifswald University Psychiatric Clinic, for example, admissions were often undertaken by assistant physicians who were there for a brief stint as part of their training. When they left the clinic, their personnel file was passed on to the next institution within their educational trajectory. The only residual document preserved in the archives was their termination contract.

117 Of all 1,424 individual case files, the following characteristics were recorded using SPPS: sex, age, place of residence, place of birth, marital status, number of children, occupation, father's occupation, reason for committal, committal pathway (Who is referring the patient—a public health officer, a family doctor, a hospital, another psychiatric establishment? Did the patient arrive without committal? Were they handed over by a court?); last place of residence before committal (Is the patient coming from home, another hospital, an old people's home, a prison, a camp?), length of stay, diagnosis, type of termination of stay (discharge, onward referral, death, prison sentence), and number of previous committals. If there were multiple committals, the criteria for the first and last were noted. All this information was recorded on the standardized admission forms.

118 I was able to do both in the following institutions: LHA Marburg, the Rodewisch Sanatorium-Nursing Home, and the Eglfing-Haar Sanatorium-Nursing Home. In the other three facilities, files were selected according to the GORT system. Of the medical records at Großschweidnitz, only those of patients whose last names begin with the letters G, O, R, or T were archived by the Saxony State Archive. The files at Bethel and the Greifswald University Psychiatric Clinic, which could not be selected by random sample, were also determined by the GORT system.

119 On the selection of medical records for a study featuring very similar questions on committal and discharge practices, in which these documents were also evaluated qualitatively and quantitatively, cf. the work of Joost Vijselaar. To cover a century, he uses a time grid of five-year intervals and selects the first five medical records in each. See Vijselaar, "Family," 279.

120 Foucault refers to the "monologue of reason about madness." Foucault, Michel, *Psychologie und Geisteskrankheit* (Frankfurt/M. 1968), 132. The patient's voice has been investigated empirically in Lachmund, Jens, and Gunnar Stollberg, *Patientenwelten. Krankheit und Medizin vom späten 18. bis zum frühen 20. Jahrhundert im Spiegel von Autobiographien* (Opladen 1995), 218; Elkeles, Barbara, "Die schweigsame Welt von Arzt und Patient. Einwilligung und Aufklärung in der Arzt-Patient-Beziehung des 19. und frühen 20. Jahrhunderts," *Medizin, Gesellschaft und Geschichte*, vol. 8, 1989, 63–91; on the power gap

between psychiatrists, asylum staff, and patients in psychiatric institutions, see Erving Goffman, who portrays individuals who have been committed as actors, but shows that ultimately they always remain the reactive party within the asylum: Goffman, *Asyle*.

121 See Bernet, Brigitta, "'Eintragen und Ausfüllen': Der Fall des psychiatrischen Formulars," in Sibylle Brändli et al. (eds.), *Zum Fall machen, zum Fall werden* (Frankfurt/M. 2009), 62–91.

122 On the value of the anamnesis with reference to sexual medicine, see Putz, Christa, "Narrative Heterogenität und dominante Darstellungsweise. Zur Produktion von Fallnarrativen in der deutschsprachigen Sexualmedizin und Psychoanalyse, 1890 bis 1930," in Sibylle Brändli et al. (eds.), *Zum Fall machen, zum Fall werden* (Frankfurt/M. 2009), 92–120.

123 See for example Goldstein, Jan, "Bringing the Psyche into Scientific Focus," in Theodore M. Porter and Dorothy Ross (eds.), *The Cambridge History of Science*, vol. 7: *The Modern Social Sciences* (Cambridge 2003), 153.

124 On this research perspective, see for example Roelcke on the history of psychiatry, Szöllösi-Janze on issues in German-German history, and Daston and Galison on the self-image of scientists in specific contemporary historical contexts. Roelcke, Volker, "Auf der Suche nach der Politik in der Wissensproduktion. Plädoyer für eine historisch-politische Epistemologie," *Berichte zur Wissenschaftsgeschichte*, vol. 33, 2010, 176–192; Szöllösi-Janze, "Wissensgesellschaft," 280 and 284; Daston, Lorraine and Peter Galison, *Objectivity* (New York 2010), 32.

125 In the 1990s, the so-called internalist approach was replaced by the "externalist" perspective. Since then, the history of science has no longer been understood primarily as an intradisciplinary field of research but has been scrutinized with regard to its origins, effects, and forms of organization within society. For the essentials of this shift, see Golinski, Jan, *Making Natural Knowledge. Constructivism and the History of Science* (Chicago 2005). A summary can be found in Greyerz, Kaspar von et al., "Einführung. Schauplätze wissensgeschichtlicher Forschung," in Kaspar von Greyerz et al. (eds.), *Wissenschaftsgeschichte und Geschichte des Wissens im Dialog—Connecting Science and Knowledge* (Göttingen 2013), 10. On the added epistemological value of a history-of-knowledge approach that embeds history-of-science themes in a broader framework to enhance our understanding of twentieth-century German history, along with as its continuities and ruptures, see Szöllösi-Janze, "Wissensgesellschaft," 280.

126 As Thomas Schlich argues, scholarly publications are a valuable source of insights into the emergence of scholarly knowledge and help us analyze the status of these insights within scholarly discourse. Schlich, Thomas, "How Gods and Saints Became Transplant Surgeons. The Scientific Article as a Model for the Writing of History," *History of Science*, vol. 33, 1995, 311–331. On the importance of access to specialist journals or conferences, see Schlich, "Fakten," 118.

127 Discourse is understood as patterns of order that are constructed and that thus reflect the distribution of power inherent in their construction. See Landwehr, Achim, "Diskurs und Diskursgeschichte," *Docupedia-Zeitgeschichte*, 11.2.2010, URL: http://docupedia.de/zg/Diskurs_und_Diskursgeschichte?oldid=84596, 6 (retrieved 22.7.2014). Many historians of psychiatry have embraced the understanding of discourse propagated by Volker Roelcke, according to which psychiatric discourses are the result of negotiation processes and thus dynamic. See Roelcke, Volker, *Krankheit und Kulturkritik. Psychiatrische Gesellschaftsdeutungen im bürgerlichen Zeitalter (1790–1914)* (Frankfurt/M. 1999), 29.

1 Historical parameters of committal practice

Psychiatry, state, and society to 1941

In 1946, the patient Martina R., whom we encountered in the introduction, was admitted to a Land sanatorium in Marburg, rather than a sanatorium-nursing home. This can be put down to historically contingent regional differences in the clinic and asylum system. In Hesse—unlike in Bavaria and Saxony, for example—it was customary to first admit patients to a Land sanatorium. Only if it was decided that a longer stay was required was the patient transferred to one of the two sanatorium-nursing homes in Haina and Merxhausen.[1] The types of clinics and asylums mentioned here will be presented in more detail in this chapter. I then shed light on the emergence of psychiatric practices and discourses as background to the mid-twentieth-century practice of committal. This includes regulations on committal, the relationship between doctor and patient, psychiatrists' expertise and scientific aspirations, the practice of psychiatric evaluations, psychiatric interpretations of society, and the relationship between war and psychiatry.[2]

Types of asylums and clinics

Most psychiatric institutions in the nineteenth century and the first half of the twentieth century were state facilities. Depending on the region, however, they were located at differing administrative levels. They could be royal or ducal institutions, as in Saxony or Mecklenburg. In other cases, they were to be found lower down the administrative hierarchy. In Hesse, asylums formed part of the newly created Prussian provincial administration from the 1870s onward, while in Bavaria they came under the district administration.[3] The character of psychiatric institutions also varied regionally. While Eglfing-Haar in Munich, Großschweidnitz, and Untergöltzsch operated as sanatorium-nursing homes, the LHA Marburg was a Land sanatorium that did not specialize in long-term residential care. The different administrative traditions continued to have an impact in the Weimar Republic, in which health care was organized by the *Länder* or states. While regional authority over the health system ended when the Nazis established a centralized administration, the traits specific to the nineteenth-century German asylum

DOI: 10.4324/9781032716237-2

system remained significant. Even after World War II, for instance, Marburg continued to focus on treatable patients.[4]

It was not until the 1870s that asylums were joined by psychiatric clinics that formed part of university hospitals.[5] These clinics constituted joint institutions for psychiatry and neurology,[6] and as part of the university hospitals they were of enormous importance to the professionalization of psychiatrists as medical practitioners. The development of psychiatry into a medical field in its own right took place in a rather unusual way in Germany that deviated from the two classical trajectories. Psychiatry emerged neither via the expansion of medical knowledge nor through processes of institutionalization. Instead, the field developed independently in the asylums and only became part of the discipline of medicine when psychiatric clinics were established within university hospitals.[7] While university psychiatry researched "mental illnesses" with the aim of curing them, successes in this area were few and far between. It was in the classification of illnesses and in prophylaxis that academic psychiatry made advances.[8] Because the university psychiatric clinics (the term used in the present book for *psychiatrische und Nervenkliniken*, literally "psychiatric and neurological clinics") were attached administratively to the university hospitals, they were—in contrast to the sanatorium-nursing homes—only designed for temporary stays. If patients required longer-term treatment, they could be referred to a sanatorium-nursing home. Nevertheless, the psychiatric clinics within the university hospitals were subject to state guidelines on admission. Both compulsory committals and committals for evaluation were possible. Much like the psychiatric asylums, the psychiatric clinics developed notable traditions of their own. For example, their diagnostic system, which was the responsibility of the head professor, played a significant role in admissions.[9] The relationship between the different types of psychiatric establishment thus entailed both collaborative elements and a parallel existence. Their differing orientations required cooperation, while the system ensured that asylums as venerable institutions and university psychiatry clinics as new ones competed and sought to distinguish themselves from one another.

In addition to state institutions, psychiatric facilities were also run by private, mostly religious, organizations. Originally, these specialized primarily in nursing care, though this changed at the turn of the twentieth century. Unlike state asylums, private institutions were not responsible for specific districts,[10] so individuals from distant regions were also committed, for example, to the von Bodelschwingh Asylums Bethel. In 1941, at the beginning of the period under investigation here, there were three types of inpatient admission of the so-called "mentally ill" (*Geisteskranke*): to state asylums, private institutions, and university psychiatric clinics as part of university hospitals.

While the university psychiatric clinics were subunits of the university hospitals, the asylums, regardless of whether they were sanatoriums or sanatorium-nursing homes, constituted a microcosm unto themselves—with their own agricultural production, slaughterhouses, fruit and vegetable gardens, workshops, laundries, festivity halls, churches, and cemeteries on the premises. Because of the space required for this and in the belief that rural tranquility promoted healing, many asylums were built outside the city centers. Toward the end of the nineteenth century, the tendency to convert old monasteries into asylums tailed off, and new ones were built in the so-called colonial style, consisting of numerous individual buildings or "pavilions" in park-like surroundings.[11] This design made it possible to distribute patients among different buildings, separated according to gender, level of care, "necessary" degree of supervision, and treatment classes.[12] Of the facilities examined in the present study, this layout was found at Eglfing-Haar, Untergöltzsch, Großschweidnitz, the LHA Marburg, and the von Bodelschwingh Asylums Bethel. All were established in the late nineteenth century as part of the so-called "lunatic boom" (*Irrenboom*). This is explained in a variety of ways in the research. While Dirk Blasius emphasizes the state's disciplinary efforts, studies produced in the English-speaking world highlight the emergence of networks on the meso-level, encompassing doctors, police, and health institutions, while also underscoring their growing power.[13]

Psychiatric institutions thus differed in three ways: function, region, and body responsible. These historically contingent differences continued to inform committal practices between 1941 and 1963, with the different facilities' orientation toward a specific clientele persisting. University psychiatric clinics mainly admitted patients for diagnostic clarification and short-term treatment, the LHA Marburg sought to admit individuals with a reasonable prospect of recovery, while the sanatorium-nursing homes focused on those who needed care only and patients who seemed likely to recover. Bethel's status as a religious institution meant that it did not have to admit compulsorily committed persons until 1963.

In addition to the administrative level, psychiatry, state, and society were related in three ways in the nineteenth century and the first half of the twentieth century. First, psychiatric institutions were places where people were housed, more or less in isolation from society, for care, cure, or safety reasons. Second, psychiatry functioned as a supplier of knowledge that was deployed by the state. Third, psychiatric knowledge served to interpret and explain social realities and problems. This was a situation of multi-layered interdependence rather than a one-sided relationship of dependency in which psychiatry functioned as an arm of the state. Comprehensive state supervision or committal of all "lunatics" was not the outcome envisaged when the asylum system was established in the nineteenth century; the aim was to make places available only for about 20 percent of the mentally ill.[14] In what follows, I outline the role of psychiatric institutions for families and the state, the function of psychiatry as a supplier of knowledge applied by the state, and psychiatric knowledge as it informed interpretations of society. I conclude by casting light on important changes that occurred during the Nazi period before 1941, the beginning of the period under scrutiny here.

The role of psychiatric institutions

Psychiatric facilities fulfilled a variety of functions. They provided long-term "quartering" and nursing care for sick individuals who could not be cured, and they were increasingly supposed to cure psychiatric illnesses as well. In addition, committals were legitimized with reference to safety considerations in the broadest of senses. These three functions of psychiatric establishments are closely related to the different groups of people involved in committals. While there was certainly a correlation between the functions of the asylum and actors' interests, this correlation involves ideal-typical ascriptions that reveal a common thread running through the web of motives for committal. For instance, committals initiated by police and the justice system were legitimized with reference to the endangerment of self and others. In certain cases, the production of security, in this case within the home, could be one of the relatives' priorities as well. Their motives for committal could also revolve around hopes of helping the sick individual or the prospect of recovery, though for a considerable period of time curing was of greater importance to the professionalization of physicians than it was to many of the committing families.

Physician and patient: cure, recovery, and quartering

For asylum physicians and the emerging profession of psychiatrists, curing took on an increasingly central role over the course of the nineteenth century. As a result, asylums ceased to be undifferentiated quartering institutions, where so-called "lunatics" were housed along with the elderly, the poor, and the sick, and became more complex.[15] Their remit now extended to people with behavior viewed as diverging from the norm, for which Foucault coined the term "deviant heterotopias."[16] The sanatorium-nursing homes, as well as the university psychiatric clinics that emerged in the final third of the nineteenth century, were responsible for both psychiatric and neurological diseases;[17] Bethel, a religious institution, also had a neurological department at the time of World War II.

Asylum physicians and university psychiatrists, subsequent to a process completed in the 1860s, saw themselves as medical professionals responsible for treating, curing, and researching "mental illness."[18] However, the families of patients from non-bourgeois backgrounds still regarded the asylum mostly as a place of accommodation and care when this could no longer be provided within the home. Hence, they regularly instigated admissions of family members whose condition was classified by doctors as incurable. In line with this, asylums sometimes went so far as to provide cost incentives to facilitate the examination of clientele from among the poor within an institution at an early stage.[19] In the final third of the nineteenth century, psychiatry was compelled to tone down its promises of cures, with the question of curability versus incurability shifting from the therapeutic to the diagnostic realm; increasingly, clinical pictures were constructed in such a way that incurability became a characteristic of a disease.[20] Dementia praecox, for example, a term used for what is now called schizophrenia, was characterized in part by its incurability,[21] according to Emil Kraepelin (1856–1926).[22]

Among relatives, hopes of a cure and/or treatment was a motive for committal typical of the nineteenth-century middle classes. Faith in cures and trust in psychiatrists distinguished the bourgeoisie from lower social classes, while helping institutionalize asylums as differentiated medical facilities in the first half of the nineteenth century.[23] Consequently, a disproportionately large number of psychiatric patients were members of the educated and economic middle class—20 percent, in contrast to an overall population share of 5 percent. Ann Goldberg shows that the many admissions of bourgeois patients were directly related to the rise of rationality within the middle class. Women made up a clear majority of those subject to bourgeois committals,[24] and Goldberg demonstrates that these were intended to educate them to ensure a better fit with society: they were to be cured of emotions that stood in the way of their social role, such as anger, "excessive" sympathy, and "social coldness."[25] Here, education and "healing" were closely related. The patient's cooperation thus proved constitutive both of successful treatment and of the asylum director's psychiatric knowledge. Goldberg shows that "medical knowledge was itself an amalgam of expert and lay opinion that was generated in large part within (and because of) his relationship with his bourgeois clients."[26] The treatment itself, then, was not based on medical expertise in the scientific sense, which the asylum directors did not possess, but on the character of the doctor and his relationship with the patient. The doctor's so-called "inner core" and the moral force emanating from it were considered decisive.[27] Here, bourgeois families were pursuing an interest different from that of the lower classes: "The bourgeois discourse on one's own mental endangerment and on deviants judged to be mentally ill must be placed in the context of the Enlightenment critique of inner and outer impediments to reason. This discourse was an active element in the attempt to get to grips with inner and outer reality and its transformation."[28]

There was no parallel to this outside the bourgeoisie. Thus, in the rural Münsterland, Doris Kaufmann finds only claims of "raving madness" (*tobender Wahnsinn*) and "insane idleness" (*verrückter Müßiggang*) as reasons for committal. In these cases, relatives expected a roof over their relatives' head rather than cure.[29] Yet doctors had expressed criticism of the use of psychiatric institutions for such prolonged "quartering" since the 1860s. Wilhelm Griesinger, the leading psychiatrist of the day, emphasized that a stay in an asylum could be counterproductive to recovery and that subsequent integration into the world outside the institution became more difficult the longer the stay lasted.[30] Despite the very different expectations of bourgeois and non-bourgeois patients regarding stints in an asylum, the rationales put forward shared a social component. Patients from both strata of origin had attracted others' attention and were no longer considered tolerable in their milieu, albeit always within their quite different class-related frames of reference. The conduct that inspired committals in the bourgeois world deviated from the norm to a far lesser extent than among the lower classes. Cornelia Brink rightly underlines that middle-class committals were for the most part socially motivated and depended on factors such as social and economic status, kin relations, gender, age, and the ability to earn a livelihood.[31]

Connections between class of origin, understandings of asylums, and doctor–patient relationships continued to shape committal practices from the 1940s to the 1960s. The category of gender was also ever present. In the course of this book, I highlight gender-specific attributions of illness as well as gender-related behavior during the committal of relatives. In addition, I bring out the role played by psychiatrists' character in their self-classification and in their attribution of expertise in the mid-twentieth century.[32]

Security, the justice system, and the police

For the police, the core function of the asylum was to avert threats and establish security.[33] Here, Robert Castel refers to the "double mandate" of psychiatry: in addition to its medical function—be it healing or, in a broader sense, caring—it also played a political-disciplinary role.[34] In Prussia, the placement of the mentally ill occurred on the basis of the General State Law (*Allgemeines Landrecht* or ALR) of 1794 until the founding of the German Empire. The ALR and the Prussian Police Administration Law (*Polizeiverwaltungsgesetz* or PVG) of 1931, which will be explained in more detail below, applied not only to Prussia, but also to northern and central Germany, including Saxony.[35] According to the ALR, only those who had previously been legally incapacitated could be committed. Although committal required incapacitation, the latter alone did not automatically result in committal. Incapacitation, which was usually requested by relatives, merely resulted in the appointment of a guardian for the person involved. Only if the guardian failed to fulfill their responsibilities was the incapacitated individual committed, with the decision to commit being made by a court and implemented by the police.

The police, however, had the option of temporarily bypassing judicial committal in cases of "imminent danger."[36] Through a ministerial decree of July 8, 1867, the care of sick individuals who constituted a danger to the public finally became the sole responsibility of the local police,[37] which began to play a key role in committals. To be sure, some regulations changed over the next eighty years after the founding of the empire. But the police retained the power to make immediate, autonomous committals if they perceived "imminent danger," a power they regularly exercised, not least in order to circumvent other, more complicated committal regulations.

One crucial change in the twentieth century was that patients no longer had to be incapacitated in order to be committed. In other words, decisions were no longer made exclusively without input from the individual involved. As a further innovation, the establishment of polyclinics—a hospital department in which outpatient examinations were performed—at the turn of the twentieth century changed the position of patients in the committal process. The Greifswald University Clinic studied in this book was one of the institutions featuring a polyclinic. In addition, health insurance companies in the Weimar Republic often operated polyclinics.[38] Here the examination was much simpler than in a sanatorium-nursing home and less stigmatized.[39] The lower admission threshold meant that—in contrast to the sanatorium-nursing homes of the nineteenth century—patients who themselves believed they needed help could also be admitted. Hence, being labeled as intolerable, either to one's family or with a view to public safety, was less often the deciding factor.[40] As part and parcel of this institutional change, then, psychiatry reached a new clientele at the beginning of the twentieth century, including lower-ranking civil servants, teachers, and white-collar employees.[41] For the first time, the psychiatric sector served all strata of the population. Within psychiatric institutions, however, a twofold distinction reflected the patient's economic circumstances. First, the sick were divided into three different treatment classes within the clinic or asylum according to their ability to pay. Second, better-off patients often used private institutions.

Contrary to the tendency advanced by the polyclinics to lower the committal threshold for those seeking help, the role of the police in cases of committal due to danger to self or others gained in importance toward the end of the Weimar Republic. This increase in power can be traced back to the introduction of the PVG on June 1, 1931, which remained in force during the Nazi era.[42] "Police authorities could, on the basis of a medical (not necessarily psychiatric) certificate, deprive mentally ill individuals who represented a 'danger to the public' of their personal liberty by forcibly placing them in an asylum, provided that 'this measure [was] necessary either to protect these persons themselves or to eliminate a disturbance to public safety or public order that has already occurred or to prevent an imminent threat to a legally protected good [*polizeiliche Gefahr*].'"[43] Hence, the police could preempt medical diagnosis and place people in an asylum without a medical consultation. The sanatorium-nursing homes were required to admit if an official physician declared it necessary in writing and the police authority ordered it in writing. Henceforth, the police played a decisive role in all cases of committal in which danger-based arguments were used. When it came to compulsory committals, psychiatrists now had less influence than the police and public health officers. While police committals had become much easier by the beginning of the "Third Reich," then, it became more difficult to get people in need of help a place in an asylum. The allocation of asylum places was, furthermore, increasingly debated in terms of expenditure, with politicians and experts questioning whether it was worth spending large sums of money on "people in need of institutional care." In the case of self-endangerment or individuals requiring treatment, the focus was no longer on intervention in the interest of society.[44] Even before the National Socialists seized power, then, the economic crisis had inspired policies intended to ensure the safety of others rather than to help the sick person.[45] This shift is fundamental to understanding forced committals during World War II.

Psychiatry as supplier of knowledge applied by the state

Psychiatrists as experts had been linked to the state in several ways since the final third of the nineteenth century. In addition to determining unsoundness of mind in court proceedings, a task long entrusted to them, their knowledge also became relevant when they were required to provide expert reports on social insurance from the 1880s onward. In addition, psychiatric knowledge gained importance as a key form of wartime knowledge.

Psychiatrists as providers of expert evaluations

Forensic assessments determining unsoundness of mind were already mentioned in the Constitutio Criminalis Carolina promulgated on the authority of Charles V in 1532, and until the eighteenth century, infancy, idiocy, and illness were considered grounds for exemption from liability, with illness here including "raving madness" (*Tobsucht*) and "insanity" (*Wahnsinn*). Free will was then introduced as the key determinant of soundness of mind in the late eighteenth century.[46] In the final third of the nineteenth century—in the wake of the rise of university psychiatric clinics—the provision of expert evaluations contributed to the rise of an independent psychiatric profession. For the university psychiatric clinics, expert assessment represented an important sphere of activity.[47] Another significant field for the young discipline of psychiatry arose through the introduction of social insurance, for which the state needed psychiatrists to provide expert evaluations. While even the newly established university psychiatric clinics were unable to make good on promises of curability,[48] the insurance system's reliance on diagnoses meant that psychiatrists could achieve great success by distinguishing and classifying psychiatric diseases.[49] Hermann Oppenheimer's concept of traumatic neurosis, for example, became established as a state-recognized diagnosis, with neurosis being conceptualized as the visible result of somatic injury to the brain or central nervous system.[50] This was a diagnosis widely used within the accident insurance system during the era of high industrialization: "Five years after Bismarck's accident insurance legislation of 1884 gave financial compensation to modernity's most visible victims, survivors of industrial and railway accidents, the Reich's Insurance Office extended this beneficence to workers who suffered from the mental and nervous effects of industrial accidents."[51] The diagnosis of traumatic neurosis was not only relevant in the context of peacetime social law, but also played a role during the war.

Psychiatric knowledge as war-related knowledge

The armed forces first showed an interest in psychiatry during the Franco-Prussian War, and as psychiatric knowledge became war-relevant knowledge the concerns of psychiatry and the state became intimately intertwined.[52] By the end of World War I, this had had three main consequences. First, penal institutions, reformatories, and even sanatorium-nursing homes had to inform recruiting authorities about patient admissions, with a comprehensive duty to report applying to all so-called "lunatic asylums" (*Irrenanstalten*) by 1906. This military interest helped more densely enmesh psychiatric institutions with other state institutions as the duty to report advanced their integration with non-military bodies, such as *Fürsorgeschulen*, schools for "difficult" children or those from "asocial" backgrounds, and civil courts.[53]

Second, an invention whose roots lay in military psychology found application far beyond this field: the intelligence test developed by Ernst Rüdin (1874–1952). The attribution of illnesses facilitated by this test was of considerable importance to the social acceptance of psychiatry, especially in view of its general inability to cure illnesses.[54]

Third, just as military psychiatry advanced the interlocking of state and civilian psychiatry, the originally "civilian" diagnoses of traumatic neurosis and hysteria in turn influenced psychiatry within the armed forces. During World War I, war veterans described as *Kriegszitterer* ("war tremblers") appeared for the first time and unexpectedly, prompting references to war neurosis, war hysteria, and nervous shock.[55] These terms in themselves highlight the coexistence of different explanations of this phenomenon, all with quite different consequences for those affected. Whether the soldiers' condition was defined as hysteria or as nervous shock and, in association with this, as traumatic neurosis, made a considerable difference to the treatment they received during the war and to whether they were granted a disability pension after the war.

German psychiatrists and neurologists disagreed in their explanations of *Kriegszitterer*. On the one hand, a kind of psychiatric "stab in the back" myth gained traction, according to which the symptoms were wishful thinking and reflected a reluctance to fight in war.[56] On this view, the "sick" soldiers were refusing to give their all to ensure victory and were thus weakening the imperial army from within. The diagnosis in such cases was hysteria. On the other hand, Hermann Oppenheimer diagnosed traumatic neurosis, which presented the symptoms as a direct, physically induced effect of shock.[57] Despite the controversy, until his death in 1926, Oppenheimer's diagnosis was crucial to the granting of disability pensions to soldiers returning from the front, who often continued to suffer from the psychological consequences of war for years or decades. Oppenheimer's analysis was then superseded by the diagnosis of hysteria.[58] Paul Lerner convincingly explains the fact that Oppenheimer's diagnosis—already recognized under insurance law before the war—was called into question due to the war and then, after the death of its originator, played virtually no role for the social insurance companies, as a specifically German development that entailed the fusion of socially racist elements with the idea of nation and state. Since traumatic neurosis was recognized under insurance law, it had undergirded pension entitlements for working-class soldiers suffering from relevant complaints. Amid the nation-alistic climate of the war, they were increasingly assailed as "pension neu-rotics,"[59] that is, they were accused of succumbing to wartime hysteria due to an unwillingness to fight and in order to claim a pension without good reason. Although the so-called "pension neurotics" were irrelevant to the national economy, the German Empire's psychiatrists generally contended that social insurance for blue-collar workers was counterproductive and inappropriate. As Stefanie Neuner shows, social Darwinist ideas about work became ever more tightly enmeshed with psychiatry and the social insurance system. In the Insurance Code (*Reichsversicherungsordnung*) of the Weimar Republic, health was finally defined as the capacity for work rather than as physical integrity; at the same time, so-called "work-shy" individuals could be punished with imprisonment.[60] In Weimar, most of those denigrated as pension neurotics were viewed as a deformity spawned by flawed social policy, and in line with this, the prevailing psychiatric doctrine declared that the welfare state had opened up space for "psychopathological parasites." In contrast, psychotherapists in the Weimar Republic espoused the opposite explanatory approach, asserting that neurotic disorders were consequences of social and economic conditions.[61] Under National Socialism, this psycho-therapeutic explanation ceased to play any role, and from 1933 onward, applications for state support due to psychological impairment had virtually no chance of success. Psychiatrists and politicians now worked closely together in the development of supply policy (*Versorgungspolitik*).[62] From 1939 on, those classified as "asocial" no longer received state benefits from the employment offices.[63]

The connections between psychiatry, war, and work were to be important to the practice of committal from 1941 to 1963 in two ways. First, the National Socialist regime wanted to avoid the "mistakes" made by the German Empire in dealing with ill soldiers: they were to be kept at the front for as long as possible without regard to psychological stress and its physical effects. The committal of soldiers that nevertheless took place during World War II must be analyzed against this background. Second, the diagnosis of "pension neurosis" remained significant in the committal context. Overall, patients' relationship to their work and the assessment of their willingness and ability to work played a major role in the practice of committal in the mid-twentieth century in a number of different ways.

Psychiatric knowledge as a foil for the interpretation of social problems

From the time of the German Empire onwards, psychiatric knowledge served to interpret social developments and self-perceptions. Two discourses can be distinguished here. The bourgeois world grappled with fear, agitation, and adjustment problems, which found expression in diagnoses mainly of hysteria and neurasthenia. The fact that no clear classification is possible here is shown by references to hysteria in the wartime context, mentioned above as a diagnosis in competition with traumatic neurosis and centered on lower-class men.[64] Following Volker Roelcke, the middle-class hysteria and neurasthenia discourse have been interpreted in part as a form of self-reflection.[65] Once again, members of bourgeois strata participated in the interpretation of their own illnesses, interacting closely with physicians as they did so. The perceptions held by doctor and patient thus remained in fairly close proximity within the bourgeois world.[66] With respect to France and Germany in the eighteenth and nineteenth centuries, Jan Goldstein concludes: "That scientific psychology ran on a double track, both academic and popular, from the very beginning is, on reflection, not very surprising."[67] However, bourgeois patients suffering from conditions such as hysteria and neurasthenia were rarely to be found in the state sanatorium-nursing homes spotlighted in the present book. When they were treated in these asylums, they were disproportionately often first- or second-class patients. For the most part, however, they made use of private sanatoriums.[68]

In contrast, the psychiatric identification and interpretation of the "problems" supposedly typical of the "lower class" were vital to the development of state psychiatric institutions. Three crucial medical phenomena converged here: the psychiatric theory of degeneration developed by Bénédict Augustin Morel (1809–1873), Emil Kraepelin's (1856–1926) biological conception of psychiatric diseases, and the rediscovery of Mendel's theory of heredity around 1900.[69] In 1886, Kraepelin published his classification of psychiatric diseases, which was based on the supposition that specific clinical pictures represented clearly distinguishable biological objects.[70] This system made a huge impact in the German Empire and in the Weimar Republic as the most important, although never the only, commonly used diagnostic approach. It was not until 1932 that the so-called Würzburg Key replaced Kraepelin's system, refining the classifications but further cementing Kraepelin's assumption of biologically separable phenomena. Yet this premise, like the theory of heredity, did not yet lead to any clear consequences for the management and evaluation of psychiatric illness. In fact, in the nineteenth century, these assumptions could potentially engender a more understanding approach to the sick: in contrast to the previously prevailing religious frame of reference, illnesses were no longer necessarily interpreted as signs of guilt or original sin.[71] However, this mode of interpretation waned in the German Empire as the medical profession embraced the doctrine of degeneration. Morel described patients suffering from minor psychiatric disorders as degenerate, as "eccentrics, emotionally labile [*Stimmungslabile*], and unreliable."[72] His explanatory approach still exhibited clear anthropological-theological traits, which no longer played any role in the general German reception of degeneration theory. Thus, Morel himself continued to regard human degeneration as a consequence of original sin. Meanwhile, the general view was that although degeneration would not lead to rapid extinction, it was a progressive condition—an important detail[73] that underpinned the argument that this was a social problem requiring medical intervention. By 1900, a discourse had become established across Europe and in the United States that branded the "underclass" a danger to the entire "nation."[74] This class was considered degenerate almost in its entirety, though just who was covered by the term was not always spelt out. A key literary text provides at least some clues. The novel *The Kallikak Family*, penned by American Henry Herbert Goddard (1866–1957) and translated into German in 1914, amounted to a kind of "myth of ancestry" for criminals, prostitutes, alcoholics, and impoverished families.[75]

Meanwhile, the term "asocial" took hold in the early nineteenth-century debate on whether individuals were worthy of support, especially when it came to welfare for the lower classes.[76] The psychiatry developed by Kraepelin and his successor Ernst Rüdin explained behaviors judged as deviant, especially in this social stratum, as hereditary degeneration that was detectable in discrete clusters of psychiatric symptoms. Physicians often diagnosed "psychopathy" and increasingly embraced the term "asocial," turning "asocial psychopath" into a common diagnosis. So-called "psychopaths" were considered degenerate and were believed to have inherited defects, conditions increasingly conveyed by the term "constitution." Yet "psychopaths" were not viewed as suffering from a hereditary disease.[77] For the most part, "psychopathy" was not viewed as a disease at all, but genetic factors were thought to play an important role in it. Rüdin, a student of Kraepelin, rose to become the most important representative of psychiatric genetics in Europe, but in Germany it was not until the Nazi period that his ideas prevailed over other scientific perspectives that remained at large.[78] For psychiatrists themselves, genetic explanations were tremendously important because they made eugenic prophylaxis possible. Originally, degeneration was linked with so-called "psychopathy," which described in a rather vague way deviations in everyday behavior, as Morel already described them. Rüdin, however, also espoused the idea of a direct genetic cause of numerous other diseases. Among other things, his research did much to advance the classification of schizophrenia as a hereditary disease under National Socialism, although he was unable to provide any empirical basis for this.[79]

The psychiatric interpretations of society, outlined above, that typified the late nineteenth century and the first half of the twentieth century, continued to exercise an effect on committals in the 1941–1963 period in three respects. First, established diagnoses remained of great importance to attributions of "degeneration," "psychopathy," and "asociality," especially among patients from the lower classes, and to the self-interpretations of bourgeois committals and the associated doctor–patient relationship. Second, these concepts illustrate the importance of scientific transfer, which was again to play a key role in debates on the role of psychiatry in society conducted in the FRG and the GDR in the 1950s. Third, the Würzburg Key continued to function in many clinics as an authoritative tool for the diagnosis of the committed well beyond the end of the war.

Changes during the Nazi era up to 1941 and the incipient murder of the sick

The conceptual amalgam of heredity theory and a social Darwinist reading of degeneration theory proved highly consequential during the Nazi period. In combination with psychiatry's proximity to the state as a result of professionalization and the debate on the cost of asylums to the welfare state, this amalgam helped exclude the sick and so-called "asocials" from the National Socialist *Volksgemeinschaft* or National Community.

Prior to the war, important innovations affecting the practice of committal occurred under National Socialism. First came the Law against Dangerous Recidivists and on Protection and Rehabilitation Measures (*Gesetz gegen gefährliche Gewohnheitsverbrecher und über die Maßregeln der Sicherung und Besserung* or GgGSB) passed on November 24, 1933,[80] which introduced a regulation on the placement of offenders of unsound mind in sanatorium-nursing homes. Section 42b of the Reich Penal Code (*Reichstrafgesetzbuch* or RStGB) provided for the admission of such offenders "if public safety so requires." This was a broad form of words that facilitated placement in forensic psychiatric institutions even for the most minor infringements of the law and interpreted unsoundness of mind to the patient's detriment.[81] Prior to this law, establishing unsoundness of mind (§ 51 RStGB) was understood as a means of protecting the "mentally ill" from punishment.[82] § 42b RStGB did away with this protective function and introduced so-called preventive detention (*Sicherheitsverwahrung*), that is, it established the *doppelter Strafvollzug*[83] still in use today. It is true that this offered non-compliant judges the possibility of using unsoundness of mind to protect the accused, but this was rendered null and void by the murder of forensic psychiatric patients.[84]

In addition, the Law for the Prevention of Hereditarily Diseased Offspring (*Gesetz zur Verhütung erbkranken Nachwuchses* or GzVeN) was enacted on July 14, 1933 and came into force on January 1, 1934.[85] It covered the following conditions: "severe hereditary physical deformities," "hereditary blindness and deafness," "hereditary St. Vitus dance,"[86] "hereditary falling sickness,"[87] "congenital imbecility," "manic-depressive insanity" (*manisch-depressives Irresein* or MDI), and schizophrenia.[88] In addition to providing for the sterilization of people afflicted by the above-mentioned diseases, the GzVeN empowered physicians to impose the same "treatment" on "those suffering from severe alcoholism," despite the fact that alcoholism was not classified as hereditary even during the Nazi era.[89] Prior to sterilization, expert assessment was carried out by the newly established hereditary health courts. In addition to sterilization reports, the Nazi conception of illness also resulted in the compiling of marriage reports, though it was already possible to divorce on the grounds that one's spouse was afflicted by a mental illness.

The Law for the Unification of the Health System (*Gesetz zur Vereinheitlichung des Gesundheitssystems*) of April 1935 established health offices nationwide, and by 1938 there were 750 of them. This went hand in hand with an enhanced status for public health officers. The resulting dense administrative network did much to ensure that committals on grounds of endangerment were carried out in a fast, uncomplicated fashion, not least because public health officers usually issued the medical certificate required for compulsory committals. In addition, during World War II, the health offices were often responsible for hospital administration,[90] and hospital patients were regularly committed to sanatorium-nursing homes. Even in the postwar period, the network of health offices remained intact, as the Allies did not classify them as specifically Nazi. In the GDR, the 1952 local government reform triggered the reorganization of the health offices, but most of them continued to exist.[91]

Finally, the Nazi state introduced support measures for "hereditarily healthy" and "racially pure" Reich citizens, such as marriage loans, child allowances, recreation for children, and educational assistance programs. At the same time, it pursued an agenda of radical exclusion, one served not just by workhouses and concentration camps but also by psychiatry and its institutions.

With the advent of war, the regime initiated the murder of psychiatric patients. In the German-Polish border areas, asylum patients were killed partly to make room for resettlers (*Umsiedler*) from Estonia and Latvia, who were now to live within the Reich in line with the National Socialists' settlement plans, their arrival in Pomerania embodying the Nazi "Home to the Reich" rallying cry.[92] The start of the war also ushered in the murder of children, which began in the asylums of the "Old Reich" in late 1939. The T4 Campaign (*Aktion T4*), the state-organized murder of adult patients, was launched toward the end of 1939. It was officially terminated on August 23, 1941, probably due in part to Bishop von Galen's public protests in the Münsterland, but it was resumed by August 1942. This second phase of the murder of the sick, however, proceeded on a decentralized basis.[93]

At least by the time the T4 Campaign was terminated, the general population was to some degree aware of the murders of the sick. Nevertheless, as Heinz Faulstich and Götz Aly observe, relatives often still facilitated their family members' long-term stays in asylums.[94] Even under these circumstances, the asylums continued to function and admitted new patients, albeit in a quite specific context. First, the murders of the sick had been resumed on a decentralized basis and had been public knowledge since 1941 at the latest. Second, committals on grounds of safety were to take priority, while patients not committed as a danger to the community were to be discharged if possible.[95] Who was responsible for the costs arising from those committed by the police as a danger to the community initially remained unclear. The potential funders were the public welfare system, the health insurance funds, and the police.[96] In 1942, this uncertainty was eliminated through the so-called Halving Decree (*Halbierungserlass*), which stipulated that the health insurance funds and welfare associations (*Fürsorgeverbände*) each had to bear half the costs, regardless of the specific reason for committal in a given case.[97] Third, the regime produced a vast amount of propaganda on the subject of psychiatry and so-called "euthanasia," which reached a huge number of people, chiefly through the medium of film.[98]

Notes

1 For a detailed account of the establishment of the asylum and how it changed over the course of a century, see Sandner et al., *Heilbar*.
2 But this is not intended as a remotely complete narrative of the history of German psychiatry up to 1941.
3 Engstrom, Eric J., *Clinical Psychiatry in Imperial Germany. A History of Psychiatric Practice* (Ithaca 2003), 18.
4 Sandner et al., *Heilbar*.
5 Engstrom, *Psychiatry*, 2.
6 The convergence of psychiatry and neurology was largely due to Wilhelm Griesinger's (1817–1868) research on mental illness as brain disease, which coincided with the founding of the first university clinics of psychiatry and neurology. See ibid., 60.
7 Ibid., 24.
8 Ibid., 12 f.
9 On the institutions studied here, see the anthology on the Psychiatric Clinic of Greifswald University Hospital: Fischer and Schmiedebach, *Direktorat*.
10 Brink, *Psychiatrie*, 142.
11 See for example Sandner, Peter et al., "Einleitung," in Sandner, Peter et al. (eds.), *Heilbar und nützlich. Ziele und Wege der Psychiatrie in Marburg an der Lahn* (Marburg 2001), 15.
12 See for example the summary in Rose, Wolfgang, *Anstaltspsychiatrie in der DDR. Die brandenburgischen Kliniken zwischen 1945 und 1990* (Berlin 2005), 16ff.
13 Andrews and Digby, "Introduction," 14ff; Blasius, Dirk, *"Einfache Seelenstörung." Geschichte der deutschen Psychiatrie 1800–1945* (Frankfurt/M. 1994). For a summary, see Brink, *Psychiatrie*, 133.
14 Kaufmann, Doris, *Aufklärung, bürgerliche Selbsterfahrung und die "Erfindung" der Psychiatrie in Deutschland, 1770–1850* (Göttingen 1995), 191.
15 Brink, *Psychiatrie*, 12.
16 Foucault, Michel, "Andere Räume," in Karlheinz Barck (ed.), *Aisthesis. Wahrnehmungen heute oder Perspektiven einer anderen Ästhetik. Essais* (Leipzig 1991), 34–46.
17 Wilhelm Griesinger, who described mental illnesses as brain diseases and thus did much to ensure the closeness and cooperation between psychiatry and neurology, made a particularly significant contribution to this. Engstrom, *Psychiatry*, 51 and 60 f.
18 Kaufmann, *Aufklärung*, 158.
19 Thus, for a certain amount of time, local authorities could be exempted from paying for residential placement if they committed patients at an early stage of illness. Following the 1891 amendment to the *Gesetz über den Unterstützungswohnsitz*, which regulated the provision of poor relief based on residency, the local poor associations (*Ortsarmenverbände*) bore one-third of the costs of residential placements. Two-thirds was paid by the Land associations for the poor (*Landarmenverbände*) and in Prussia by the equivalent provincial associations (*Provinzialverbände*). See Brink, *Psychiatrie*, 114.

20 This shift had much to do with the close connection between psychiatry and brain anatomy at the time. Diseases could be identified more easily after death as the brain could be examined for changes. See Walter, Bernd, "Fürsorgepflicht und Heilungsanspruch. Die Überforderung der Anstalt (1870–1930)," in Franz-Werner Kersting et al. (eds.), *Nach Hadamar. Zum Verhältnis von Psychiatrie und Gesellschaft im 20. Jahrhundert* (Paderborn 1993), 83 f.

21 On the challenge to Kraepelin's concept of diagnosis by Eugen Bleuler (1857–1939) and the introduction of the term schizophrenia, see Bernet, Brigitta, *Schizophrenie. Entstehung und Entwicklung eines psychiatrischen Krankheitsbildes um 1900* (Zürich 2013), 12 f.

22 Kraepelin was a very well-known and influential German psychiatrist whose ideas on the classification of psychiatric diseases continue to make an impact today. He was also the founder of the German Research Institute for Psychiatry (Deutsche Forschungsanstalt für Psychiatrie) in Munich, a Kaiser Wilhelm Institute. On Kraepelin's relevance, which is now contested, see Engstrom, Eric J. and Matthias M. Weber, "Introduction to Special Issue: Making Kraepelin History. A Great Idea?" *History of Psychiatry*, vol. 3, 2007, 267–273.

23 Kaufmann, *Aufklärung*, 140.

24 Goldberg, "Conventions of Madness," 178.

25 Ibid., 186. Doris Kaufmann also highlights the significance of moral practice in the psychiatric and philosophical discourse of the time: Kaufmann, *Aufklärung*, 36.

26 Goldberg, "Conventions of Madness," 180.

27 Kaufmann, *Aufklärung*, 178 and 199.

28 Ibid., 20.

29 Ibid., 245.

30 On this phenomenon, typically labeled "hospitalism," see Huppmann, Gernot, "Milieuschäden intramural untergebrachter Geisteskranker: eine historiographisch-medizinpsychologische Studie zum 'Anstaltssyndrom,'" in Huppmann, Gernot (ed.), *Prolegomena einer medizinischen Psychologie der Hoffnung* (Würzburg 2006), 455–502.

31 Brink, *Psychiatrie*, 116ff.

32 In the present book, see esp. the section "The psychiatrist as expert: diagnostic classifications and the clinical picture of schizophrenia in the Nazi era and early FRG" in Chapter 4.

33 Brink, *Psychiatrie*, 198.

34 Castel, Robert, "Vom Widerspruch der Psychiatrie," in Franco Basaglia and Franca Basaglia-Ongaro (eds.), *Befriedungsverbrechen. Über die Dienstbarkeit des Intellektuellen* (Frankfurt/M. 1980), 81.

35 See Schwegel, Andreas, *Der Polizeibegriff im NS-Staat* (Tübingen 2005), 26.

36 There were numerous regional additions to the ALR: Brink, *Psychiatrie*, 50.

37 Ibid., 52.

38 Ernst, *Sozialismus*, 333.

39 As early as the 1860s, Wilhelm Griesinger fought at the Charité in Berlin to simplify the admission procedure at the university psychiatric clinic and to put doctors rather than the police in charge of it. See Engstrom, *Psychiatry*, 70.

40 Ibid., 191.

41 Brink, *Psychiatrie*, 194.

42 In Bavaria, Article 80/II of the Bavarian Police Penal Code (*Polizeistrafgesetzbuch* or PStGB), which is comparable to the PVG, was authoritative. On the reach of Prussian police regulations, which extended, for example, to Saxony, and on the more independent policing tradition in the southern German states (though this entails no major differences from the Prussian tradition when it comes to

"protection against threats" [*Gefahrenabwehr*]), see Schwegel, Andreas, *Der Polizeibegriff im NS-Staat* (Tübingen 2005), 25 f.

43 Brink, *Psychiatrie*, 259.

44 For details, see ibid., 263.

45 Elke Hauschildt makes the same point about sanatoriums for the alcohol-dependent (*Trinkerheilanstalten*), which were closely related to the psychiatric institutions: Hauschildt, Elke, *"Auf den richtigen Weg zwingen ... ." Trinkerfürsorge 1922–1945* (Freiburg 1995), 105.

46 Kaufmann, *Aufklärung*, 306ff.

47 Engstrom, *Psychiatry*, 195.

48 The problem of curability is a venerable one that runs through the entire history of psychiatry, no matter which geographical area we consider. See for example Goldstein, Jan, *Console and Classify. The French Psychiatric Profession in the Nineteenth Century* (Chicago 1992).

49 Engstrom, *Psychiatry*, 167.

50 Hence, the diagnosis of traumatic neurosis did not imply a psychological consequence of an accident or event, as trauma has been understood since the 1970s in connection with Vietnam veterans. For more detail, see Lerner, Paul, *Hysterical Men. War, Psychiatry, and the Politics of Trauma in Germany, 1890–1930* (Ithaca 2003).

51 Lerner, Paul, "Psychiatry and Casualties of War in Germany, 1914–18," *Journal of Contemporary History*, vol. 1, 2000, 14.

52 See Quinkert, Babette et al., "Einleitung," in Quinkert, Babette et al. (eds.), *Krieg und Psychiatrie 1914–1950* (Göttingen 2010), 12.

53 Lengwiler, Martin, "Auf dem Weg zur Sozialtechnologie. Die Bedeutung der frühen Militärpsychiatrie für die Professionalisierung der Psychiatrie in Deutschland," in Eric. J. Engstrom and Volker Roelcke (eds.), *Psychiatrie im 19. Jahrhundert. Forschungen zur Geschichte von psychiatrischen Institutionen, Debatten und Praktiken im deutschen Sprachraum* (Mainz 2003), 245 and 253 f.

54 Ibid., 251.

55 Quinkert et al., "Einleitung," 14ff.

56 The drastic treatment methods, which were aimed at getting the soldier back to the front by all available means, were also based on this interpretation. These treatments are still evaluated in contrasting ways in present-day research; see ibid.

57 The term trauma, whose roots lie in ancient Greek, originally means "wound" and was used in this somatic sense until the twentieth century. Oppenheimer was thus referring to a wounding of the nervous system, which manifested as a neurosis.

58 Lerner, *Men*, 9.

59 Ibid., 32.

60 Neuner, Stephanie, *Politik und Psychiatrie. Die staatliche Versorgung psychisch Kriegsbeschädigter in Deutschland 1920–1939* (Göttingen 2011), 71 and 77.

61 Ibid., 149.

62 Ibid., 166 and 253.

63 Ibid., 298.

64 For a detailed account of these diagnoses in the German Empire, see the works of Paul Lerner and Doris Kaufmann; on the Anglo-Saxon debate, which goes into more depth, see the studies by Jonathan Andrews and Anne Digby: Lerner, *Men*; Kaufmann, *Aufklärung*; Andrews and Digby, "Introduction."

65 Roelcke, *Krankheit*, 30.

66 For overviews of the neurasthenia discourse as a predecessor to the notion of "stress" and on the discussion of gender in relation to hysteria and neurasthenia, see for example Kury, Patrick, *Der Überforderte Mensch. Eine Wissensgeschichte vom Stress zum Burnout* (Frankfurt/M. 2012), 46ff; Nolte, Karen, "'So ein Gefühl,

als wenn sich jeder Nerv im Kopf zusammenziehe.' Die 'moderne' Diagnose Nervosität—Zum Konzept der Marburger Anstalt am Beispiel der Behandlung 'nervöser' Patientinnen (1876–1918)," in Peter Sandner et al. (eds.), *Heilbar und nützlich. Ziele und Wege der Psychiatrie in Marburg an der Lahn* (Marburg 2001), 184.

67 Using the example of mesmerism—a nineteenth-century theory situated between popular belief and science, which explained psychological responses with reference to magnetic forces flowing through the body, a practice that was forbidden in France but permitted in Prussia—Goldstein shows that conditions in Germany were particularly favorable to the development of this "double track." Goldstein, "Psyche," 139ff. and 153.

68 Nolte, "Gefühl," 186.

69 The Mendelian theory of heredity was first published in 1866 but made its impact in the field of psychiatry only around 1900. On the history-of-science context in France, especially on the connections between the theories of Pinel, Esqirol, and Morel and the French development of the theory of degeneration, see Weber, Joachim, "Von der 'moral insanity' über die Psychopathie zur Persönlichkeitsstörung. Ein psychiatriegeschichtlicher Rückblick," in Reinhard Steinberg (ed.), *Persönlichkeitsstörungen. 22. Psychiatrie-Symposium* (Regensburg 2002), 16ff.

70 Roelcke, Volker, "Die Etablierung der psychiatrischen Genetik, ca. 1900–1960. Wechselbeziehungen zwischen Psychiatrie, Eugenik und Humangenetik," in Christine Wolters et al. (eds.), *Abweichung und Normalität. Psychiatrie in Deutschland vom Kaiserreich bis zur Deutschen Einheit* (Bielefeld 2013), 112.

71 Eirund, Wolfgang, "Auswirkungen biologischer Krankheitsmodelle auf die psychiatrische Behandlung—eine medizin-historische Studie am Beispiel von Krankenakten aus zwei Jahrhunderten," in Christina Vanja et al. (eds.), *Wissen und irren. Psychiatriegeschichte aus zwei Jahrhunderten—Eberbach und Eichberg* (Kassel 1999), 96.

72 Weber, "Insanity," 19.

73 Ibid.

74 Roelcke, "Etablierung," 119.

75 Ayaß, *Asoziale*, 13.

76 Eberle, Annette, "Sozial—Asozial. Ausgrenzung und Verfolgung in der bayerischen Fürsorgepraxis 1934–1945," *München und der Nationalsozialismus. Menschen, Orte, Strukturen* (Berlin 2008), 209.

77 Until National Socialism, various "constitutional" theories existed side by side, all of which revolved around the classification of people into types and were intended to explain susceptibility to certain diseases. In doing so, they drew to some extent on ancient tropes found in the work of Hippocrates and Galen, as in the constitutional psychology of Ernst Kretschmer (1888–1964), which enjoyed success under Nazism.

78 From 1931, Ernst Rüdin also headed the German Research Institute for Psychiatry (Kaiser Wilhelm Institute) in Munich.

79 Roelcke, "Etablierung," 121.

80 Wagner, Patrick, *Hitlers Kriminalisten. Die deutsche Kriminalpolizei und der Nationalsozialismus* (Munich 2002), 56ff.

81 § 42b remained in force in this form until 1975. § 63, which replaced § 42b, then formally made placement more difficult. Since then, significant criminal acts must have been committed and an overall evaluation of all the circumstances must be made. See http://dejure.org/gesetze/StGB/63.html (retrieved 27.1.2014).

82 Brink, *Psychiatrie*, 275.

83 There are two forms of imprisonment in Germany: in ordinary prisons (*Gefängnisse*) and in prisons especially designed for criminals categorized as mentally ill. This

means that while there is no official way to send someone to prison for the rest of their life—as *lebenslang* in the judicial context refers to fifteen years—people can be detained (*sicherheitsverwahrt*) until they die if they are criminals considered mentally ill and are therefore viewed as a threat to public safety.

84 Ibid; Aly, *Belasteten*, 214.
85 Ibid.
86 Now known as Huntington's disease.
87 Now known as epilepsy.
88 Ernst Rüdin, who did much to advance the understanding of schizophrenia as a hereditary disease, also contributed to the commentary on this law, though he knew it was not based on empirical research. Roelcke, "Etablierung," 129.
89 Hauschildt, *Trinkerfürsorge*, 142.
90 In Munich, this was not the case until 1944; see Christians, *Amtsgewalt*, 57 and 59.
91 See Süß, *Volkskörper*, 36; Ellerbrock, Dagmar, *"Healing Democracy"—Demokratie als Heilmittel. Gesundheit, Krankheit und Politik in der amerikanischen Besatzungszone, 1945–1949* (Bonn 2004), 159; specifically on reorganization and psychiatry, see Hanrath, *Euthanasie und Psychiatriereform*, 351.
92 The first to be affected were patients in Danzig (Gdańsk), Gdingen (Gdynia), Swinemünde (Świnoujście), and Stettin (Szczecin); see Rieß, Volker, "Zentrale und dezentrale Radikalisierung. Die Tötungen 'unwerten Lebens' in den annektierten west- und nordpolnischen Gebieten 1939–1941," in Klaus-Michael Mallmann and Bogdan Musial (eds.), *Genesis des Genozids—Polen 1939–1941* (Darmstadt 2004), 127–145.
93 For a summary, see Pohl, *Verfolgung*; for more detail on the decentralized murder of the sick, see ibid., 30 f and Süß, *Volkskörper*, 320ff.
94 Aly, *Belasteten*, 281; Faulstich, Heinz, *Von der Irrenfürsorge zur Euthanasie* (Freiburg 1993), 327.
95 See Götz Aly on the potential to discharge patients destined to be murdered during their stay in an "intermediate institution" (*Zwischenanstalt*): Aly, *Belasteten*, 281.
96 Brink, *Psychiatrie*, 255.
97 Ibid., 386, footnote 58.
98 Benzenhöfer, Udo and Wolfgang Eckart, *Medizin im Spielfilm des National-sozialismus* (Tecklenburg 1999); Roth, "Entstehungsgeschichte."

2 The state and psychiatric institutions

Parameters and committal decisions

When Martina R. was committed in the spring of 1946, her mother-in-law provided an explanation for the new patient's condition that highlighted personal blows of fate, which she related directly to prevailing historical realities. But what did Martina R. herself make of her situation? Upon admission to the LHA Marburg, she described the following scenario:

> My husband has been in a political camp since May 14 [1945] and we had to leave the house at the beginning of July. We live in [Giessen]. I was able to send my children to [Marburg] and then I cleared what I could out of the house. The previous year I had a miscarriage and was physically done in. At the time of the eviction, I was three months pregnant, and my youngest was born in December. After that I went to [Marburg]. But I'm desperate to go back to [Giessen]. If I stay away for eight weeks, my right to move there [*Zuzugsrecht*] expires. I want to get a room. And if I have to claim support, [Giessen] is the only option.
>
> (When did you start to have trouble coping with things?) I've been struggling the whole time. The first three months I heard nothing at all from my husband and officially I still have no news of him.[1]

This reference to status and housing problems not only dovetails with the mother-in-law's statements but was a specific feature of admissions in the first few postwar years. Martina R. had suffered a double loss of status. As described in the introduction, her family had lost its assets, and her husband, who had enjoyed prestige and power as an SS officer, was immediately taken captive by the Americans when the war ended. The confiscation of her house was directly related to this. The search for housing, which for the time being had concluded with Martina and her children moving in with her mother-in-law, was a widespread problem. The situation tended to be particularly urgent for displaced persons,[2] who were often among those committed between 1945 and 1947. This was because—unlike Martina R.—they did not necessarily have relatives or friends in their new place of residence.

This chapter traces how these era-specific conditions interacted with committal practices by analyzing committal pathways, actors, and

DOI: 10.4324/9781032716237-3

negotiation processes. The chapter is based on the qualitative analysis of patient records and also scrutinizes sources pertinent to debates on committal practices. At the same time, I use the sample taken for this study to reconstruct different committal pathways. With respect to the Eglfing-Haar Sanatorium-Nursing Home, I combine analysis of the sample with the institution's own statistics, found in its detailed annual reports.[3] My overall goal is to trace major changes in the practice of committals.[4]

The murder of the sick and shortages: the practice of committal during World War II

Committals between 1941 and the end of the war took place under very specific conditions. First, asylums changed as a result of the Todt/Brandt Campaign (*Aktion Todt/Brandt*). Transfers and the takeover of ever larger parts of the asylums as ersatz and military hospitals left ever less room for psychiatric and neurological admissions from among the civilian population, although attempts were made to compensate for this through overcrowding.[5] Second, the murder of the sick had to some degree been public knowledge at least since the termination of the T4 Campaign.[6] In addition, committals took place against the backdrop of vociferous propaganda against "life unworthy to live" and in favor of "euthanasia."[7]

How did patients and their relatives conduct themselves against the backdrop of war, the murder of the sick and "euthanasia" propaganda, and what does this behavior tell us about Nazi society during the war? How did patients and their relatives deal with the knowledge of these murders if they or a person in their social milieu were to be admitted to a clinic or asylum? Did people still seek help from clinics and asylums in the first place? The following remarks are based on the observation that—regardless of war-specific changes, the particular way in which the state made use of psychiatric institutions, and the murder of the sick—committals did not take place only or even primarily on an inter-institutional basis. Patients, and above all their social milieu, remained key actors.

Between 1941 and 1945, for the majority of patients in all asylums and in the Greifswald University Psychiatric Clinic, their own home was the last long-term place of residence before committal, as revealed by evaluation of the sample taken for the present study. It is true that the number of patients who had been living permanently at home was lower during the war than in later periods. Yet the committal of such individuals continued to occur regularly despite the war-related repurposing of psychiatric institutions and the murder of the sick described above. Hence, private actors, that is, the committed themselves, as well as their families and friends, also played a role in committal decisions, and not just institutions, be they hospitals, old people's homes, nursing homes (the latter two sometimes combined under one roof) or prisons. In the case of the Untergöltzsch Sanatorium-Nursing Home near Chemnitz, for example, until the end of the war, 58 percent of patients lived at home before their committal, while 33 percent were admitted without the involvement of another institution, such as a university psychiatric clinic.[8] The proportion of patients admitted from home increased steadily in Untergöltzsch/Rodewisch until 1963, a pattern also found in all the other institutions studied here. Between 1950 and 1955, no less than 76 percent of those admitted to Rodewisch had previously lived at home.[9] The figures were similar in Eglfing-Haar and Marburg, and they were higher still in the religiously based von Bodelschwingh Asylums Bethel and in the Psychiatric Clinic of Greifswald University Hospital. I elucidate the reasons for this in the course of this chapter.[10] The frequency of committal from within the domestic sphere indicates that in many of these cases, members of the patient's immediate environment may have been involved. The fact that patients almost never visited a clinic or asylum alone but were usually accompanied by someone from their social milieu, points to the same conclusion. These committals of patients from their home environment were by no means mainly compulsory committals carried out by the police, in which the family may not have been involved at all.

The proportion of compulsory committals varied considerably among the different institutions. Between 1941 and the end of the war, these made up almost 45 percent of admissions to Eglfing-Haar, about 25 percent to Untergöltzsch, and only about 7 percent to Marburg. The latter can be explained chiefly in light of the specific type of clinic involved, namely, the sanatorium (*Heilanstalt*), which was intended for short stays. Bethel as a religious institution and Greifswald as a university clinic, meanwhile, were not typical places of accommodation in cases of compulsory committal. In principle, formal compulsory committals must be distinguished from other forms of committal for two reasons. First, in the Nazi era, the executive branch, in the shape of the police or health office, was involved in compulsory committals, while in the FRG the judicial branch played a major role. This shifted power toward state decision-making bodies. Second, the negotiation of compulsory committals usually took place over patients' heads. I explore compulsory committals in the next chapter, while focusing on their civil equivalent in this one.

The first issue I consider here is the relationship of trust between physician and patient, before turning to relatives' behavior with respect to the committal decision. The term "trust" is important in both contexts. As an individual, partly emotion-based phenomenon, trust is difficult to pin down historically. The advantage of the term is that it enables us to get at the heart, conceptually, of individuals' emotional motivation for entering or avoiding a clinic—which the sources do not allow us to grasp in detail—without claiming to reconstruct individual decisions. Precisely because of its relative vagueness, the concept of trust highlights the complexity of individual emotionality, which eludes precise historical parsing. Following Ute Frevert, the present study thus works with a broad understanding of trust. Her definition draws in turn on the terminology proposed by Russel Hardin: "Trust exists when one party to the relation believes the other party has incentive to act in his or her interest."[11] For the context under investigation here, this means that when an individual decided to see a doctor or attend a clinic, or when relatives sought the best possible residential option for a family member—which they by no means always did—it is assumed that they placed a certain amount of trust in the relevant doctor or medical institution.

Patients and physicians in cases of committal

In an era featuring the murder of the sick and war, committal was no easy step for patients. This is illustrated by the case of Elisabeth F.[12] In March 1941, the 18-year-old was admitted to the Greifswald University psychiatric clinic via a polyclinic with suspected encephalitis. At Greifswald, however, the diagnosis was multiple sclerosis.[13] Since Elisabeth F., according to the staff responsible, "very much wanted to go home,"[14] she was discharged at the beginning of April at her parents' request.[15] When her symptoms returned in January 1942, the family doctor tried to recommit her, but the patient refused. The doctor went into the background to this resistance in a letter to the physician responsible at the Greifswald clinic of January 23, 1942:

Dear Professor,
   I advised Miss [F.] to consult you personally. She had fallen ill on January 13, 1941. At the time, I believed she was suffering from influenza and ensuing encephalitis. The diagnosis of multiple sclerosis was then made in the clinic. The *neo-Solgankur* [sic] begun at the clinic was completed here. During the summer she was in excellent shape, and after a vacation in Leba in August/September she began working again, could ride a bike, and no longer felt sick.
   She has been showing symptoms again since December 7, 1941, namely abnormal sensations affecting the skin on the left side of her face, plus shakiness of the left arm and leg.
   Unfortunately, the film that is currently [being widely shown], the content of which she had read about, caused her to feel deeply depressed. I could only tell her that I have seen many a patient who had been declared incurable regain their health. She is still anticipating an inunction treatment, which she was promised at the clinic. She is terribly afraid of being admitted to the clinic.
   My sincere thanks in advance for a brief reply, your obedient servant and Heil Hitler![16]

Although the name of the film is not mentioned, it stands to reason that it was *Ich klage an* ("I Accuse"), which was shown in movie theaters from August 1941 and made a considerable splash. The movie is about a woman suffering from multiple sclerosis who is killed by her husband at her own request due to the incurable, progressive nature of the disease. The patient's murder is presented as a difficult but understandable act and is portrayed against the backdrop of the "problem" of the large number of "incurably ill people in the Reich."[17] Elisabeth F.'s resistance to committal seems to have been nourished by her reception of this film. Her case exemplifies the fraught nature of the decision-making process for those involved, a predicament also apparent in many other committal files. People in this situation acted within a field of tension between *hope* of and *fear* of treatment. Attending a clinic held out the prospect of medical help, yet this was countered by knowledge of the murder of the sick and euthanasia-focused propaganda. In Elisabeth F.'s case, this problematic reality prompted her to consult her family doctor about her ailments but to reject his proposal to refer her to the university psychiatric clinic when she realized that the illness she had been diagnosed with was one that, as shown in the film, rendered the sufferer "unworthy of life." When it comes to the relationship between doctor and patient during the war, it is striking that Elisabeth F. informed her family doctor of the reasons for her reservations. Other doctor's letters enclosed with her medical records, moreover, point to regular visits to the doctor's office.[18] Both pieces of evidence indicate that in this case greater trust was placed in the family doctor than in the university psychiatric clinic. Only when her symptoms worsened did Elisabeth F. decide to attend that establishment after all.

Elisabeth F.'s story highlights the complexity of patients' and their families' relationship with physicians, among other things with respect to the latter's institutional affiliation. There is some evidence that patients and their social milieu distinguished between different physicians and medical institutions and had different levels of trust in them. They also seem to have differentiated between psychiatric institutions, that is, between university clinics and sanatorium-nursing homes. Significantly more people were committed to the Psychiatric Clinic of Greifswald University Hospital from home during the war than to the asylums examined in this study. In 89 percent of cases, those admitted to the university clinic during the war lived permanently at home prior to their admission, while 68.5 percent were not in an inpatient facility, such as a hospital, old people's home, or reserve hospital (*Reservelazarett*), even immediately prior to their committal.[19] Of patients at Eglfing-Haar, Untergöltzsch, and LHA Marburg, only between 55.1 and 59 percent were living at home prior to their admission.[20] However, about half of them were in another medical facility or a "home" (that is, the institution known as a *Heim*) immediately before committal and thus already in an institutional context in which their own views did not necessarily carry weight.[21]

This high number of patients at Greifswald who lived at home before admission is only partly due to fundamental differences in the number of those making use of university psychiatric clinics and asylums.[22] This is evident in the fact that the difference in numbers between the Greifswald university psychiatric clinic and the other institutions studied in this book decreased after the end of the war,[23] a convergence suggesting that patients and some relatives tried to avoid asylums in particular during the war. The committal figures for the LHA Marburg, which was similar to Greifswald in terms of function but was nonetheless an asylum, also indicate that patients, their social environment, and perhaps also physicians in private practice distinguished between the psychiatric clinics of university hospitals and asylums during the war. At Marburg, a significantly smaller proportion of those admitted during the war lived permanently at home prior to their committal (59.3 percent) and the proportion of patients coming directly from home to the institution was also much lower (27.5 percent) than at Greifswald (88 percent). The findings for Marburg during the war thus correspond to those for the two sanatorium-nursing homes of Untergöltzsch and Eglfing-Haar. In the postwar period, this changed again: the LHA Marburg once again operated more in line with its original character, namely, similar to a university psychiatric clinic and less like a sanatorium-nursing home.[24]

Independent physicians (niedergelassene Ärzte) and committal decisions

In addition to the finding that patients, along with their social milieu, distinguished between different physicians and medical institutions, there is also evidence of differentiating practices among family doctors.

Between 1941 and 1945, independent physicians issued fewer committal certificates for asylum stays than in the postwar period.[25] Does this mean they were reluctant to implement Nazi policies due to a long and close relationship with their patients? This interpretation seems plausible in the context of committals, but it does not explain everything.[26] The behavior of Elisabeth F. and that of other patients not discussed here suggests that intact relationships of trust did in fact exist between family doctors and patients. But we should bear in mind that it does not necessarily show up in the files if this was not the case. Among independent physicians, moreover, there may have been differences between general practitioners and psychiatrists. In the case of medical specialists, there is less likely to have been a lengthy relationship with the committed and their families. Especially in the case of psychiatric patients, we cannot generally assume a relationship of trust that prompted the psychiatrist to protect their interests—though in individual cases there may well have been. Crucially, we can work on the assumption that most of those committed to a public institution were of a lower-class background: since the days of the German Empire, psychiatrists had styled themselves as experts on the threats posed by a "degenerate lower class."[27] As "better-off" patients were more likely to be referred to private sanatoria, it hardly seems logical to postulate a special interest among independent psychiatrists in protecting potential asylum patients. It is more likely that during the war patients placed less trust in these psychiatrists than in general practitioners. Of the almost 400 medical records I reviewed for the Nazi period, examples comparable to Elisabeth F.'s committal, in which a sick person confided in a physician, can be found only with respect to general practitioners, not psychiatrists. In any event, as we will see, committed persons were far from always able to make independent decisions; these often fell to relatives, who may have been pursuing interests that differed from those of the patient.

Beyond the question of trust, however, it is essential to consider practical factors that affected people's access to independent physicians—whether psychiatrists or general practitioners. The lower numbers of referrals are congruent with a shortage of independent physicians in the Reich, a large number of whom were at the front.[28] In addition, the switchover to company-based health care reached its peak when the war began. All day-to-day health care was increasingly linked to and geared toward the enterprise. For example, in firms important to the war effort, only company doctors were allowed to write sick notes from 1940 onward. In addition, "the DAF [Deutsche Arbeitsfront or German Labor Front] worked systematically to ensure that the sick were cared for in company-operated facilities rather than within the family, in order to gain greater control over them."[29] The company doctors were recruited from among independent physicians,[30] which meant that a visit to the doctor could be difficult to arrange, especially for those who did not work outside the home. This lends credence to the argument that reduced access to independent physicians played a role in the decreasing number of committals initiated by them.

Hence, neither the behavior of independent physicians nor that of relatives can be straightforwardly interpreted on the basis of the figures alone. More detailed analysis does, however, show clearly that in some cases relatives did attempt to avoid state asylums. Conversely, in what follows I briefly touch on the fact—which is fleshed out in the subsequent chapters—that some relatives and other individuals in the social milieu of the committed initiated or supported (compulsory) committals with chiefly pragmatic or self-interested aspects in mind. In this context, I also cast light on interactions with physicians of varying institutional affiliations.

Initiation of committals by relatives

Relatives cooperated less often with state asylums during World War II than in the postwar period, though such cooperation did not cease during that conflict. If we look at the committals of those whose last abode was the family environment, we find that those in which family members were directly involved occurred continuously during the war.[31] It is also apparent that the initiation of committals to asylums after the war was once again more often carried out by families or, to shift perspective, that families again more often cooperated directly with the asylum.

The limits of patients' and their families' cooperation with state asylums during the war are illustrated by several committals to the von Bodelschwingh Asylums Bethel, a private Protestant institution. Although Bodelschwingh himself was "loyal to the new state,"[32] he rejected the murder of the sick. In addition, at Bethel, Pastor Paul Gerhard Braune in particular opposed the surrender of patients within the framework of the T4 Campaign.[33] There is some evidence that families considered Bethel and private asylums in general to be safer, although this was by no means always true.[34] During the war, for example, significantly more patients who had lived permanently at home (69 percent) and whose last abode was their own home (42 percent) were committed to Bethel than to Marburg, Munich, or Untergöltzsch.[35] These figures continued to rise at Bethel as elsewhere after the war; even before the founding of the FRG, they stood at 75.8 and 72.7 percent.[36] What is particularly noteworthy here is that the proportion of patients living permanently at home and those admitted from home was almost congruent at Bethel after the war, whereas it diverged by more than 20 percentage points during the war.[37] This gap may indicate that during the war period, more patients (or their families) who would have turned to a state institution under other circumstances consciously sought a place at Bethel. On this premise, the difference in the number of patients living permanently at home and those admitted to the institution from home was due to the fact that patients (and their families) tried to secure a place at Bethel following their admission to a university psychiatric clinic or state asylum. That some relatives avoided state asylums in favor of what they perceived as "comparatively safe church-run or private nursing homes"[38] can be demonstrated by two further examples.

First, in February 1942, the governor (*Oberpräsident*) of the Province of Westphalia noted that relatives were bypassing state institutions in favor of private ones. In a letter to the Reich Minister of the Interior of March 5, 1942, he elaborated on this:

> When it comes to sick people in need of help who are accommodated at the expense of the public welfare system, I have the right to determine the institution. In order to avoid this, the public—no doubt partly on the advice of private institutions—is increasingly resorting to the expedient of placing the sick in religious establishments, initially as self-payers. After just a short time—often a few days—the relatives stop paying, prompting the private institutions to apply for public welfare for the sick person. Since the conditions for this do indeed pertain, these requests must almost always be granted. However, the decree of December 22, 1941, prevents the transfer of the patient to a provincial institution. Signed by order of the Landesrat.[39]

The decree of December 22, 1941 prohibited transfers in the absence of "compelling factual grounds."[40] Herbert Linden (1899–1945), the Reich Commissioner for Sanatorium-Nursing Homes, responded with reference to the situation in Westphalia that this had not been the intention of the decree. In this case, the patient could be transferred, but "without the use of long-distance trains, automobiles, etc."[41] It should be noted that although Linden was keen to avoid the undesirable effect of increased admissions to private institutions, his restriction on the use of cars and long-distance trains will have made this considerably more difficult: transfers were usually carried out by car. Long-distance trains, which the decree also prohibited, were used only for very long journeys.

Second, patients and relatives tried to obtain admission to Bethel in an unofficial way by making inquiries to Pastor Bodelschwingh and/or making much of earlier dedication to the institution in their admission requests. These unofficial inquiries accounted for 20.5 percent of committals from 1941 to the end of the war; later they were no longer made.[42] In such cases, relatives pressed for admission or transfer to Bethel, never explicitly stating why the sick person would be better off there, but always underlining why this particular patient deserved to be admitted. For example, Mrs. N. wrote to Pastor Bodelschwingh in 1942 requesting that her "mentally disturbed" (*nervenkrank*) sister-in-law be admitted, pointing out that the latter had collected donations for the Bethel *Ährenlese* charitable program for years.[43] Mrs. N's sister-in-law was in fact subsequently admitted to Bethel. Dieter M., who was transferred from the Leipzig-Dösen Sanatorium-Nursing Home to Bethel in the summer of 1944 at his wife's request, was admitted in a similar way. The 64-year-old's wife wrote to Bethel:

> I am writing to enquire whether you can accommodate a sick individual and what this would cost. At the moment, my husband is staying at the university psychiatric clinic (*Nervenklinik*). Unfortunately, I cannot bring him home because of the risk of air raids and attacks. My husband has done a great deal for Bethel and I would be glad if you would take him in.[44]

Mrs. M. did not state explicitly in her letter why she preferred to place her husband in Bethel instead of Leipzig-Dösen, but her request was successful, and Dieter M. was admitted three months later.[45] As in the previous example, reference was again made to the patient's earlier dedication to Bethel. After his admission, the friends of this man expressed doubts to the staff there as to whether he required institutional care in the first place; they suspected that his wife was pursuing the committal due to domestic strife.[46] The Bethel doctors did not share this view.[47] His wife too reported family problems but stated that her husband struck her and their children when in a delusional state.[48]

I found many similar cases at Bethel. In some of the rationales for committal that ultimately led to placement in a state asylum, it is also clear that the relatives had initially tried to place their family member in a private establishment. For example, patient Martin C. was admitted to Eglfing-Haar after a neighbor woman had called the police at his mother's behest, informing them of "worsening mental disturbances" and aggression toward his mother.[49] The patient was first admitted to the Munich university psychiatric clinic and then to Eglfing-Haar. His mother had requested that her son be placed in Schönbrunn, a Catholic institution, though if necessary she would consent to Eglfing-Haar.[50] The background to this committal was that the mother had been taking care of her son—long considered "mentally disturbed"—at home, but now she was too ill to do so and he was becoming violent.[51] As recent research has shown, however, it was a misconception that Schönbrunn was trying to protect its patients.[52]

Common to both admissions is female family members' reference to an acute physical threat. They sought to place the husband or son in a religious institution and did not see it as an option to continue caring for them at home. This shows that even in wartime, from the point of view of those committing the patient, the asylums retained their peacetime functions and proved urgently necessary or unavoidable in certain familial situations. The presence of a male family member who was violent toward the family is typical of committals as a whole.[53]

However, people did not always make an effort to find the safest possible residential option for their family members and regularly initiated committals without taking the murder of the sick or conditions in the asylums into account. Such cases sometimes reveal an odd ambivalence in family members' behavior, as when they initiated committals in a proactive way, partly for reasons that the public health officer did not consider compelling, but then wrote to the asylum following the committal requesting that their family member be treated well. This is illustrated in more detail below through the case of Hans A.'s placement. Other committals did not proceed in exactly the same way. This example, however, is representative of a common phenomenon—relatives acting in an inconstant way but without deciding to bring a family member back home or, for example, arranging for them to stay with other relatives.[54] Hans A. was admitted to Eglfing-Haar in March 1944 with the consent of his son. At first, an attempt had been made to initiate compulsory committal "on grounds of danger" in accordance with Article 80/II of the Bavarian Police Penal Code (*Polizeistrafgesetzbuch* or PStGB). However, the district medical officer (*Bezirksarzt*) did not consider this necessary and rejected compulsory committal.[55] Nevertheless, the university psychiatric clinic transferred the patient to the sanatorium-nursing home with the son's consent. Strictly speaking, committals against the will of the person concerned had to be certified by the police or the public health officer. Officially, this could only be circumvented in the case of underage patients. Time and again, however, as in this case of committal, patients who were in fact of age were admitted solely with the consent of their relatives. The 72-year-old man's son had first taken his father to the Munich university psychiatric clinic. His case history there contains a note on his transfer to Eglfing-Haar:

Today the patient's son came to see us and further informed us that it is not possible to leave the patient at home. He himself is on active service, and the patient's daughter-in-law is herself in poor health (pulmonary tuberculosis) so it is impossible for her to care for the patient. The air-raid precautions are a particular source of trouble. There is no air-raid shelter in the home itself, and the patient, who is bedridden, must always be carried across a courtyard fifty meters away. As far as the patient's relatives are concerned, there is no reason why he cannot be committed to the Eglfing Sanatorium-Nursing Home.[56]

The man's son thus portrayed a situation in which it was impossible to keep his father at home due to the war. In the medical records of the Munich university psychiatric clinic, Hans A.'s afflictions were described in more detail. The patient had "clubfoot" and thus problems walking. Regarding his mental condition, the physician stated: "Nothing particularly noticeable psychologically. His memory is said to have diminished somewhat recently. Patient feels lonely and has become quieter lately."[57] He further noted that the patient had never been in hospital before and had been working in an office just three weeks earlier. The explanation mentioned for his foot trouble was that Hans A. used to be a salesman and had to do a lot of walking.[58] The description of his condition in the letter of referral reads more drastically than the statement that Hans A. had problems walking, while the fact that the public health officer rejected compulsory committal also suggests that his admission to Eglfing-Haar was not urgent or inevitable. After the decision was made to transfer him to this sanatorium-nursing home, his son sent a letter to the doctors there asking that his father be treated well, since he was "harmless."

He is a harmless fellow who is generally of regular habits and inconspicuous. The only thing is that he imagines that his left—healthy—foot is so weak that he can no longer walk without two sticks or without someone helping him. [...] In the opinion of the attending physician, Dr. St., this is a psychogenic superimposition that can be remedied by appropriate treatment. [...]

I would therefore ask that you place him, if possible, in a room with harmless cases only at Haar. As soon as I am granted leave—I have been on active service as a member of the Luftwaffe since September 24, 1939 and am currently in northwest France—I will call on you and will be glad to provide any explanations.

I ask you to take care of my father—who in earlier years, as a very comfortably-off merchant, was always extremely generous when it came to social and charitable matters and gave valuable help to many a needy person—to the best of your ability,

Yours sincerely,
Heil Hitler.[59]

There were no further personal statements by this man's son: Hans A.'s death was recorded in his file just two months later.[60] In this case, the son expedited his father's committal by emphasizing that—as long as he was at the front—his wife could not take care of him. This reference to immediate wartime circumstances is very common and crops up again in many cases of committal in the following chapters. Nor was it unusual for relatives to play an instrumental role in initiating committals. The letter indicates that the son was concerned about what was happening to his father and how he was getting on in the asylum. Yet there were clear limits to this concern, as he never considered arranging another placement for his father, let alone bringing him back home. Whatever worries may have plagued him, ultimately, they failed to unsettle his assessment that his father's behavior was intolerable to his family under the circumstances. The son's conduct, which may seem paradoxical at first glance, can be explained, I argue, in light of the radicalization of everyday life on the "home front." Asylums were used to "solve" the problems of everyday coexistence with sick family members, as we will see for the postwar period as well. In general terms, committal to an asylum on such grounds had long been an essentially "normal" process. During the war, however, the social microcosm featured particularly high expectations when it came to its members' compliant behavior and problem-free integration into everyday wartime life. People were expected to act quickly and correctly, especially in the context of bombing raids, a norm that comes up time and again in the next chapter as well. Apart from making it to the air-raid shelter, often the priority was to maintain the blackout. The argument that sick or elderly people posed a risk during bombing raids was usually accepted unquestioningly by physicians. At the same time, the murder of the sick was certainly no secret in 1944.[61] Many rumors circulated about the killing of the elderly in particular.[62] People's acceptance that the murder of the sick might well be happening but failure to see that this might have implications for their own behavior can be read as a particularly powerful sign of radicalization. Some families still tried to avoid committals or sought to place relatives in what they saw as safer asylums, while others regarded the use of these institutions as a normal step despite their perversion by the regime. Radicalization in this sense means that decisions and actions leading to the potentially lethal exclusion of certain individuals could be legitimized and thus fell within the realm of "normal" behavior.[63]

In summary, we can identify three aspects central to actor constellations, power relations, and scope for action between 1941 and the end of the war. First, there was a practice of committal that was specific to the wartime situation, a practice constrained by transfers and the repurposing of parts of psychiatric institutions; the position of hospitals and independent physicians within the committal process had also changed.

Second, in the committal situation, patients and their relatives operated within a space that was quite specific to the Nazi era and to the war. Propaganda films and knowledge of the murder of the sick had an impact on whether patients went to clinics or asylums and to which ones, while patients and relatives distinguished state asylums from both university clinics and confessional establishments.

Nevertheless, third, from the layperson's point of view, the function of the asylum had not changed completely. It still served to resolve problems in the home that were viewed as having become intolerable, above all those involving domestic violence. But as the last example shows, family members by no means always made an effort to find a positive solution for their sick relative.

Committal practices in a "society in a state of collapse" (*Zusammenbruchgesellschaft*), 1945–1949

The situation in the asylums and psychiatric clinics remained catastrophic in the immediate postwar period, not least due to the Allies' lack of interest, the murder of the sick having failed to prompt either them or the Germans to consider making changes or improvements to psychiatric establishments.[64] Death rates were often even higher than during the war,[65] while food rations for psychiatric patients remained extremely meager in the occupation zones.[66] In the FRG, supply chains and general economic life only began to return to normal around four years after the war had ended.[67] In contrast, the GDR continued to struggle with its public finances even in the 1950s.[68] Throughout Germany, patient numbers reached a low point in the first two postwar years. In the Soviet occupation zone in particular, too few places were available due to the use of asylums for other purposes.[69]

In line with conditions in the psychiatric clinics, the documentation of committals became more difficult during the occupation due to material shortages. Old folders were reused in every clinic and asylum examined in this book: names and dates noted in relation to former patients were crossed out and replaced by the details of newly admitted ones. At times, medical histories were summarized in a cramped space on the back of pieces of paper that had already been used for other purposes, or information about those committed was noted on an envelope and inserted into the file. The administration and documentation of committals thus took place under more challenging conditions. This material undersupply eased in West German asylums from about 1948 but persisted at the Greifswald university psychiatric clinic and at Rodewisch until 1951–1952.

Committal practices changed in the immediate postwar years at different levels and for various reasons: committal pathways took new forms and there were also changes in the groups of patients involved. Finally, problems specific to the era emerged, and these were often mentioned by those committed. The process unfolding here cannot, therefore, be described uniformly as rapid "normalization" or as a "state of emergency."

Psychiatric establishments' rudimentary functioning in this period is reflected in the temporary suspension of committals for psychiatric evaluation— to determine capacity for work, the "need" for sterilization, or unsoundness of mind. The provision of expert assessments was almost discontinued at the LHA Marburg, Untergöltzsch, and Eglfing-Haar;[70] only at Greifswald did physicians continue to provide regular expert evaluations during the occupation. Between the end of the war and 1949, about 7 percent of committals in the latter establishment were used to assess capacity for work and about 4 percent to determine unsoundness of mind.[71] University psychiatric clinics were, however, specialized in this field.

In sharp contrast to committals for evaluation, civil committal pathways normalized fairly quickly in many cases. After the end of the war, for example, more patients were again admitted from domestic settings. At Marburg and Greifswald, a greater number of individuals who had previously lived at home were committed during the occupation than in wartime. For a correspondingly larger proportion of those committed in these two institutions, the last place of abode was their own home. At Eglfing-Haar, a similar number of patients lived at home before their committal in the postwar period (about 58 percent) as in wartime (about 55 percent).[72] In the postwar years, however, only about half of them arrived following a stay at other institutions, such as hospitals.[73] The figures for Untergöltzsch defy clear interpretation. It is true that there, in contrast to all the other establishments studied in this book, the number of committed persons previously living at home decreased in the first postwar years. But what this means is hard to determine, since a large number of patient files fail to state the last abode.[74]

The Marburg Land Sanatorium in particular was characterized by the admission of a greater number of people from their family environment.[75] There, the number of patients committed from home during the war roughly corresponded to the percentage at the two sanatorium-nursing homes of Eglfing-Haar and Untergöltzsch. After the war, then, the LHA Marburg again had more in common with a university clinic than with a sanatorium-nursing home, in line with its original conception. At the LHA, the few committals by physicians during the war were related to its war-specific transformation: large parts of the institution were used for new purposes, and its psychiatric patients included soldiers, prisoners of war, and forced laborers.[76] In addition to this problem of space, the reluctance of some families to entrust their relatives to state establishments, as discussed earlier, must also be taken into account. Against this background, the changes that occurred after the war can be read as an indication that the relationship between the institution on the one hand and independent doctors and families on the other was returning to normal under the Allied occupation.

There were many patients in the first few postwar years about whom virtually no information can be found. This is especially true of the years 1945–1947 but also applies to many committals in the following three years. The files are often sparse and contain no or only a very brief medical history. A strikingly large number of these poorly documented committals were of elderly people[77] and/or displaced persons.[78] At the end of the war, the latter were admitted chiefly to psychiatric establishments near the border. Many of them were committed because there were no known family members who might have looked after them, and they could no longer live on their own. The admission of 24-year-old Anna M. to Greifswald in 1949 is exemplary of many other cases. The only information available about the patient, who had fled the Sudetenland, is that the rest of her family was either dead or living in the Czechoslovak Republic (ČSR). Her landlady had arranged for Anna M. to be committed because she felt that living with her had become intolerable.[79]

Since the admission forms did not record the status of "displaced person," it is impossible to quantify exactly how many there were. We can, however, gain some sense of this from the mostly rudimentary medical records. In particular, information on the last abode is often helpful in this regard, since this was typically in areas that now formed part of the ČSR or Poland. In the immediate postwar period, displaced persons were present in greater numbers in the establishments near the border in Greifswald and Saxony than in the other areas under occupation.[80] The allocation of hospital beds to displaced persons, as well as to the elderly, meanwhile, was often criticized as a "waste" in the postwar period, and not only in the Soviet occupation zone. In 1948, for example, the district president of Kassel wrote a letter denouncing the "use [of beds] for purposes other than those for which they were intended."[81] In addition, in the early 1950s, the "repatriation" and admission of mentally ill Germans in Czechoslovakia was a vexing problem discussed jointly by West Germany and the ČSR.[82]

Finally, certain key problems were mentioned frequently by patients and those in their milieu: loss of "homeland,"[83] lack of housing, and the fall of the Nazi regime. These unsurprising themes continued to be mentioned regularly in the early 1950s in both the FRG and GDR. The end of the war and the end of National Socialism were still highlighted by some patients years later as triggers for subsequent illnesses. The 24-year-old journeyman saddler Markus W., who was admitted to Greifswald in 1951 after visiting the clinic, "of his own accord" as noted in his file, stated that he had "previously been an avowed National Socialist."[84] "As he had then experienced the collapse [of the Nazi regime], flight, etc., he had succumbed to severe mental conflicts, and had struggled to cope mentally with the collapse of his fatherland."[85] The end of the Nazi era also played a role in Martina R.'s committal, cited at the beginning of the book. She too regretted the "downfall of the Reich."[86] However, she did not present her disappointment at political realities as the only reason for her distress but also highlighted the general living conditions, her husband's imprisonment, and the fact that she and her children had had to move in with her mother-in-law.[87] Such accounts referring to immediate postwar circumstances had become much rarer by the early 1950s. However, the emotional upheaval triggered by the end of National Socialism long figured as a causal factor in the self-attribution of psychological distress, as in the case of Markus W. He mentioned flight as well: his family had lived near Stettin (present-day Szczecin in Poland) and had then fled to the Baltic Sea island of Usedom.[88] No further details were provided in this case about the expulsion or about integration into the new place of residence; the focus was on getting over the fall of the "Third Reich."

On the whole, however, when it came to displaced persons, it was often concrete circumstances in the wake of their arrival that tipped the scales in favor of committal. This is exemplified by the admission, also in 1951, of Magdalena T., a 44-year-old widow who presented herself for admission to the LHA Marburg accompanied by one of her sons. The family hailed from the vicinity of Warsaw.[89] Her son stated:

In the Herfa camp, she had attracted attention since November of last year due to her great irritability and frequent vocal complaints. She had been particularly angry and had quarreled with a district nurse because it had not been possible to give her a place to live. She had also cried a lot, then went back to ranting, until finally the district nurse had said: 'I'll take you somewhere you've never been before.'[90]

The sample collated for this book reveals many examples of patients mentioning problems obtaining housing. This was a major issue highlighted by displaced persons but also came up repeatedly in the Soviet occupation zone and East Germany when patients had lost their homes due to the bombing raids. Karin S., for example, who had been compulsorily committed to the Untergöltzsch Sanatorium-Nursing Home by the Reichenbach Health Office in 1948, was considered a "troublemaker" because she did not want to settle for the apartment allocated to her, having lost her home in the bombing of Dresden.[91] The Health Office emphasized that if Karin S. were to be discharged, the "constant harassment of all public agencies is sure to ensue."[92] In a letter two months later, the chief physician at Untergöltzsch urged the authorities to assign the patient another dwelling after all, so she could then be discharged from the asylum:

The querulous behavior she is currently exhibiting was triggered by the allocation of a dwelling that [S.] claims is impossible for her to live in. Miss [S.] no longer has any immediate relatives. She would, therefore, potentially have to stay permanently in the asylum.

As a result, the health office has requested that checks again be carried out to determine whether the dwelling assigned is suitable for Miss [S.] and, if necessary, that she be provided with another one. This is another attempt to rein in the patient's querulous tendencies outside the asylum, rather than allow Miss [S.] to become a burden on the community, possibly for many years to come, by placing her in an asylum.[93]

In this committal dating from the time of the Soviet occupation zone, beyond the housing problem—which crops up particularly often in files from the 1940s—two issues are highlighted that also played a role time and again in the 1950s. First, we can discern differing ideas about the functions of an asylum. The term "troublemaker" (*Querulantin*) in itself indicates that Karin S. became a patient because she was viewed as disruptive. The municipality and the health office considered her persistent complaints about the dwelling she had been allocated intolerable and believed that committal was an appropriate means of remedying the disruption to everyday administrative business. The doctors at Rodewisch, on the other hand, saw no medical reason to keep the patient under their care and thus appealed to the municipality, as the responsible authority, to resolve the housing issue. Given the asylums' parlous state, the psychiatrists had no interest in admitting more patients than absolutely necessary. The assumption that Karin S. would spend the rest of her life in the asylum because she had no close relatives was based on experience,[94] and it was clear to the physicians that social factors weighed heavily in the decision to admit her and in the length of her stay. Moreover, to make the second key point, they cited the cost to the "community" (*Allgemeinheit*). This was a discourse already at large in the Weimar Republic.[95] In the GDR, the debate on which patients' clinics and asylums ought to serve intensified once again under conditions of sustained underfunding.

New pathways and lack of places: the practice of committal in the GDR

In what follows, I scrutinize the function of the asylum and the actor constellation involved in committals in East Germany in the light of three key characteristics. First, psychiatric institutions were typified by a lack of places and structural underfunding. Second, the reorganization of the health care system induced changes in the power relations between different groups of physicians within the practice of committal, though it should be noted that psychiatric establishments played only a very marginal role in the construction of the new state. Third, compulsory committals in the GDR were not reformed until 1968. In practice, this led to major shifts in power when it came to decisions to commit.

Underfunding and lack of places

Until the 1960s, the Soviet occupiers used the premises of psychiatric institutions for other purposes.[96] At the same time, the territorial reform of 1952 exacerbated the undersupply of the asylums, entrenching it over the long term.

With the abolition of the states (*Länder*), asylums came under the jurisdiction of the districts (*Kreise*).[97] Compared to the FRG, then, they were at the lowest level of the administrative hierarchy rather than in the middle. The municipalization of the sanatorium-nursing homes weakened their position, as it made cooperation between them more difficult. It also meant that the district administrations "struggled to keep track of fields of health care extending far beyond their own municipal boundaries."[98] Moreover, the asylums' transfer to the municipal level entailed no increase in staff or funding for the district administrations under whose jurisdiction they now came. In both respects, then, asylums represented a major burden on the districts. From 1952 onward, the asylums in Brandenburg complained that the restructuring had hit their finances so hard that they were struggling to provide for patients and pay their staff.[99] Things were much the same in Saxony. Not only was it becoming difficult to pay staff, but it was extremely hard to find doctors for the asylums in the first place; they were hopelessly understaffed. The response of the two asylums—now called specialist hospitals (*Sonderkrankenhäuser*)—of Großschweidnitz and Rodewisch to an inquiry from Dr. Lammert of the Ministry of Health, Department of Health Protection Organization, in 1962 is revealing. Lammert had contacted the asylums because she desperately needed a psychiatrist for the Facklam Sanatorium in Gernrode. Like all other specialist hospitals, the two institutions gave a negative response because they were already suffering from staff shortages of their own. The medical director of Großschweidnitz, Dr. Fabian, explained in his letter of July 5, 1962, that the asylum had only three medical specialists, since it had lost four doctors "due to death or illness" in recent years. He had been trying to replace these four for years without success.[100] The Rodewisch Specialist Hospital explained its negative answer as follows:

Dear Dr. Lammert,

In reply to your letter of June 26, 1962, which arrived here today, I regret to have to respond in the negative. Our medical staffing has deteriorated greatly in recent weeks, as one colleague was detained for attempted flight from the republic (*Republikflucht*) and another colleague is about to be certified as an invalid due to Parkinson's disease. As a result, we had to close our polyclinic, which provides psychiatric care for 5 districts [*Landkreise*], on July 1, 1962, until further notice.

You will no doubt understand that in light of this we cannot give up any of our doctors to Dr. Hörmann. I remain respectfully yours, Dr. Walther.[101]

These two letters addressed two crucial problems, namely, the aging of psychiatrists and the urgent need for replacement staff. Finding new personnel was hampered by the fact that many physicians had left the GDR: as a group, they were particularly unlikely to identify with the new political system.[102]

The Greifswald university psychiatric clinic also complained of sustained overcrowding.[103] The provision of care in the district of Rostock, in which the Greifswald clinic was located, was in fact particularly overstretched. In the entire district, there were for a time only the two university psychiatric clinics of Rostock and Greifswald, but there was no sanatorium-nursing home, in other words no option of admitting patients for lengthy stays. The

Ueckermünde Sanatorium-Nursing Home, which had previously served this area, had been closed in 1954 due to "untenable conditions." In 1953, a tuberculosis sanatorium in Stralsund was at least converted into a psychiatric unit, though it had just 210 beds.[104] In comparison, the several asylums in Saxony had between 400 and 1,000 beds,[105] pointing to serious regional differences in the provision of psychiatric care in East Germany. Despite this strained situation, however, in discussions on how to deal with the lack of admission capacity, the university psychiatric clinics in the Rostock district successfully insisted that the main tasks of institutions of their type were teaching and research. Admitting long-term patients, they contended, was thus out of the question.[106] Indeed, in contrast to the immediate postwar period, in the 1950s very few people were admitted who were then referred to other establishments for long-term stays. The sample analyzed for the present book reveals that the Greifswald university psychiatric clinic itself referred only 3 percent of admitted patients between 1950 and 1963.[107] It thus insisted on sticking to its traditional areas of activity, which distinguished it from sanatorium-nursing homes.

With the founding of the GDR, the function of the asylum within the state also became a significant topic of discussion, one debated in the early 1950s, for example, in the journal *Psychiatrie, Neurologie und medizinische Psychologie* ("*Psychiatry, Neurology and Medical Psychology*"). Hermann Nobbe (1894–1970), director of the Uchtspringe Land Sanatorium, identified five key tasks: treatment; reintegration, care, and accommodation of "mentally ill" patients classified as posing a threat to others; and research on the physical bases of mental illness.[108] The latter imperative distinguished Nobbe's vision of the role of asylums in the GDR from that typical of the "Third Reich" and FRG: sanatorium-nursing homes, unlike university psychiatric clinics, were not usually sites of research. The research Nobbe had in mind here represented the empirical underpinning of Pavlovian theory.[109] However, the author correctly noted that there was likely no prospect of asylums pursuing such research. They were, he acknowledged, already so overburdened that taking on this new role was out of the question.[110] Their most pressing problem was in fact a lack of places.

A huge number of people were waiting for a place in an inpatient facility.[111] As the individual case files show, Greifswald did not immediately admit even patients at acute risk of suicide but instead sent them home, informing them that they would be contacted as soon as a place became available. The delayed admission of Hanna S. provides an example of this. This patient was examined at the polyclinic in 1950 but was not admitted as an inpatient. The polyclinic wrote to the referring physician: "..., [the patient] admitted having suicidal thoughts. We consider it necessary to admit her as an inpatient and will contact her ourselves if a place becomes available."[112] Finally, in 1954, due to the scarcity of inpatient places, "at the suggestion of the Ministry of Health, the colonization [*Kolonisierung*] of the mentally ill was launched. Mentally ill persons capable of work who posed no risk to those around them were placed in state-owned estates."[113] The reasoning of Rostock district in this specific case was that this was a pragmatic way of dealing with the lack of places. No connection was made here with the system of noninstitutional care (*offene Fürsorge*) in the Weimar Republic, though the 1948 guidelines for psychiatric care had already emphasized the goal of orienting psychiatry toward Weimar's progressive health care system.[114] Placing asylum patients outside the institution for pragmatic reasons was not a new measure or one specific to the GDR. In the postwar period, it was also deployed in the FRG and exhibited a degree of continuity with Nazi-era policies.[115]

Given the asylums' limited functioning due to underfunding, staff shortages, and repurposing, the expert assessment system functioned remarkably well at the Greifswald university psychiatric clinic, whose district was hit particularly hard by these problems. In the 1950s and early 1960s, evaluations at Greifswald eventually accounted for over 20 percent of committals. Most of these are related to patients' ability to work.[116] Despite the serious lack of psychiatric beds, then, evaluations involving inpatient admissions took place on a significant scale, which tells us something about the role of psychiatry in the state (and in the Soviet occupation zone). Just as the scarce resources within an underfunded health system were earmarked for citizens who contributed to "economic and biological productivity,"[117] the very few places in the university psychiatric clinic were also used to a considerable extent to assess capacity for work. This fits into a picture of East Germany in which the welfare system was designed to exploit labor power to the maximum, in some resemblance to the Nazi state.[118] Hence, old-age insurance was by far the weakest part of the social security system.[119] Furthermore, enterprise-based health care played a major role. This had been introduced in the Soviet occupation zone,[120] and the enterprise (*Betrieb*) had been involved in everyday health care ever since.[121] The socialist welfare state's one-sided orientation toward the working population is also evident in who was allocated the available places in psychiatric institutions.[122] At the same time, in some cases medical assessments were carried out to establish whether an individual had reduced working capacity due to war-related ailments. Keeping the number of people recognized as having this status low was an explicit concern of the Ministry of Labor and Vocational Training (Ministerium für Arbeit und Berufsausbildung), due to fears that they could become a major burden on the state.[123]

In the early GDR, then, university psychiatry at Greifswald was guided by institutional self-interest, which chiefly meant prioritizing teaching and research, and by the state's interest in deploying psychiatric expertise to maximize the exploitation of labor power. The provision of comprehensive care for patients in the district was not the top priority. Despite the structural undersupply of psychiatric institutions, however, committals in East Germany were more regulated and better documented than they had been in the Soviet occupation zone.

Changes in committal pathways associated with the role of polyclinics and specialist boards (Fachärztegremien)

How exactly did the now more regulated admissions in the GDR unfold? To elucidate this, it helps to take a look at the reorientation of the health care system. While it would be wrong to claim that the 1950s saw the "Westernization" of health care in the FRG or its "Sovietization" in East Germany,[124] this does not mean there were no major changes. In the Soviet occupation zone, the Germans had a relatively free hand when it came to organizing health care. In the first instance, they built on elements from the Weimar Republic as well as demands articulated by the workers' movement since the time of the German Empire.[125] In the course of this restructuring, changes specific to the GDR occurred that had major consequences for committal pathways, though they were not aimed specifically at the psychiatric sphere.

A letter of referral from the Zittau Polyclinic from 1954 provides an insight into typical committal procedures in East Germany. Anne K.[126] was committed by that institution to the Großschweidnitz Land Asylum.

> Dear colleague,
>
> We would like to refer our patient, Mrs. [Anne K.], to you for specialist assessment and, if necessary, for inpatient observation.
>
> Regarding her previous history, we wish to draw your attention to the following indicators.
>
> Mrs. [K.] was treated for neuralgic complaints [...] in 1951. After two to three months her condition improved. In the autumn of last year, the patient visited the clinic again and complained of severe depression, which escalated into suicidal thoughts. In addition, neuralgia-like ailments reappeared. After a brief attempt at treatment with vitamin B complex and sedative medication, the patient reported no improvement. This prompted us to refer Mrs. [K.] to the psychiatric outpatient clinic of the Karl Marx University, Leipzig, which informed us of its findings as follows: This is essentially a case of climacteric complaints with corresponding psychological changes amounting to a depressive state.
>
> In light of the proposed treatment, we administered propaphenin or megaphene tablets[127] and vitamin E. Temporary improvement was then reported by the patient.
>
> One of the attending physicians in this case, Dr. S., Zittau, who could find nothing pathological in gynecological terms except changes in the internal genital organs corresponding to the menopause, also prescribed hormone preparations.
>
> A few days ago, the patient came to see us again complaining of a new bout of severe depression, and also expressed suicidal thoughts. This has led us to conclude that the therapy deployed so far is producing no useful results. In order to rule out a different etiology, we believe a specialist

neurological-psychiatric evaluation to be advisable, and possibly inpatient observation, and kindly ask you to undertake these. With collegial greetings.[128]

This referral letter reveals both general characteristics of committals and procedures specific to the GDR. Consulting a gynecologist was typical of committals beyond that state. Psychiatry had constructed connections between female corporeality and mental illness or attributions of unacceptable behavior as early as the nineteenth century.[129]

In contrast to the Nazi era, it became increasingly common to prescribe psychotropic drugs in both successor states in the 1950s,[130] though these were less often available in East Germany than in the FRG.[131] In both states, the intake of these substances could alter committals in two ways. First, patients were sometimes committed later because—as in this case—an attempt was first made to treat them as outpatients. Second, people were discharged from asylums earlier—as physicians noted—but also readmitted more frequently.[132] The referral of the patient to various specialists is another aspect not specific to a particular sociopolitical system.

Unlike the referral letter we saw earlier from the Nazi period concerning the admission of a woman suffering from MS to the Greifswald university psychiatric clinic, the above letter was not issued by an independent physician, but by a polyclinic.[133] Another institution of the same type played a role in the committal decision, namely, the Psychiatric Polyclinic of Karl Marx University. This in itself shows that committal mechanisms in the GDR differed to some extent from earlier procedures and from those in West Germany. This was not due to new regulations governing psychiatry but to the general reorientation of the health care system. In addition to committals by polyclinics, however, they were still regularly made by independent physicians in private practice. While no new private practices had been allowed since 1949,[134] many still existed. Greifswald had been home to a polyclinic before the existence of the GDR, but now medical records more often noted that the patient was committed by this polyclinic or by rural outpatient clinics in the surrounding area. Furthermore, many private physicians initially referred patients to a polyclinic, which then transferred them to another institution, as revealed by the almost 500 medical records from the GDR reviewed for the present book.[135] In any case, it is clear that for the patient a polyclinic often represented a step on the path to committal. Even in the case of referrals and transfers from hospitals, often the patient at Greifswald was first examined in its own polyclinic and then transferred again to its department of neurology/psychiatry.[136] In light of this, it is worth considering how polyclinics contributed to changes in the constellations of actors and power involved in committal practices.

First, polyclinics often formed part of inpatient institutions. It was not only Greifswald that had its own polyclinic; so did most psychiatric institutions. We should bear in mind that the thinking of physicians who came into direct contact with the admitting institution is likely to have been influenced by this. We can also assume that they simultaneously anticipated the asylum's capacity when deciding on inpatient committals, and that communication, at least between polyclinics and the inpatient facility to which they were attached, went more smoothly than the generally poor or non-existent communication between independent physicians and hospitals in West Germany.[137]

As exemplified by Anne K.'s committal to Großschweidnitz, polyclinics often represented key intermediate stages within psychiatric committals. This not only shifted the balance of power within the medical profession, but also shaped the patient's position vis-à-vis the committal decision. Second, polyclinics expanded patients' room for maneuver simply because those slated for examination were not immediately admitted as inpatients. This meant that they did not have to decide whether to enter an asylum in an institution in which they might well struggle to make their voices heard while interacting with established experts on their complaints.

Third, the possibility of outpatient examinations in polyclinics could lower the psychological barrier to seeing a doctor, as has already been observed for the polyclinics of the German Empire and the Weimar Republic.[138]

While polyclinics and rural outpatient clinics played an important role in the GDR, committals via university psychiatric clinics had already decreased significantly in the Soviet occupation zone. At Untergöltzsch, they dropped to about 6 percent and remained at this level in the 1950s and 1960s.[139] During the war, by contrast, these referrals had accounted for about 20 percent of all admissions. It was in the university psychiatric clinics in particular that key decisions had been made by medical specialists and assessments had been carried out to determine whether a patient required a lengthy stay in an institution. These decisions were now more often made by polyclinics and the specialist medical boards in the asylums. Patients whose medical status was unclear, as in the case of Anne K., were sent "for specialist assessment and, if necessary for inpatient observation"[140] to a specialist psychiatric hospital, as the asylums were now called, in order to determine whether they required institutional care.[141] In both West Germany and the "Third Reich," meanwhile, medical decisions on committal were made at an earlier stage in the vast majority of cases and did not take place in the institution. This was especially true of first-time committals.[142]

Overall, the role of the polyclinics and the medical boards in the specialist hospitals shows that state health care institutions played a much greater role in committal practices in the GDR than during the war or in West Germany. Their powers often extended to the formal committal of patients who had been living at home prior to their admission and had not come from another institution. The position of psychiatrists, meanwhile, was enhanced by the making of decisions within asylums. This assessment is congruent with Sabine Hanrath's finding that in the debate on a new law on placement in psychiatric institutions (*Unterbringungsgesetz*) in the GDR, in contrast to the FRG, psychiatrists managed to strengthen physicians' position in decision-making procedures relating to forced committals.[143]

Relatives remained important within the committal process in East Germany. Since there were fewer formal compulsory committals, their opinion came to play a key role in committal decisions. Many committals proceeded as in the case of Karin F. and Albin H., two civil admissions. 31-year-old Karin F. came to Großschweidnitz in 1958, having suffered from "spastic paresis of the hip" since childhood.[144] Her parents explained that an ever-greater number of nursing tasks were required as the paresis worsened. Her mother had first contacted the local polyclinic about this, which referred daughter and mother to the specialist medical committee at the Großschweidnitz asylum. There, her mother spoke in favor of inpatient placement.[145] The doctors agreed: "Admission to inpatient care would be advisable in this case. However, this is not feasible for reasons of space—at least in the next few months. For the time being, we can only pencil this case in and return to it in due course."[146] This shows once again that there were too few places available for admission. A short time later, however, Karin F. was in fact admitted as an inpatient. Three weeks after her admission, following a decrease in spasticity, she was discharged at her parents' request.[147] The decision in favor of inpatient admission was thus made by the parents and the doctors at Großschweidnitz. While the patient in this instance was ambivalent about admission, there were also cases in which doctors and relatives clearly instigated committal against an individual's will. One example is the committal of 71-year-old Albin H. in 1958. He was living with his son, who sought admission after his father began wandering around the house in the evenings and physically attacking other household members, including his son.[148] What both committals, for all their differences, had in common was that the home situation was the deciding factor for the relatives, whether due to an increased need for care or in connection with violent behavior.

Summary: state and psychiatric institutions in the GDR

Overall, compared to the wartime period, we can identify two major changes in framework conditions, actor constellations, and the scope of action enjoyed by individual groups of actors in committal practices in East Germany.

The stages of the committal pathway had been altered by the GDR-specific restructuring of the health care system. Polyclinics gained importance as a new institution, while university psychiatric clinics no longer played much of a role at all, and doctors in private practice only a secondary one.

Asylum physicians also occupied a key position in committal decisions, the deliberations of the specialist medical committees strengthening their voice.

Despite these ruptures, we can also identify continuities. For example, there continued to be an acute shortage of space in psychiatric institutions, although the reasons for this had changed compared to the Nazi period.

In addition, the provision of expert reports remained an important field of activity for psychiatrists, especially at the Greifswald university psychiatric clinic, and also continued to be a reason for temporary committals. Of course, there is a fundamental difference between an expert assessment intended to facilitate sterilization and one meant to establish the capacity for work. The common ground lies at the structural level: in both systems, short-term committals were an opportunity for the state to draw on psychiatric expertise.

The contested role of psychiatric institutions and controversial committal practices in West Germany

The institutions in the western occupation zones too suffered from every conceivable kind of shortage.[149] In order to cope with the overcrowding, North Rhine-Westphalia, similar to Rostock District, began to place the sick in the so-called "family assistance"[150] program or leave them with their families. On July 2, 1949, the *Westfälische Zeitung* newspaper described these measures in an article titled "For the Poorest of the Poor":

> Less known is the fact that [the authorities] have gone over to putting some of the less severely ill in the so-called "family assistance" program. These sick individuals are placed, with a care allowance, in families of rural and artisanal employers as workers; they are under constant medical observation and are familiarized with normal conditions. The individual asylums care for between fifty and ninety patients each in this way.
>
> Some sick individuals—who strictly speaking require institutional care—behave in a placid way and are left with their families, which entails the provision of an allowance of up to 30 DM. This saves on the higher costs of institutional care and eliminates the need for accommodation. There are about 190 cases of this kind in Westphalia.[151]

Although the situation in West German psychiatric institutions remained strained in the 1950s, this was less of a problem than in the GDR. There was no long-term outside use of asylums, and the psychiatric facilities were located at an intermediate administrative level, sparing them the financial problems that had arisen in East Germany when asylums were transferred to the district level without an increase in funding. Unlike in the GDR, the administrative system took its lead from the pre-Nazi period.[152] Moreover, in contrast to the eastern portion of Germany, its western counterpart was not affected by a continuous exodus of medical specialists. The FRG, in addition, restored the old German health care system almost completely. Diverging from East Germany, physicians could once again organize themselves autonomously, while the social insurance system was built on traditional distinctions between blue-collar workers, white-collar workers, and privately insured persons.[153] Since there were no major upheavals in the health care system, unlike in the GDR, no new institutional actors entered the committal process, such as polyclinics or rural outpatient clinics. In West Germany, new decision makers entered the scene not as a result of changes in the health care system, but in connection with new regulations on compulsory committals.

Who belongs in an asylum? Debates on costs and the relationship between security and illness

What were asylums for, or what should they be for? Though the FRG picked up the threads of venerable structures, on practical grounds this question was raised there as well. Analogous to the GDR and its debate on whom the few available places should be allocated to, this issue was rooted in the problem of costs. The western discourse, however, took a different course. While in East Germany the core issue was those who caused costs, in other words, the question of who could and should be admitted in the first place, in the FRG the debate revolved around those who bore the costs, that is: Who should pay for asylum stays and why? These contrasting discussions were a reflection of the fact that there were even fewer places available in the GDR than in the FRG.

It is true that there were discussions in the west among top asylum staff and welfare associations (*Fürsorgevereine*) about who the asylum was intended for, as Sabine Hanrath has brought out.[154] However, this involved dividing patients into various groups that might be accommodated in different ways. In North Rhine-Westphalia, for example, consideration was given to separating "healing" and "care" institutionally.[155] The main question in West Germany was therefore how, and in which medical institutions, psychiatric and neurological patients should be treated, and who should pay for inpatient stays.

The discussion on costs was originally sparked by the so-called Halving Decree of 1942, which regulated the assumption of expenses for almost all committals.[156] The regulations stated that in cases of committal the welfare associations were to pay half the costs and the health insurance funds the other half, regardless of whether the patient was committed primarily for treatment or for long-term residential care for reasons of public safety. The Halving Decree was issued for pragmatic reasons, since it was no longer necessary to carry out checks to establish the grounds for committal or to vet the payer. This entailed both simplification and standardization, a shift whose pragmatism nevertheless reveals that in the Nazi era all patients could be labeled with little ado as potentially dangerous. The decree continued to apply in the FRG throughout the period under study; it was even reaffirmed in 1960.[157]

However, there were discussions from 1949 onward about whether the Halving Decree made sense and what a different arrangement might look like. This cost-centered debate provides a good indication of who the asylum was intended for. Individual asylums, health insurance schemes, and welfare associations, as well as the views advocated by affected persons' organizations and the justice system, were all significant within the debate. It was initiated by the health insurance companies, which argued that the Halving Decree had in practice encumbered them with unjustified costs. In May 1949, the Hamburg Association of White-Collar Workers' Health Insurance Funds (Verband der Angestellten Krankenkassen e. V., Hamburg) wrote to the ministries of labor and social affairs of the *Länder* (the West German states) as follows: "In light of the requirement for health insurance providers to bear half the costs in cases of purely residential care, they should, as a *quid pro quo*, receive a guarantee that they will be charged only half the costs in all other cases as well."[158] In practice, this was not always the case: at times, the welfare associations reclaimed their expenses from the persons concerned, who could then file a claim with their health insurer. Via this circuitous route, then, the health insurance funds ultimately bore the entire cost after all.[159] It should be noted that these practices varied from region to region. For example, some Bavarian district administrations, to which the welfare associations were subordinate, stated that the difficulties mentioned by the Hamburg Association of White-Collar Workers' Health Insurance Funds had never arisen in their districts.[160]

For years, a variety of actors debated whether or not the Halving Decree and the ways it had been implemented were legal and whether its regulations placed reasonable demands on the health insurance funds. Another point is of interest here, namely, the ideas—always present between the lines of this discourse—about what purpose asylums had and ought to have. The Halving Decree took up a pre-existing classification of motives for committal, which was discussed in the course of the debate on costs. The Association of Health Insurance Funds (Krankenkassenverband) referred to "safeguarding cases" (*Bewahrungsfälle*) and "other cases," thus differentiating between committals for "quartering" and for treatment. This distinction was interpreted, adopted, or challenged in the 1950s and early 1960s. Numerous binary pairings, such as cases of "safeguarding" and treatment, somatic and mental illness, and police and judicial committals—but less often the need to question them—were discussed in the early FRG to determine who ought to pay in light of the grounds for committal.

Exemplary of the majority opinion at the beginning of the debate in 1949 is the assessment of the Günzburg District Welfare Association (Bezirksfürsorgeverband), whose spokesman proposed the following procedure in June 1949:

> The basic thrust of my proposal is that: 1) In the case of admission to an asylum chiefly on grounds of treatment for an illness, the health insurance fund liable to pay the costs should do so within the framework of the provisions of the RVO,[161] 2) In the case of admission on grounds of public safety and need for assistance, the competent welfare authority should pay the costs. The cause of the committal must of course be determined in a

given case. Based on my cooperation with the local sanatorium-nursing home, it is clear that patients admitted for treatment for an illness are far more numerous than cases of treatment on grounds of public safety.[162]

Four aspects of this statement deserve emphasis. The first is the assumption that there was an isolable cause for each committal, and the second is the notion that the payer should be determined in the light of this cause. Third, it was taken as read that the two possible causes were illness and safety issues. Fourth and finally, the association assumed that illness as grounds for committal led to treatment in the asylum, while safety issues led to long-term residential placement. All four points were contested over the next ten years, with the differing concerns of the institutions involved playing a key role in this regard. The health insurance funds were keen to annul the Halving Decree in order to save costs,[163] while the welfare associations argued for its retention for the same reason, but also put forward substantive arguments.[164] Thus, in July 1949, the Bavarian Association of Administrative Districts (Landkreisverband Bayern) wrote in defense of requiring the health insurance funds to pay in "cases of long-term residential placement."

> But even in the so-called safeguarding cases, that is, those in which the mentally ill person was admitted to the asylum primarily for reasons of public safety, it cannot be disputed that an illness is involved, even if it is not of the kind identified in the RVO. Moreover, since the patient is insured, it does not seem unreasonable that in these cases, too, the insurance provider should pay half the costs from the outset, since it has collected the mentally ill person's contributions prior to his admission.[165]

The welfare associations thus argued that grounds of illness and safety converged and that there were no committals that occurred solely for "reasons of public safety."

Once it had arisen, the question of who ought to pay was not only addressed by the health insurance funds and welfare associations. Since this was partly a matter of "public safety," and in the western occupation zones and the FRG the district courts (*Amtsgerichte*) played a crucial role in this, the Judicial Treasury (*Justizfiskus*) could potentially be viewed as responsible for payment. Here, with respect to committals that took place on "grounds of public safety," a further internal distinction was made between temporary residential placement and long-term accommodation. The Bavarian State Ministry of Justice opined that the welfare associations should be responsible for long-term placements and that the Judicial Treasury should pay for temporary stays, as these were the equivalent of pretrial detention.[166]

In 1952, the sanatorium-nursing homes were asked to give their views on the Halving Decree. For these institutions, the key issues included how they were perceived against the background of the Nazi era and their relationship to the university psychiatric clinics. At the request of the Bavarian State

Ministry of the Interior, the director of Eglfing-Haar, Dr. Braunmühl (1901–1957),[167] commented on the debate on the Halving Decree and emphasized that it could only be understood in light of the consistently negative attitude toward the mentally ill during the Nazi era. As a result, Braunmühl stated, the asylums had been regarded as detention centers, a notion on which the Halving Decree drew.[168] This understanding, he went on, was also the root of the different approach to covering costs arising in the clinics, which in his opinion ought to be changed:

> It is impossible to agree with the position of the health insurance funds that they should assume in full the costs arising in university psychiatric clinics, even if the public welfare system might potentially pay, while declining to cover the costs arising in the sanatorium-nursing homes, despite the fact that there the sick are not only cared for in the same way as in the clinics, but often receive the most modern treatment as well.[169]

The director of this Upper Bavarian sanatorium-nursing home was making his case against the backdrop of the competition between university psychiatric clinics and sanatorium-nursing homes.[170] One of his key concerns here was that the latter ought to be perceived and accepted as medical institutions; he demanded that health insurers recognize that the "mentally ill" (*Geisteskranke*) were always treatable cases.[171] He thus did away with the dichotomy of safety and illness that had undergirded the debate, instead calling for the asylum to be viewed unambiguously as part of the medical sector. This line of argument is typical of psychiatrists' self-presentation in the early FRG. Sabine Hanrath has noted that physicians in North Rhine-Westphalia stylized themselves as the profession that considered the whole person and was less politically corrupt than the administrative authorities.[172] The medical argument was presented as the ethically correct one—with psychiatrists' integrity and impartiality taken as read. By dissolving the functional dichotomy, many physicians thus sought to lend medical interpretations an absolute authority.[173] In this context, Braunmühl opened up an intra-medical dichotomy, indignantly declaring that "It is quite unfathomable why it has proved impossible to convince the administrative authorities that the mentally ill should be treated no differently than the physically ill (...)."[174] According to Braunmühl, the distinction between mentally and physically ill patients was crucial to the coverage of costs: physically ill people undoubtedly came under the medical field, such that the health insurance funds bore the costs without further ado.

As the debate progressed, the internal distinctions that were considered relevant became ever finer. In an expert evaluation by Dr. Schulz, a member of the German Association for the Mentally Disabled (Deutscher Verein für psychisch behinderte Personen), he declared two far-reaching intra-psychiatric distinctions to be fundamental to determining the coverage of costs. Schulz argued that health insurance funds should not be responsible if patients were "psychopaths," "suffering from geriatric disorders" (*Alterskranke*), or "feeble-minded" (*Schwachsinnige*).[175] Two key criteria came into play here: the somatic/physical cause of an illness and age. "Psychopaths" were located on the borderline of somatic disorders; for many physicians, this placed them at the margins of medicine, because postwar German psychiatry overwhelmingly saw itself as somatically oriented.[176] "Feeble-mindedness" and "geriatric disorders" (*Alterserkrankungen*) were undisputedly thought to have somatic causes but were located at the extremes of the age scale. Since feeble-mindedness was seen as hereditary or at least always as an early childhood phenomenon, according to Schulz a "mentally full-fledged personality" (*geistig vollwertige Persönlichkeit*) never developed.[177] Only those who did not behave "normally" for somatic reasons, without this being attributed to "normal" physical development, were regarded as "mentally ill" and thus as falling within the remit of the health insurance funds. The isolated consideration of geriatric phenomena is parallel to the discussions in the GDR, where, for example, the university psychiatric clinics in Rostock district refused to deal with the elderly and those dependent on care so they could focus on teaching and research, despite the absence of alternative venues for inpatient treatment.

The debate on costs features three points that tell us much about the understanding of the asylum in the postwar period. First, the course of the debate was characterized by increasingly specific internal distinctions. In light of the illness-safety dichotomy, illness was first divided into the categories of somatic and mental. Psychiatric disorders were then further differentiated. Yet these increasingly elaborate classifications in no way resulted in agreement. Quite the reverse. All those involved in the discussion laid claim to interpretive sovereignty by making their own field the starting point for their ideas about who should be housed in sanatorium-nursing homes and why. Hence, in the 1950s there was no new regulation and practices remained unchanged, that is, highly fragmented. Theoretical attempts at classification and practical diversity are found side by side in the psychiatry of the 1940s and 1950s and in a virtually dialectical relation with each other. The attempt to overcome ambiguities by means of the clearest possible classification schemes, and the constant failure of this project, will be further explored in the following chapters.[178]

Second, the debate was characterized by a diversity of viewpoints. Depending on the institution, opinions differed as to what the asylum was there for. Should safety issues or medical considerations be to the fore? What exactly should these entail in a given case? A range of questions emerges here, which I explore in more detail in the course of this book.

Finally, and directly related to the second point, substantive and interest-driven arguments intermingled. In the debate on costs, psychiatry was always defined in light of the interests and function of particular institutions. But this does not mean that we must view substantive arguments solely as strategic attempts to legitimize particular interests.[179] In fact, both levels are intertwined and must be examined together. This interweaving of content and function is significant to psychiatry as a whole and will be even more evident in the reasoning of relatives of those committed. In their thinking, too, pragmatic concerns were intermeshed with substantive assessments.

Patients between doctors, relatives, and overcrowded clinics

How families made use of the asylum depended on various factors, which, as in the GDR, were of an essentially pragmatic nature. Let's look at the example of Miranda L., a patient who was committed several times in the 1950s. In December 1952, she was committed for the third time. This was not an official measure; her brother and sister-in-law brought her to the asylum without a doctor's referral. In such cases, an asylum doctor undertook the formal committal. Unlike in East Germany, in the vast majority of cases these direct admissions by the asylum in West Germany only occurred if the patient had already been in the same asylum once or several times before.[180] In her previous admissions, Miranda L. had been committed by her family doctor.[181] In this respect, the third admission stands out: not only was there no committal certificate, but no medical referral at all. Congruent with this, at the beginning of her case history, where the statement of the referring physician usually appears, we find one by her sister-in-law:

> ... Then she began to rant and rave—for example at her mother, whom she said had allowed her to be put in the asylum—about the [electroconvulsive] shock [therapy] in the asylum, etc.
>
> Things got really bad about fourteen days ago. Since then, she has been ranting for a while, then talking in a chaotic, muddled-up way, interspersed with times when she is quite level-headed.
>
> About eight days ago, she herself said that an [electro-]shock would have been good after all.
>
> She has also come with us to the asylum quite willingly today [...]
> Patient signs consent form for admission.[182]

This pattern was repeated during her next admission in 1954, when it was noted that "after initial reluctance [the patient] agreed to return to the LHA" and then signed the admission form. She was again brought by relatives, once again with no medical referral. Instead, one of her relatives stated, "We know what's wrong with my sister-in-law. There's nothing a doctor can do for her."[183]

Miranda L.'s committals highlight the gray area of voluntariness and coercion in which many non-official committals took place. It was not just in Miranda L.'s case that relatives decided on an asylum stay in advance: this was typical of committals in the FRG and GDR—and to a lesser extent also during World War II. Bringing the patient directly to the asylum put the family in a particularly powerful position, as this allowed them to bypass the otherwise antecedent negotiation process with an independent physician.

With regard to families' expectations of the asylum, a similar pattern emerges in the case of Miranda L. as in that of Karin F. and Albin H: relatives hoped not so much for medical help as for a solution to a problem of care and supervision. Miranda L.'s relatives explained that they could not supervise the patient during her states of agitation because all of them were engaged in farming from dawn till dusk.[184] Hence, their goal was in no way to "lock up" the patient over the long term. Analogous to Karin F., following each of Miranda L.'s committals the doctors discharged her back into the care of her relatives after a few weeks, when her condition suggested she could be better integrated into everyday family life. But it is not entirely clear whether we can interpret this situation wholly as a problem of supervision, since the reference to shock therapy at the asylum is bound up with expectations of improvement. Such multi-layered expectations, which fused hopes of solutions to practical problems with vague hopes for improved health, often characterized the attitudes of relatives in both German states. During World War II, meanwhile, the use of asylums was shaped primarily by security concerns and less by hopes of health improvements.

Overall, there were more admissions via medical practices and the psychiatric departments of university hospitals in the FRG than in the GDR. At both the Marburg LHA and Eglfing-Haar, in the 1950s committals by independent physicians increased compared to the wartime period, while admissions via university psychiatric clinics decreased.[185] Eglfing-Haar's 1959 annual report listed the number of committals from university psychiatric clinics for every year between 1950 and 1959. This was 23 percent of all admitted patients in 1950, but only 1.7 percent in 1959.[186] In communication with the Upper Bavaria Land Welfare Association (Landesfürsorgeverband Oberbayern), Haar's director, Dr. Braunmühl, attributed this to the overcrowding of the university psychiatric clinic. In January 1953, he stated: "At the moment, 50 percent of all admissions originally intended for the university psychiatric clinic in Munich are going through every day in Haar in the absence of admission by the university psychiatric clinic ([patients are] effectively turned away by the doorman of the clinic and told to go to Haar) because the clinic declares itself overcrowded and in no need of any new admissions."[187]

At the LHA Marburg, the individual case files point to the same problem.[188] It is noted repeatedly that the patient was only admitted to the LHA because the Marburg University Psychiatric Clinic had turned them away due to overcrowding. These could be committals for diagnostic clarification as well as acute emergencies. An example of the former is the committal of Katrin H., who was referred to the university psychiatric clinic by her family doctor in 1950. According to the certificate he provided, he thought the patient might be suffering from schizophrenia but was not certain. This was to be clarified in the clinic through inpatient observation.

Ms. H was in fact admitted to the LHA Marburg, her medical file containing both the certificate referring her to the university psychiatric clinic and the note "committed here due to lack of space."[189] Lisa Z., meanwhile, was an acute case. With regard to her admission in February 1954, her medical record notes: "Patient arrived here during the night, brought by her husband, after many hours on the road. They had been sent on from St. Joseph's Hospital, Olsberg, to Marburg, to the Marburg University Psychiatric Clinic, because of overcrowding. Sent here from there for the same reason."[190] The admission of Lisa Z. to the LHA was thus preceded by two rebuffs. There was no disagreement about the fact that she was in urgent need of inpatient treatment. She was later referred back from the LHA to the university psychiatric clinic when beds finally became available there.[191]

Here, we can discern a dual functional equivalence between university psychiatric clinics and asylums. Both were responsible for diagnostic clarification and admission in case of immediate need for treatment. These two institutions, asylum and university psychiatric clinic, which were still very different when the latter was established, thus moved closer together.[192] This functional equivalence, a result of referral due to overcrowding rather than genuinely medical factors, was underlined by the director of Eglfing-Haar. After stating that a large number of patients were admitted to his establishment rather than the university psychiatric clinic, he wrote: "The situation as it stands is that the Haar asylum is clearly acting as an independent specialist hospital, one in no way subordinate or secondary to the clinic."[193] The asylums' desire not to be seen as professionally less competent "quartering institutions" (*Verwahranstalten*) shines through clearly here.[194] Braunmühl's self-confident account is not the only possible interpretation of these transfers. As we will see in the next section, on the subject of compulsory committals, the redirecting of patients to the asylums on purely pragmatic grounds was typical of the wartime period and de facto consolidated their role as "quartering institutions" before the end of the war.[195]

In order to scrutinize the decrease in referrals from university psychiatric clinics from different angles, beyond the issue of overcrowding, we would have to evaluate the files of a university psychiatric clinic in the early FRG in the same way as I have done for the Greifswald university psychiatric clinic in the GDR.[196] In the West German asylums I studied, the decrease in committals from university psychiatric clinic was accompanied by an increase in committals by independent physicians. Some of these were in fact committals to a university psychiatric clinic, but as in the examples cited, due to overcrowding they culminated in admission to an asylum. In addition, however, independent physicians simply initiated more committals to the asylums studied here than during the war. We are thus dealing partly with the normalization of committal processes in the postwar period—though this does not fully explain the rapid decrease in committals from university psychiatric clinics. The developments mentioned at the beginning of the chapter, which I have described in detail as causes of the low number of committals by independent physicians during the war, also come into play here as explanatory factors: reduced access to independent physicians under the "Reich" due to their deployment at the front, the switch to company-based medicine, and a loss of trust among patients.

As a private institution, Bethel recorded particularly high numbers of committals by independent physicians. These made up just over 50 percent of committals between 1950 and 1955 and almost 65 percent between 1956 and 1963.[197] Such committals were less common at the LHA Marburg: between 1950 and 1955, they accounted for 28.7 percent of all committals, and 36.6 percent between 1956 and 1963.[198] In all the establishments considered in this book—except Bethel from 1945 onwards—there was a difference of about 20 percent during World War II, in the FRG, and in the GDR between the number of patients who had lived permanently at home before committal and the number of those who had not been resident in another institution even immediately prior to their admission. This is because almost 90 percent of patients came to the von Bodelschwingh Asylums from their own homes, and only about 6 percent from a hospital.[199] In the postwar period, then, patients and relatives negotiated committals to Bethel much less frequently with the involvement of other institutions.

The Bodelschwingh Asylums differed from the LHA Marburg in another respect. At Bethel, a particularly large number of expert assessments were carried out in the 1950s and early 1960s, especially to determine capacity for work (about 18 percent dealt with the latter topic).[200] At the LHA, too, expert evaluations were again being produced in the 1950s, but fewer than at Bethel (about 5 percent).[201] In addition, at Marburg these expert reports more often sought to determine unsoundness of mind than capacity for work.[202] Bethel's religious character is no longer particularly reflected in committals by relatives in the postwar period, whereas this factor was highly significant during World War II.

Between voluntariness and coercion, assistance and long-term residential placement: committals from the perspective of patients in the Nazi era, the GDR, and the FRG

In my analysis of committal practices so far, the patient as an actor has appeared rather sporadically, although they were the central figure around whom the whole process revolved. In the negotiation of committal, patients played a dual role: they were always both the object of decisions and the subject who participated in or could react to them. I now analyze the patients' perspective during World War II, in the GDR, and in the FRG, since there was a fair amount of common ground despite the different political systems.

Patients could evaluate committals in a wide variety of ways. It is beyond doubt that some of them chose to go to a clinic or asylum and signed a declaration of voluntariness,[203] even in the Nazi period. During the war, as revealed by a review of the files, these cases were less common than in the

1950s, but they did occur. Once again, it is evident that patients distinguished between different types of inpatient psychiatric treatment. While it was the absolute exception for a person to push for admission to Eglfing-Haar, this occurred more frequently in the case of the von Bodelschwingh Asylums as a Protestant institution and Greifswald as a university psychiatric clinic. Amelie F., for example, was transferred to Greifswald at her own request in 1942. The wife of a business owner had undergone surgery at a hospital on the island of Rügen. From there, at her own request, she was transferred to the Greifswald university psychiatric clinic after insisting that there was something wrong with her nerves.[204] According to her medical records, she expressed a profound sense of relief upon admission: "I am so glad I ended up here with you, where one can really talk things through. The other doctors merely perform an operation, but here I can really talk about how I feel in my heart of hearts."[205]

But even if the patient agreed to admission, it is not always as clear as in the example just given whether they wanted to enter the institution or not. In the end, this question cannot always be answered: both the sources and the categories are problematic. For one thing, even ego documents in medical records do not allow us to look into patients' minds.[206] Furthermore, the categories of "voluntariness" and "coercion" are not unchanging and clearly defined.[207] I address them in this book, but always while factoring in their contingency and constructedness. Still, it seems useful to approach the question of voluntariness from several different angles—not to answer it, but to make the issue more comprehensible. With this aim in mind, I now turn to a number of exemplary committal scenarios.

First of all, I scrutinize the reasons for civil committals, which raises the question of what significance the asylums might have had for those committed. I show that the formal classification of "voluntary" or "with force" may not have dovetailed with patients' self-perception; the next chapter then focuses on power relations and the reasons for compulsory committals. There were fluid transitions between "coercion" and "voluntariness," suggesting a continuum rather than a clear dichotomy.

With respect to both questions, I deliberately refrain from commenting on the extent to which, following Foucault, even formally "voluntary" admissions can be traced back to internalized coercion. Foucault's claim is that the "insane" internalize the "surveilling gaze" and thus exercise self-censorship and self-control.[208] This might apply, for example, to people who remained "voluntarily" in the asylum for fear of harming themselves or others due to visual, auditory, or haptic hallucinations. This cannot, however, be proven definitively on the basis of sources. Such an interpretation would also run the risk of trivializing the anguish that may precede a stay in an asylum on the part of the patient. I argue that the circumstances of committal, which could be associated with extreme suffering for the individual, cannot be entirely resolved into socially induced internalized constraints. Whether and, if so, to what extent internalized coercion played a role in individual cases will not be my focus in what follows. However, we can productively contemplate the reasons given by patients who formally entered an asylum "voluntarily" and seek to assess whether and, if so, why these reasons changed according to historical era; whether the original impetus for an asylum stay was internalized coercion remains a moot point.

In the asylum records I reviewed, the reasons given did in fact change over time. During World War II, patients mostly mentioned existential fears—the example from Greifswald, in which the patient wanted to "talk things through," is not the rule, though not a complete exception either. Typical of committal to an asylum, as opposed to admission to a clinic, was the case of 23-year-old Herbert M. He came to Bethel in 1941 without a referral and was able to stay there. According to his medical history, as soon as he had a knife in his hand, he was haunted by the idea of killing himself or others; he had previously received outpatient treatment but had felt no better afterward.[209] His statements are reproduced in his medical record as follows:

It was [, he said,] a terrible state to be in. He had cried for days at home. [...] Above all, he wants to know if cardiazol therapy might help him. He [emphasizes that he] must finally be cured. Patient is friendly, polite, but extremely insistent and restless, and subjectively appears greatly tormented."[210]

The patient was given several leaves of absence from the asylum and was collected by his relatives, but returned before the end of the leave or did not take it at all because he felt a persistent fear of harming his relatives.[211] The tremendous psychological strain and the safety aspect were this patient's key concerns. Such cases occurred between 1941 and 1963 in all three systems. When it comes to the GDR, an analogous line of argument can be seen, for example, in the admission of a 62-year-old widow to Rodewisch. She had thrown her grandson out the window because she believed she had to sacrifice him. She herself had no wish to return home. Her medical file notes: "It is quiet here, [she states,] but if she goes home, she fears the problems will kick off again. Since the death of her husband, she has had frequent turns, during which she had to be restrained by five siblings."[212]

However, in the postwar period on both sides of the Iron Curtain, in addition to such scenarios, an increasing number of patients cited less drastic concerns. It was not uncommon for people to write to an asylum and request admission because they believed it could help them. During the war, this occurred mainly at Bethel and the Greifswald university psychiatric clinic; in the postwar period, it was a more widespread phenomenon. The patient Miranda L., for example, whom we have already encountered, is expected to benefit from committal to the LHA Marburg through the use of electroshock treatment.[213] Another example is documented in a 1953 letter by a former Bethel patient to the doctor who had treated him for melancholy (*Schwermut*) when he was first committed in 1947. A married farmer, now 60 years old, he was considering returning to the asylum. In his letter to the doctor, he explained that he had been unwell for three months and was contemplating whether his illness might be "something hereditary."[214] He had heard about hypnosis as a new method of treatment and asked:

> Dear Dr., could you perhaps try this on me? I would so much like to be free of this ailment and help my family with the work (which there is no lack of). My wife has said to me several times that I should apply for a disability pension; but if I go to the responsible health insurance doctor (*Kassenarzt*) here, he will likely find nothing wrong with me because I am physically healthy. Or could you, Dr., perhaps issue me a certificate? No one can understand this disease apart from those unfortunate enough to suffer from it themselves, and I wouldn't wish it on my worst enemy. May God help me battle my way through it! Dear Dr., you told me that if it got worse again, I could come and see you. If I don't get an answer to my letter, I might pay you a visit on October 7.[215]

Unlike the patients mentioned above, this was not a case of fears of harming a family member or oneself. Although a subjectively intense state of suffering is also front and center here, for the patient this evokes less dramatic concerns, such as worry over his inability to help out with the work that needs to be done.

Patients' self-perceptions were not necessarily congruent with the formal status of committal, a point illustrated by Miranda L.'s committal in the early 1950s. Although she entered the LHA "voluntarily," the states of agitation that were crucial to this move revolved in part around her reproaching her mother for having allowed her previous asylum stay. Rather than a "voluntary" act, on the occasion of her next admission the file notes that the patient signed the admission form only "after initial reluctance."[216] At the same time, on each occasion of admission her relatives insisted that caring for her at home would make it impossible to manage the farm. All three aspects indicate that the patient herself, at least temporarily, did not feel that she was in the asylum "voluntarily," though she had signed a declaration of voluntariness in each instance. In the case of a committal such as this, then, it makes little sense to seek to determine whether the person involved was in the institution on a subjectively "voluntary" or "coerced" basis. It seems more apposite to underline that the committed individuals themselves often moved within a persistent state of tension between voluntariness and coercion.

This is reinforced by the fact that there are cases in which the patient's feelings differed from those of Miranda L. Despite often not being involved in the negotiation process surrounding a compulsory committal, some of them had a positive view of their stay in the asylum. Given the shortage of space that persisted in all three states from 1941 to 1963, in fact, physicians sometimes facilitated an admission desired by the patient by initiating a compulsory committal with reference to the supposedly acute risk faced by the individual or their milieu.[217] In addition, self-perceptions could change: patients brought to the asylum by force sometimes remained there voluntarily. Just how ambivalent compulsory committals could be for the patient, even during the war, is apparent in the 1943 case of Walther M.[218] In view of noisy quarrels with his wife, he was admitted—and not for the first time—to the LHA Marburg as a danger to the public. At least in retrospect, however, the patient in no way perceived this compulsory committal as a problem: according to his medical history, during his stay he was glad to be receiving treatment. He stated that he was in urgent need of prolonged rest, which is why he referred to the LHA as a "convalescent home for the nerves."[219] When he was discharged after about six months, the same length of stay as in his previous committals, he even expressed thanks for the successful treatment, according to his file.[220] This can be explained in part by the fact that the patient and his family knew the asylum and individual doctors well due to his frequent stays. Walter M. was compulsorily committed to the LHA Marburg a total of nine times between 1927 and 1945; between these stays, his wife corresponded with the asylum to solicit advice.[221]

The attitude of the individuals concerned also depended on how the committed were treated in a given institution and thus on its physicians. Hence, there is no evidence of cases comparable to that of Walther M. in Marburg at Eglfing-Haar between 1941 and 1951. His case should not, therefore, be viewed as exemplary of patients' perception of compulsory committals but as illustrative of the broad spectrum of responses. Yet however diverse patients' motives and expectations could be, their reasoning was partly bound up with the political and social context. In the following chapters, I explore this more systematically by examining separately the complexes of security, illness, and work.

Summary: framework conditions, actors, and the role of the asylum in comparative perspective

All three systems featured room for maneuver, which expanded and contracted significantly in line with political and institutional circumstances. When it came to civil committals, the decision to commit never rested solely with institutional actors. The practice of committal during World War II, in the GDR, and in the FRG can in fact be summarized in the light of three comparative parameters. First, the specific situation of psychiatric asylums as admitting institutions; second, the stages of the committal process and, in connection with this, actors and their room for maneuver; and third, the function or role of the asylum.

The admission situation between 1941 and 1945 was war-specific in multiple ways: due to knowledge of the murder of the sick, propaganda films on "euthanasia," plus the relocating and repurposing of parts of the asylums in the course of the Brandt Campaign. Nevertheless, the asylums remained functional, while in the immediate postwar period they often operated only in rudimentary fashion. Certain tasks, such as expert evaluations, ceased almost entirely during this period, while the documentation of committals also deteriorated significantly compared to the wartime period. This was a result both of material shortages and the admission of many displaced persons and elderly people about whom no one was able to provide information. Meanwhile, during the war and in the immediate postwar period, a particularly large number of people who had not previously lived at home were admitted. They came from hospitals, both civilian and military, forced labor camps, old people's homes, nursing homes, and refugee camps. Into the 1950s, the admission situation remained particularly strained in East Germany. To be sure, overcrowding in university psychiatric clinics was an issue in the FRG as well, influencing committal pathways as, for example, these institutions ceased to function as intermediate facilities. In the GDR, however, the problem was more deeply rooted in structures and more severe. The use of parts of asylums by third parties contributed to this, but in Rostock district especially the key problem was the lack of relevant establishments. The systemic underfunding of the specialist psychiatric and neurological hospitals due to their transfer to district authority control in 1952 played a role as well.

Certain stages of the committal pathway were consistently relevant, with hospitals and independent physicians playing a significant role in all three political systems. While hospitals remained important everywhere, the relevance of independent physicians within the committal process changed depending on a number of factors. Doctors of this type played a markedly greater role in the FRG—above all at the private establishment of Bethel—than during the war or in the GDR. In the latter, state-employed physicians in the polyclinics, as well as the directors of the asylums and their in-house medical boards, more frequently decided on admissions. The polyclinics also altered the relationship between doctors and patients, with the realities of outpatient treatment and consultation often strengthening laypersons' hand. During the war period, by way of contrast, families' sense of trust eroded due to knowledge of the murder of the sick and the poorer medical care on the "home front." As a result, more referrals were made via the university psychiatric clinics during this period.

The patient's position was frequently bound up with the attitudes and conduct of their relatives. For the wartime period, I have shown that the latter sometimes tried to place family members in institutions they considered safer. It has also become clear, however, that at times certain family constellations eclipsed such considerations and led to rapid committal to the next available asylum. The main reason for this was violence within the family—regardless of the sociopolitical system involved. In addition, one of the cases we have considered has already hinted at a phenomenon that I will be fleshing out in the next chapter: while they often tried to help patients, relatives sometimes used their room for maneuver to initiate compulsory committals or at least tolerated such committals.

The patient acted within a field of tension between voluntariness and coercion that was far more complex than suggested by the distinction between civil and compulsory committals. In any case, it is evident that the reasons patients stated for their committal changed in the postwar period—regardless of whether they perceived their admission as voluntary or imposed. Whereas in the wartime period most patients articulated existential questions and anxieties, such as the fear of committing suicide or killing other people, in the postwar period in both East and West additional rationales came into play, such as the hope of treatment or regaining the ability to work.

This shift in emphasis from security issues to aspects of medical treatment took place on several levels. In the first few postwar years, psychiatric establishments responded almost exclusively to the practical functional requirements of a society in a state of collapse (*Zusammenbruchgesellschaft*) and, in a relatively unregulated way, admitted people who, under these specific circumstances, were disruptive or could not be cared for anywhere else. The pragmatic use of these facilities—already prevalent during the war—now became even more pronounced. In the 1950s, this pragmatic approach continued to play a role in both East and West, but there were concurrent debates on the orientation and function of psychiatric clinics and asylums in society, debates that were linked with their financing. In the GDR, the main issue was the contrast between treatment and long-term residential placement; in the FRG, the discussion presupposed a dichotomy between illness and security. This was linked with the fact that compulsory committals in East Germany often took place below the threshold of state regulations, so that there was little inducement to problematize the relationship between security and treatment. The political sphere, however, did contemplate new regulations on compulsory committal, as analyzed by Sabine Hanrath. But since no new legal regulations came into force until 1968 and the regulatory vacuum was filled by the circumvention of official compulsory committals, the questions of such relevance in West Germany did not arise.

Notes

1 LHA Marburg, Patient file sign. 16K10740F, Entry, March 15, 1946, LWV Hesse, 16.
2 In the following, the term "displaced persons" is used, though it was not necessarily the phrase used at the time. The choice of term does not imply a value judgment.
3 The statistics in the annual reports incorporate all admissions in a given year and thus provide a valuable supplement to the sample compiled for this book. They list both patients' last abode and the institutional route of admission. However, the last long-term abode, which was recorded for the present study, is not indicated. In addition, the categories are sometimes problematic because some of them were changed several times between 1941 and 1949, and a number of the relevant places of admission were not listed individually. For example, old-age homes are listed separately only for 1946. See HPA Eglfing-Haar, Annual Report 1941, Table: Movement of Patients, AB Upper Bavaria, EH; HPA Eglfing-Haar,

Annual Report 1942, Table: Movement of Patients, AB Upper Bavaria, EH; HPA Eglfing-Haar, Annual Report 1943, Table: Movement of Patients, AB Upper Bavaria, EH; HPA Eglfing-Haar, Annual Report 1944/45, Table: Movement of Patients, AB Upper Bavaria, EH; HPA Eglfing-Haar, Annual Report 1946, Table: Movement of Patients, AB Upper Bavaria, EH; HPA Eglfing-Haar, Annual Report 1947, Table: Movement of Patients, AB Upper Bavaria, EH; HPA Eglfing-Haar, Annual Report 1948, Table: Movement of Patients, AB Upper Bavaria, EH; HPA Eglfing-Haar, Annual Report 1949, Table: Movement of Patients, AB Upper Bavaria, EH.

4 The variable archiving and corresponding selection of files do not permit sociologically precise statements. See also my remarks in the introduction to the present book.

5 On the use of psychiatric facilities as special hospitals in the Todt and Brandt campaigns, see Süß, *Volkskörper*, 284 and 330ff. See the same text on transfers within the Reich after the T4 Campaign. Specifically on the Marburg asylum, which is examined in the present study, see Müller, Roland, "Militärpsychiatrie im Zweiten Weltkrieg. Die Reservelazarette III und IV in der Landesheilanstalt," in Peter Sandner et al. (eds.), *Heilbar und nützlich. Ziele und Wege der Psychiatrie in Marburg an der Lahn* (Marburg 2001), 305–314.

6 For a summary of knowledge about the murder of the sick, see for example Brink, *Psychiatrie*, 327ff.

7 Benzenhöfer and Eckart, *Medizin*; Klee, *Euthanasie*; Roth, "Entstehungsgeschichte."

8 Appendix: Statistical Analysis of the Committal Pathway: T2 and T7.

9 Appendix: Statistical Analysis of the Committal Pathway: T32.

10 For exact figures on "Permanent Abode prior to Committal" for all the asylums and clinics studied in this book, see Appendix: Statistical Analysis of the Committal Pathway, T1–5 for the wartime period and T16–20, T31–34, and T43–46 for the postwar period.

11 See Frevert, Ute, *Does Trust have a History? Max Weber Lecture No. 2009/01*, URL: http://cadmus.eui.eu/bitstream/handle/1814/11258/MWP_LS_2009_01. pdf;jsessionid=43C3D99861F422AC1B3ED3BF0897FE25?sequence=1 (retrieved 2.7.2014) 2; specifically on trust in experts and institutions, see Frevert, Ute, "Vertrauen—eine historische Spurensuche," in Ute Frevert (ed.), *Vertrauen—Historische Annäherungen* (Göttingen 2003), 7–66.

12 PsychN Greifswald, Patient file prov. sign. 1941/26/874, UA Greifswald, PsychN.

13 As briefly outlined in the introduction, multiple sclerosis is a disease that can lead to neurological dysfunctions of all kinds due to inflammation of the brain and spinal cord. See Murray, *Multiple Sclerosis*, 2.

14 PsychN Greifswald, Patient file prov. sign. 1941/26/874, Letter from Dr. K. to PsychN Greifswald, January 23, 1942, UA Greifswald, PsychN.

15 Since the age of majority was twenty-one, the decision was up to the patient's parents.

16 Ibid.

17 Roth, "Entstehungsgeschichte," 97.

18 PsychN Greifswald, Patient file prov. sign. 1941/26/874, Letter from Dr. Kohnert to PsychN Greifswald, July 29, 1942, UA Greifswald, PsychN.

19 See Appendix: Statistical Analysis of the Committal Pathway: T1 and T6.

20 See Appendix: Statistical Analysis of the Committal Pathway: T2–T5.

21 27.5 percent in the LHA, 17.9 percent in EH and 33 percent in Untergöltzsch. At Bethel, as a private institution, more people entered from their family environment: 46 percent were admitted directly from that context and 69 percent also lived at home. See Appendix: Statistical Analysis of the Committal Pathway: T6–T10.

22 It is true that generally more people checked in voluntarily to a university clinic than to an asylum, since from the patients' and their social environment's point of view it was more easily accessible and a stay there was considered less stigmatizing. In addition, a stay at a university hospital's psychiatric clinic was usually of shorter duration. See Engstrom, *Psychiatry*, 191.

23 Between 1956 and 1963, the difference between Greifswald (88 percent) on the one hand and Marburg (74 percent) and Großschweidnitz (74 percent) on the other was only about 15 percent (in contrast to about 30 percent during the war). All relevant figures for the postwar period can be found in Appendix: Statistical Analysis of the Committal Pathway: T16–20, T31–34, and T43–46.

24 Between 1956 and 1963, of those committed to the LHA Marburg, about 74 percent had previously lived at home. For all clinics and asylums between 1941 and 1963, see the tables listed in the previous endnote.

25 This is especially true of facilities that were intended for longer stays, and thus to a lesser extent of Greifswald and the LHA Marburg. In Untergöltzsch/Rodewisch, for example, about 18 percent of patients were committed via a doctor's office during the war, and about 28 percent from 1950 to 1955. For all figures on committal by physicians in private practice, see Appendix: Statistical Analysis of the Committal Pathway: T11–14, T26–30, T39–42, and T51–54.

26 Winfried Süß speculates that the low level of implementation of Nazi ideology by family doctors was due to a special relationship of trust between them and their patients. Süß, *Volkskörper*, 373.

27 Roelcke, "Etablierung," 119; for a summary, see also my remarks in Chapter 2.

28 By 1944, only half as many doctors were available to the civilian population as previously: Süß, *Volkskörper*, 372.

29 Ibid., 261ff.

30 Süß considers the implementation of company-based health care a development of no less import than the hereditary-biological turn at the start of Nazi rule: ibid., 263.

31 However, this is not an unambiguous indicator. People who lived permanently at home could of course also be committed by the police without the involvement of their social milieu. However, the vast majority of people living at home were committed either by a physician in private practice or via the Health Office. In both cases, their social environment was almost always involved.

32 Klee, *Euthanasie*, 204.

33 Ibid., 205 f. The ambivalent attitude of the Bodelschwingh Asylums to the Nazi regime also manifested itself in relation to the postwar legal response to its crimes. For example, the Bethel directors composed an appeal for clemency for Karl Brandt, who was sentenced to death at Nuremberg. See Aly, *Belasteten*, 290.

34 See Christians, *Amtsgewalt*. Overall, there is a lack of research on private asylums and their possible involvement in the decentralized murder of the sick.

35 See Appendix: Statistical Analysis of the Committal Pathway: T10 and T15.

36 See Appendix: Statistical Analysis of the Committal Pathway: T20 and T24; on the further increase in committals from the home environment in the 1950s and early 1960s, see ibid., T34, T38, T46, and T50.

37 In all other asylums, these figures consistently diverge by about 20 percentage points.

38 Aly, *Belasteten*, 284.

39 Governor of the Province of Westphalia, Letter to RMI, March 5, 1942, StAM, District Administrative Office Munich/59141.

40 The Reich Commissioner for Sanatorium-Nursing Homes, Decree, December 22, 1941, StAM, District Administrative Office Munich/59141.

41 Reich Commissioner for Sanatorium-Nursing Homes, Letter to the Governor of the Province of Westphalia, May 20, 1942, StAM, District Administrative Office Munich/59141.
42 See Appendix: Statistical Analysis of the Committal Pathway: T15, T30, T42, and T54.
43 vBS Bethel, Patient file sign. 34/485, Letter from Mrs. N. to Pastor Bodelschwingh, March 5, 1942, HAB, Patient files Mahanaim 1.
44 vBS Bethel, Patient file sign. 133/1918, Letter, June 5, 1944, HAB, Patient files Morija I.
45 Ibid., Letter to Pastor Wörmann, September 2, 1944.
46 Ibid., Letter from Senior Medical Officer (*Obermedizinalrat*), Dr. W., October 26, 1944.
47 Ibid., vBS Bethel letter of reply, November 25, 1944.
48 Ibid., Statement by wife, April 25, 1944 in Leipzig-Dösen.
49 HPA Eglfing-Haar, Patient file sign. EH 486, Letter from Municipal Health Office, November 29, 1941, AB Upper Bavaria, EH.
50 Ibid.
51 Ibid., under "Statement by neighbor."
52 Christians, *Amtsgewalt*.
53 Gründler, *Armut und Wahnsinn*, 119.
54 See for example HPA Eglfing-Haar, Patient file sign. EH 10389, AB Upper Bavaria, EH.
55 HPA Eglfing-Haar, Patient file sign. EH 778, Entry, March 7, 1944, AB Upper Bavaria, EH.
56 Ibid., Entry, February 29, 1944 in the medical record of the Psychiatric Clinic of Munich University Hospital.
57 Ibid.
58 Ibid.
59 Ibid., Letter from son, March 5, 1944, to Eglfing-Haar Sanatorium-Nursing Home.
60 Ibid., Entry, May 6, 1944.
61 Aly, *Belasteten*, 259ff.
62 Ibid., 263.
63 The tacit, self-evident acceptance of exclusion is described in a similar way by Ulrich Herbert with reference to Germans' treatment of forced laborers. Herbert, Ulrich, *Fremdarbeiter. Politik und Praxis des "Ausländer-Einsatzes" in der Kriegswirtschaft des "Dritten Reiches"* (Berlin 1985), 358.
64 Brink, *Psychiatrie*, 361.
65 They reached their peak in 1946. For more detail, see Faulstich, *Hungersterben*, 671ff.
66 In the British occupation zone, patients of sanatorium-nursing homes received less food than the physically ill. This was also the case during the Nazi era. In the Soviet occupation zone, physically and mentally ill people were treated equally, but both were placed in the lowest food ration category because they did not work. Hanrath, *Euthanasie und Psychiatriereform*, 53 and 164.
67 Brink, *Psychiatrie*, 362.
68 On the enduringly precarious situation in the asylums of Brandenburg, see Rose, *Anstaltspsychiatrie*.
69 Hanrath, *Euthanasie und Psychiatriereform*, 161.
70 See Appendix: Statistical Analysis of the Committal Pathway: T27, T28 and T29.
71 Ibid., T26.
72 Ibid., T3 and T18
73 Ibid., T8 and T23.

74 Ibid., T17.
75 In line with this, the number of people referred by a medical practice at Marburg was also very high during the occupation, at 41.5 percent, about twice as high as during the war. Ibid., T14 and T29.
76 Soldiers 5 percent and prisoners of war/forced laborers 6 percent. Ibid., T4.
77 It is known that the average age and mortality in the first three postwar years were higher than during the war and that this was related to the refugee flows. Many old people were left behind at various points along the way and became patients of sanatorium-nursing homes. For a summary, see Hanrath, *Euthanasie und Psychiatriereform*, 162; for more detail on many asylums, including those discussed in the present book, see Faulstich, *Hungersterben*; on the establishments studied here, see also the annual reports of Eglfing-Haar: admission figures by age were recorded in its annual reports, divided into four groups: 16–30, 31–45, 46–60, and over 60 years of age. Between 1946 and 1949, the over-60 category was the second largest, and between 1941 and 1945 the third largest. In the 1950s, people over 60 made up the third- or fourth-largest group. See HPA Eglfing-Haar, Annual Report 1941, Table: Movement of Patients, AB Upper Bavaria, EH; HPA Eglfing-Haar, Annual Report 1942, Table: Movement of Patients, AB Upper Bavaria, EH; HPA Eglfing-Haar, Annual Report 1943, Table: Movement of Patients, AB Upper Bavaria, EH; HPA Eglfing-Haar, Annual Report 1944/45, Table: Movement of Patients, AB Upper Bavaria, EH; HPA Eglfing-Haar, Annual Report 1946, Table: Movement of Patients, AB Upper Bavaria, EH; HPA Eglfing-Haar, Annual Report 1947, Table: Movement of Patients, AB Upper Bavaria, EH; HPA Eglfing-Haar, Annual Report 1948, Table: Movement of Patients, AB Upper Bavaria, EH; HPA Eglfing-Haar, Annual Report 1949, Table: Movement of Patients, AB Upper Bavaria, EH.
78 Both groups had specific "institutional careers." Elderly people often died quickly in the poorly supplied asylums. Displaced persons usually stayed for a long time. This was partly due to the fact that individuals without families generally spent longer periods in asylums: the ground was laid for discharges by checking whether the patient had someone to go to. In most cases, the person to be released was first given a probationary "leave of absence" to stay with relatives. Since many displaced persons became asylum patients because they had no relatives to look after them, the latter were also absent as a source of help to prepare for their discharge.
79 PsychN Greifswald, Patient file prov. sign. 1949/1106, UA Greifswald, PsychN. The reason for the committal was that Anna M. no longer left her bed. Since she no longer used the toilet, urine eventually dripped into the landlady's rooms below, prompting the latter to arrange for her committal.
80 In the postwar period, the number of persons living permanently at home before committal decreased in Untergöltzsch, while it remained about the same in Eglfing-Haar and increased in the other asylums. This was probably due to Rodewisch's location in the region bordering the later Czechoslovak Republic. A large number of people about whom little was known were admitted there. Judging by their last abode and the statements in the medical records, many of them were displaced persons. The same phenomenon can also be observed at the Psychiatric Clinic of Greifswald University Hospital, which was located near the border with the Polish People's Republic. These asylums and clinics near borders were stretched so thin in the early occupation period due to the large number of displaced persons that there was simply less room for patients who could be accommodated elsewhere. Of course, there were also refugees in Eglfing-Haar and in Marburg, but not on the same scale. On the problems faced by institutions in the border regions, see Rose, *Anstaltspsychiatrie*, 29ff.

81 The District President of Kassel, Department of Public Health, Letter to the district's public health officers, March 9, 1948, Re: Use of hospital beds for other purposes, StA Marburg, 401.15/83.

82 Commissioner for the Furth im Wald Border Crossing Point, Reports on the committal of displaced persons in West German territory and the Land of Hesse, 1950–1951, StA Marburg, 401.17/219.

83 This fits into a picture of displaced persons themselves feeling uncomfortable in their "new home" and receiving no warm welcome. The medical records reflect conditions with which researchers are already familiar, but they add no new details and open up no new perspectives. On the integration of displaced persons in East and West, see for example Kossert, Andreas, *Kalte Heimat. Die Geschichte der deutschen Vertriebenen nach 1945* (Bonn 2008); Schwartz and Goschler, "Kriegs- und Diktaturfolgen," 600ff.

84 PsychN Greifswald, Patient file prov. sign. 1951/1332, Entry, November 8, 1951, UA Greifswald, PsychN.

85 Ibid.

86 LHA Marburg, Patient file sign. 16K10740F, Entry, March 15, 1946, LWV Hesse, 16.

87 Ibid.

88 PsychN Greifswald, Patient file prov. sign. 1951/1332, Entry, November 8, 1951, UA Greifswald, PsychN.

89 LHA Marburg, Patient file sign. 16K12161F, Entry, July 4, 1951, LWV Hesse, 16.

90 Ibid.

91 KA Rodewisch, Patient file sign. 7523, Letter from the Reichenbach Municipal Health Office, January 9, 1948, SächSta, 32810.

92 Ibid.

93 Ibid., Letter from Head Physician KA Rodewisch to Reichenbach Municipal Health Office, March 10, 1948.

94 As described earlier, the ground was usually laid for discharge with the help of relatives.

95 Brink, *Psychiatrie*, 208ff.

96 Rose, *Anstaltspsychiatrie*, 64.

97 Ibid.

98 Ibid., 65.

99 Ibid., 66 f.

100 KA Großschweidnitz, Letter to MfG, Department of Health Protection Organization, Sector General Health Protection, Dr. Lammert, July 5, 1962, BAB, DQ1/21600.

101 Ibid., see Rodewisch Special Hospital to Ministry of Health, Department of Health Protection Organization, Dr. Lammert, July 4, 1962.

102 On the large number of fugitive physicians and the unsuccessful attempts to reduce it, see Ernst, *Sozialismus*, 87.

103 Department of Health, Report: "On the Situation with respect to the Care of Psychiatric and Neurological Patients" [n. d., 1957], LA Greifswald, 200 9.1/14.

104 Rostock District Council, Department of Health, Report on the Work of the Department of Health 1953–54, LA Greifswald, 200 9.1./56.

105 While it should of course be borne in mind that the population density in Saxony was higher than in Western Pomerania, the evidence shows a clear difference in basic psychiatric care. According to the homepage of the Federal Statistical Office, in 1950 about three times as many people lived in Saxony as in Mecklenburg-Western Pomerania. https://www.destatis.de/DE/Publikationen/Thematisch/Bevoelkerung/Bevoelkerungsstand/

Bevoelkerungsfortschreibung2010130107004.pdf?__blob=publicationFile (retrieved May 2, 2014).

106 District Assembly and Council of the District of Rostock, Department of Health, Letter to the Central Commission for State Oversight, Commissioner for Rostock District, June 7, 1957, Re. Placement of the mentally ill, LA Greifswald, 200 9.1/14.

107 See Appendix: Further Statistical Analyses: T55.

108 Hermann Nobbe: "Über eine Erweiterung der Aufgaben der Landesheilanstalten," *Psychiatrie, Neurologie und medizinische Psychologie. Zeitschrift für Forschung und Praxis*, 1951, vol. 3, no. 1, 25–28, 25 f.

109 Ibid., 26.

110 Ibid.

111 District Assembly and Council of the District of Rostock, Department of Health, Letter to the Central Commission for State Oversight, Commissioner for Rostock District, June 7, 1957, Re. Placement of the mentally ill, LA Greifswald, 200 9.1/14.

112 PsychN Greifswald, Patient file prov. sign. 1956/290, Letter, May 23, 1950, UA Greifswald, PsychN.

113 District Assembly and Council of the District of Rostock, Department of Health, Letter to the Central Commission for State Oversight, Commissioner for Rostock District, June 7, 1957, Re. Placement of the mentally ill, LA Greifswald, 200 9.1/14.

114 In addition, the document primarily dealt with the internal reorganization of the asylums. In this regard, Sabine Hanrath summarizes that—much as in the FRG—the inner realm of the asylum was to be more differentiated, that is, a distinction was to be made between curable and incurable, calm and restless, and capable and incapable of work. See Hanrath, *Euthanasie und Psychiatriereform*, 351 f.

115 There was a similar solution for people committed by the police at Eglfing-Haar during the Nazi era. The asylum granted "leave of absence" to such patients so they could be placed in "suitable families" outside the institution. Rather than a clever circumvention of the rules, this was officially possible thanks to an amendment to Article 80 II of the PStG, which regulated police committals in Bavaria. Government of Upper Bavaria, Letter to the district police authorities, June 18, 1933, StA Munich, 116848.

116 1946–49: 7.4 percent assessment of incapacity for work, 4.3 percent assessment of unsoundness of mind; 1950–55: 21.5 percent assessment of capacity for work, one individual assessed for need for care and one for unsoundness of mind. See ibid., T26, T39, and T51. 1956–63: 17.8 percent assessment of capacity for work, 7.8 percent assessment of unsoundness of mind: T51.

117 Fulbrook, *Leben*, 113.

118 Hockerts, "Einführung," 15.

119 At the same time, the pension system, with its ultimately seventeen additional systems, pointed up the limits to equality in the GDR; ibid., 17.

120 Schagen and Schleiermacher, *Gesundheitswesen*, 411. The enterprise-based health system resulted in greater supervision of the sick. Sick leave lasting more than ten days could only be authorized by a so-called advising physician (*Beratungsarzt*), and disputed cases had to be brought before a medical commission. In 1953, the advising physician system was abolished and subsequently the decision was always made by a medical advisory committee (*Ärzteberatungskommission*). See Ernst, *Sozialismus*, 96.

121 There were, for example, health workers in the enterprise and it was not unusual for its members to visit the sick and bring them food and drink. See Hübner,

Peter, "Betriebe als Träger der Sozialpolitik, betriebliche Sozialpolitik," in *1949–1961 Deutsche Demokratische Republik. Im Zeichen des Aufbaus des Sozialismus* (*Geschichte der Sozialpolitik in Deutschland seit 1945*, vol. 8, Berlin 2004), 770.

122 This provides confirmation of the work-centered character of the GDR *Versorgungsstaat* or "all-providing state," a trait whose presence researchers have mostly identified in light of the inadequate financial benefits for those not in employment—from pensioners to single-parent widows. See for example Conrad, "Alterssicherung," 114; Hoffmann, Dierk, "Sicherung bei Alter, Invalidität und für Hinterbliebene, Sonderversorgungssysteme," in *1949–1961 Deutsche Demokratische Republik. Im Zeichen des Aufbaus des Sozialismus* (*Geschichte der Sozialpolitik in Deutschland seit 1945*, vol. 8, Berlin 2004), 347–387.

123 Boldorf, Marcel, "Rehabilitation und Hilfen für Behinderte," in *1949–1961 Deutsche Demokratische Republik. Im Zeichen des Aufbaus des Sozialismus* (*Geschichte der Sozialpolitik in Deutschland seit 1945*, vol. 8, Berlin 2004), 467.

124 Hockerts, "Einführung," 10.

125 One such demand now fulfilled in the GDR was the establishment of a discrete Ministry of Health for the first time. However, this should not obscure the fact that health policy in the early GDR, just as in the FRG, was not an especially high priority. Other ideas originating in the imperial era were blanket insurance (*Einheitsversicherung*) and the orientation of the health care system toward social hygiene. Unlike in the FRG, in the 1950s all citizens in the GDR were fully covered in the event of illness. See Schagen and Schleiermacher, *Gesundheitswesen*, 401ff.

126 KA Großschweidnitz, Patient file sign. 2726, HSta Dresden, 10822.

127 Propaphenin was used in so-called healing sleep therapy (*Heilschlaftherapie*) to treat "mania" (*erregte Psychose*). On production problems in the GDR and the great importance attributed to the drug, see Klöppel, Ulrike, "1954. Brigade Propaphenin arbeitet an der Ablösung des Megaphen. Der prekäre Beginn der Psychopharmakaproduktion der DDR," in Nicholas Eschenbuch et al. (eds.), *Arzneimittel des 20. Jahrhunderts. Historische Skizzen von Lebertran bis Contergan* (Bielefeld 2009), 199–223.

128 KA Großschweidnitz, Patient file sign. 2726, Letter from Zittau Polyclinic, April 7, 1956, HSta Dresden, 10822.

129 See for example Kaufmann, Doris, "Nervenschwäche, Neurasthenie und 'sexuelle Frage' im deutschen Kaiserreich," in Christine Wolters et al. (eds.), *Abweichung und Normalität. Psychiatrie in Deutschland vom Kaiserreich bis zur Deutschen Einheit* (Bielefeld 2013), 197–199. On gender-specific diagnoses in this context, see my remarks on medical and lay diagnoses in the chapter "Illness and Diagnosis" in the present book.

130 On the introduction of psychotropic drugs in the FRG, see Balz, Viola, *Zwischen Wirkung und Erfahrung—eine Geschichte der Psychopharmaka. Neuroleptika in der Bundesrepublik Deutschland, 1950–1980* (Bielefeld 2010).

131 See Klöppel, "Brigade Propaphenin"; the patient files of Rodewisch and Großschweidnitz provide evidence of this: relatives often offered to obtain psychotropic drugs for patients from the West. See the section "Knowledge circulation between East and West" in the chapter "Illness and Diagnosis."

132 HPA Eglfing-Haar, Annual Report 1959, AB Upper Bavaria, EH, 6.

133 In contrast to the Weimar Republic, the health insurance schemes were no longer responsible for running the polyclinics; this task was entrusted to the local authorities. The restructuring of the health care system had already taken place to a large extent before the founding of the state. Thus, many polyclinics had already been established in the 1940s. Ernst, *Sozialismus*, 25 and 30.

134 Ibid., 33.
135 Physicians in private practice, rural outpatient clinics, and polyclinics that were not affiliated with asylums or hospitals were not recorded separately in the statistics because physicians could not always be clearly assigned to a particular institution.
136 See for example PsychN Greifswald, Patient file prov. sign. 1951/1196, UA Greifswald, PsychN.
137 On the early FRG, see Lindner, *Gesundheitspolitik*, 91.
138 Ibid., 30.
139 Accordingly, we find virtually no referrals to asylums in the records of the Psychiatric Clinic of Greifswald University Hospital. It should, however, be noted that there were very few establishments in Rostock District to which they might have been referred. See Appendix: Statistical Analysis of the Committal Pathway: T12, T27, T40, and T52.
140 KA Großschweidnitz, Patient file sign. 2726, HSta Dresden, 10822.
141 This was a regular occurrence in cases of committal to Rodewisch and Großschweidnitz. In Großschweidnitz, admissions were systematically noted by the in-house panel of medical specialists and could therefore be recorded statistically. They accounted for approximately 10 percent of admissions. See Appendix: Statistical Analysis of the Committal Pathway: T51.
142 In the case of committals of individuals who were admitted to the same institution on multiple occasions, in the FRG, too, patients were sometimes committed directly by the asylum. However, this was not due to West German committal structures, but to the fact that relatives and patients sometimes bypassed these structures if they were familiar with the establishment and its doctors.
143 The 1968 law did not limit the power of doctors to the same degree as in the FRG. The courts were involved only in the case of placements of more than six weeks' duration. Hanrath, *Euthanasie und Psychiatriereform*, 366 f.
144 KA Großschweidnitz, Patient file sign. 2577, Entry, November 14, 1958, HSta Dresden, 10822.
145 Ibid.
146 Ibid.
147 Ibid., Entry, December 4, 1958.
148 KA Großschweidnitz, Patient file sign. 3854, Certificate of committal, May 28, 1958, HSta Dresden, 10822.
149 Faulstich, *Hungersterben*, 686ff; for details on the postwar situation in North Rhine-Westphalia, see Hanrath, *Euthanasie und Psychiatriereform*, 50ff.
150 *Westfälische Zeitung*, July 2, 1949, "Für die Ärmsten der Armen," HAB, Sar 1–378.
151 Ibid.
152 In the newly founded federal Land of Hesse, the LHA Marburg formed part of the Land Welfare Association (*Landeswohlfahrtsverband*) based on the tradition of the Prussian provincial associations. Eglfing-Haar came under the district of Upper Bavaria.
153 Hockerts, "Entscheidungen," 37.
154 Hanrath, *Euthanasie und Psychiatriereform*, 249ff.
155 Ibid., 250.
156 On the Halving Decree, see Brink, *Grenzen*, 386. What the debate on the Halving Decree shows is that there was no consistent understanding of whether or in which cases it should or should not be applied, and on what grounds.
157 H. E. Schulz, Lohr am Main, Statement on the following issues: application of the Halving Decree, "mental illness as understood from a medical point of view" and "which regulation ought to be proposed to the health insurance funds," undated, November 1960, BayHSTA, Minn 80914.

158 Association of White-Collar Workers' Health Insurance Funds, Letter to the Ministries of Labor and Social Affairs, April 13, 1949, BayHSTA, Minn 80911.
159 Ibid.
160 See for example District Administration, Welfare Association (Landsratsamt Bezirksfürsorgeverband), Letter to the Government of Swabia, June 24, 1949, BayHSTA, Minn 80911.
161 Insurance Code or *Reichsversicherungsordnung.*
162 Günzburg District Administration, Welfare Association, Letter to the Government of Swabia, June 22, 1949, BayHSTA, Minn 80911 (original emphasis).
163 Association of White-Collar Workers' Health Insurance Funds, Letter to the Ministries of Labor and Social Affairs, April 13, 1949, BayHSTA, Minn 80911.
164 See for example Augsburg Municipal Administration, Letter to the Government of Swabia, June 15, 1949, BayHSTA, Minn 80911.
165 Bavarian Association of Administrative Districts, Letter to the Bavarian State Ministry of the Interior, July 27, 1949, BayHSTA, Minn 80911.
166 Bavarian State Ministry of Justice, Letter to the Bavarian State Ministry of the Interior, August 8, 1949, BayHSTA, Minn 80911.
167 Anton von Braunmühl had been an assistant physician (*Assistenzarzt*) at Eglfing-Haar since 1927, becoming director in 1946. He himself stated that he had refused to take part in the Nazi killing campaigns during World War II. On Eglfing-Haar during the war, see Siemen, Hans-Ludwig, "Die bayerischen Heil- und Pflegeanstalten während des Nationalsozialismus," in Michael von Cranach and Hans-Ludwig Siemen (eds.), *Psychiatrie im Nationalsozialismus. Die Bayerischen Heil- und Pflegeanstalten zwischen 1933 und 1945* (Munich 1999), 445.
168 HPA Eglfing-Haar, Letter to the Upper Bavarian District Welfare Association, February 14, 1953, 1, BayHSTA, Minn 80911.
169 Ibid., 2
170 Since the foundation of the first university psychiatric clinics, there had been frictions between asylum physicians and clinicians, which manifested themselves, among other things, in disputes over educational trajectories. See Engstrom, *Psychiatry*, 46 f.
171 HPA Eglfing-Haar, Letter to the Upper Bavarian District Welfare Association, February 14, 1953, 2, BayHSTA, Minn 80911.
172 Hanrath, *Euthanasie und Psychiatriereform*, 256. Psychiatrists made similar arguments in the debates of the late Weimar period. They argued against the discretionary powers granted to the police by the new regulations of 1932, rejecting the concept of "danger to the public" (*Gemeingefährlichkeit*) and seeking to establish illness as the basis for every kind of committal to an asylum. For more detail, see Brink, *Grenzen*, 260 f.
173 The reasoning of laypeople, as elaborated in the following sections, shows that committals can by no means be grasped solely in light of medical criteria. The problems and limits of a primarily medical interpretation of asylums are also highlighted in Meier et al., *Zwang zur Ordnung*, 34. While the cost discussion of the 1950s revolved around psychiatrists' attempts to expand their medical competence, however, *Zwang zur Ordnung* foregrounds society's ceding of competence and responsibility to medicine. "By favoring therapeutic-medical motives and simultaneously tabooing coercion to disciplinary ends, societal coercive mechanisms are delegated to medicine, thus transforming sociopolitical problems into what seem to be purely medical-diagnostic issues."
174 HPA Eglfing-Haar, Letter to District Welfare Association, February 14, 1953, BayHSTA, Minn 80911.
175 H.E. Schulz, Statement on the Halving Decree [n.d., late November 1960], BayHSTA, Minn 80914.

176 For a detailed treatment of psychiatrists' somatic orientation, see Chapter 4, "Disease and Diagnostics."

177 H.E. Schulz, Statement on the Halving Decree [n.d., late November 1960], BayHSTA, Minn 80914.

178 See esp. my remarks on diagnostic practice in Chapter 4, "Disease and Diagnostics."

179 The dangers of rushing to apply the so-called "interest model" to explain scientific change have rightly been underlined, as has the fact that is often impossible to convincingly demonstrate that interests, as factors not intrinsic to science, are *per se* more explanatory than the reasoning of physicians. See Schlich, "Fakten," 112 f.

180 This occurred particularly often at the LHA Marburg, as it was an asylum designed for short stays and there were therefore many instances of multiple committal.

181 LHA Marburg, Patient file sign. K12962F, Entry, December 1951, LWV Hesse, 16.

182 Ibid., Readmission, December 8, 1952.

183 Ibid., Readmission, April 7, 1954, fol. 1.

184 Ibid.

185 From 1950 to 1955, 21 percent of those admitted to Marburg were still committed via a university psychiatric clinic; from 1956 to 1963, the figure was about 12 percent. See Appendix: T41 and T53; HPA Eglfing-Haar, Annual Report 1959, AB Upper Bavaria, EH, 6.

186 Ibid.

187 HPA Eglfing-Haar, Letter to Upper Bavarian District Welfare Association, February 14, 1953, BayHSTA, Minn 80911 (original emphasis).

188 Statistics are not available for the LHA.

189 LHA Marburg, Patient file sign. 16K10919F, Entry, June 12, 1950, LWA Hesse, 16.

190 LHA Marburg, Patient file sign. 16K12972F, Entry, February 20, 1954, LWV Hesse, 16.

191 Ibid., Entry, February 22, 1954.

192 Engstrom, *Psychiatry*, 51 and 60 f.

193 HPA Eglfing-Haar, Letter to Upper Bavarian District Welfare Association, February 14, 1953, BayHSTA, Minn 80911.

194 On the origins of this competitive situation, see Engstrom, *Psychiatry*, 51.

195 See Chapter 3, "Danger and Security," section 1.2, "The elderly as a threat."

196 This was my original intention. Despite intensive efforts, however, the archive of Cologne University has not allowed access to the medical records of the university psychiatric clinic.

197 See Appendix: Statistical Analysis of the Committal Pathway: T42 and T54.

198 Ibid: T41 and T53.

199 Cf. ibid: T1–10, T16–25, and T43–50. On Bethel from 1956 to 1963, see ibid: T50.

200 Ibid: T54.

201 Ibid: T53.

202 Again, for more precise comparison with the provision of expert evaluations at the Greifswald university psychiatric clinic, the examination of files from the same kind of institution would have been informative.

203 On the decision of patients to seek medical treatment, see also Porter, Roy, "Introduction," in Porter, Roy (ed.), *Patients and Practitioners. Lay Perceptions of Medicine in Pre-Industrial Society* (Cambridge 1985), 1–22.

204 PsychN Greifswald, Patient file prov. sign. 1942/1149, Entry, August 7, 1942, UA Greifswald, PsychN.

205 Ibid.
206 See also Jureit, Ulrike, "Motive—Mentalitäten—Handlungsspielräume. Theoretische Anmerkungen zu Handlungsoptionen von Soldaten," in Christian Hartmann et al. (eds.), *Verbrechen der Wehrmacht. Bilanz einer Debatte* (Munich 2005), 165.
207 On the many possible definitions of coercion, see Meier et al., *Zwang zur Ordnung*, 31ff. The authors state: "There are pronounced areas of friction and partly irreconcilable contradictions between the different definitions. This ambiguity must be factored into a historical perspective." Ibid., 32.
208 Foucault, Michel, *Wahnsinn und Gesellschaft* (Frankfurt/M. 1969); Raffnsøe et al., *Foucault*, 102.
209 vBS Bethel, Patient file sign. 9/152, HAB, Patient files Morija I.
210 Ibid., patient's own statement on 1941 committal.
211 See for example ibid., Entries of April 1944.
212 KA Rodewisch, Patient file sign. 4772, Entry, September 15, 1953, SächSta Chemnitz, 32810. To explain cases like these solely with reference to the phenomenon of hospitalism is, in my opinion, short-sighted. First, patients are then denied all autonomy. Second, as in this case, committed patients often stated immediately after admission that they were glad to be in the asylum. Hospitalism, conversely, assumes that the fear of life outside the asylum is generated by the stay in it. On hospitalism, see Huppmann, "Milieuschäden."
213 LHA Marburg, Patient file sign. K12962F, Readmission December 8, 1952, LWV Hesse, 16.
214 vBS Bethel, Patient file sign. 4877, HAB, Gilead III.
215 Ibid., Letter, September 23, 1953.
216 See for example LHA Marburg, Patient file sign. K12962F, LWV Hesse, 16.
217 On this practice at the LHA Marburg, see Nolte, "Gefühl," 186. On this practice in the FRG as a whole, see Brink, *Grenzen*, 396.
218 LHA Marburg, Patient file sign. K10563M, LWV Hesse, 16.
219 Ibid., Admission 1943, fol. 1.
220 Ibid., Admission 1943, fol. 2.
221 In December 1948, for example, one of the senior physicians wrote to the patient's wife that she could indicate to the housing office that he considered it appropriate to allocate another dwelling to the family due to her husband's illness. Ibid., Admission 1945, Letter, December 15, 1948.

3 Danger and security

On the practice of compulsory committal

As we saw in the last chapter, irrespective of the type of committal, patients themselves often operated within the ambivalent field of tension at the interstices of voluntariness and coercion. In this context, we have also touched on the importance of security and danger in rationales for committal. Both concepts—security (or "safety") and danger (or "threat")—often played a key role in legitimizing committals. The actors involved either used these terms or fell back on a form of words that implied them: her family "could no longer bear responsibility for her,"[1] was how Martina R.'s mother-in-law quoted the words of the family doctor in the course of her committal in the spring of 1946. Her outburst of rage toward her own child mentioned by her mother-in-law served as a key piece of evidence here.[2] Martina R. herself did not deny this incident, but expressed a critical view of its consequences: "I admit all that, but none of it justifies putting me in a sanatorium-nursing home."[3] What behavior was viewed as unacceptable? At what point was someone considered dangerous? And who decided all this? Such assessments depended heavily on the social and political conditions of the war and postwar period. Two aspects, however, were common to all three socio-political systems and the occupation period. First, certain themes cropped up time and again: physical violence, sexuality, and the ability and willingness to work. Second, the assessments put forward by the actors involved diverged substantially. These gaps are evident between the affected person and their social environment, as in the case of Martina R., as well as between the doctors and other parties involved, such as neighbors and landlords.

Arguments featuring danger and security played a crucial role in the context of compulsory committals (I use this term and "forcible committals" interchangeably). These committals were undergirded by the rationale that there existed a "danger to the safety" (*Gefahr für die Sicherheit*) of the patient or the public. Alternatively, the terms "self-endangerment" (*Selbstgefährdung*) and "danger to others" (*Fremdgefährdung*) were used.

The term "compulsory committal" covers a spectrum of practices, all of which excluded consideration of the patient's wishes. We can distinguish two basic types. First, there were committals "on grounds of danger" (*auf Grund von Gefahr*) in accordance with the PVG of 1931 and the comparable Art. 80/II

DOI: 10.4324/9781032716237-4

of the Bavarian Police Penal Code and its later iterations. A person could be committed immediately on the grounds that they represented an acute danger. I scrutinize these compulsory committals in what follows. Second, there was the possibility of preventive detention (*Sicherungsverwahrung*).[4] Such forensic committals were imposed as a result of a crime if the offender was judged to be of unsound mind and was transferred from pretrial detention (*Untersuchungshaft*) to forensic psychiatric care. The justice system and psychiatric profession were both involved in the decision-making process in such cases. Preventive detention committals are not examined in this book for two reasons. First, they are not the result of a negotiation between institutional and noninstitutional actors, but between the judiciary and psychiatric professionals. They do not, therefore, tell us anything about the understanding of security within the societal microcosm, nor about the interaction between private and public spheres. Second, the sample taken for this study contains so few forensic committals that they do not allow us to make inferences about typical lines of reasoning or actor constellations. Furthermore, they were far less common than forcible committals executed according to the PVG of 1931 and its successor regulations. This will be briefly illustrated by looking at the figures in the annual reports of the three sanatorium-nursing homes of Eglfing-Haar, Rodewisch, and Großschweidnitz. At Eglfing-Haar, the yearbooks record both the number of forensic committals and of forcible police committals. Forensic committals to this asylum were always relatively few in number and in the postwar period, their share of both forcible committals and total annual committals declined further. In 1942, 522 police committals contrasted with 31 committals for preventive detention under § 42b of the RStGB (of the kind not examined here)—out of a total of 881 committals. A similar finding applies to the following year: in 1943, 601 committals were carried out by the police and 43 were forensic, out of a total admission figure of 1,427.[5] In 1956, Eglfing-Haar admitted 17 persons in accordance with Sec. 42b of the Criminal Code on Preventive Detention (StGB zur Sicherheitsverwahrung) and 541 on the basis of the Detaining Act (*Verwahrungsgesetz*), the successor regulation on police committal in the FRG.[6] The figures available for the same year on forensic committals to Rodewisch and Großschweidnitz are comparably low. At Rodewisch, 34 out of 348 patients were committed according to § 42b StGB, and 44 out of 782 at Großschweidnitz.[7] The legal basis for these committals was also § 42b StGB in the East German asylums, since the penal code of May 15, 1871 applied in all three German states. Comprehensive reforms did not take place until 1968 in East Germany and 1970 in the FRG.

The following analysis of compulsory committals refers primarily to the sanatorium-nursing homes of Eglfing-Haar in Munich, Untergöltzsch near Chemnitz, and Großschweidnitz near Görlitz. Unlike university psychiatric clinics (such as Greifswald), private asylums (such as Bethel), or Land-run asylums (such as the Marburg Land Sanatorium), these sanatorium-nursing homes were partly—though by no means only—geared toward compulsory committals.[8] At these institutions, the numbers of compulsory committals "on grounds of danger" (*auf Grund von Gefahr*) during the war outstripped those of the postwar period. At Eglfing-Haar, meanwhile, they were significantly higher than at Rodewisch, exceeding 40 percent. We thus find considerable regional differences. While 25 percent of wartime committals at Untergöltzsch were compulsory committals by the authorities, this applied only to about 10 percent of later committals.[9] In Munich, the number of compulsory committals decreased from 1947 onward, whereas no decrease can be observed after the war in 1945 or 1946. In 1946, 461 of 660 admissions were still carried out under Art. 80/II of the PStGB, but in 1949 this was true of only 48 of a total of 1,638 admissions.[10] However, with the introduction of judicial placement, which I discuss in detail in this chapter, the numbers rose again significantly. Following the introduction of the Bavarian Detaining Act in 1952, judicial committals accounted for about a quarter of all patients.[11]

"A threat to public safety"? Compulsory committals during World War II

The issue of security was of considerable importance to the National Socialist health care system in general and to the practice of committal in particular. The concept of security within health policy during the Nazi era was, however, Janus-faced. Families classified as "Aryan" were granted social security, while the sick were increasingly excluded from society. The police saw themselves as the "physician to the national body" (*Arzt am Volkskörper*) tasked with ensuring its survival and protecting it from "hereditarily sick" minorities.[12] Accordingly, in the psychiatric field, too, committals on grounds of security were prioritized. Patients not committed as a danger to the community were to be discharged if possible, while relatives' discharge requests were generally to be granted.[13]

At the same time, the police and the health offices carried out official compulsory committals in large numbers. These had two main characteristics during the war. First, forcible committals fell within the purview of the police. Normally, the police could only have an individual committed by obtaining a medical certificate, which was usually issued by the health offices.[14] However, in case of danger, committal was at the police officers' discretion. Second, this means that the decision-making power over compulsory committals did not lie with the asylum doctors and that the judiciary played no role at all in such committals—in contrast to compulsory forensic committals.[15]

A large number of compulsory committals were made to the two sanatorium-nursing homes of Eglfing-Haar and Untergöltzsch during the war.[16] Nevertheless, what was specific to the war was not necessarily their number, but rather the committal pathway, the constellation of actors involved, and the reasoning used to frame committals. The higher number during the war was bound up with the role of health offices and the police in forcible committals, a role that had already grown considerably before World War II. Since the period under investigation in this book begins in 1941, here I will touch only briefly on the case of Eglfing-Haar, which shows that a relatively large number of committals were already being undertaken by the authorities before the war began.

In a letter to the district president of Munich of September 1939, Eglfing-Haar's director stated that there were now almost no direct admissions.[17] Committals, he explained, now virtually always took place either via the psychiatric departments of the Munich hospitals or according to Art. 80/II of the Police Penal Code. Committals from the catchment area around Munich, he went on, were almost exclusively compulsory committals not involving a judicial decision. The large number of committals on security grounds at the beginning of the war suggests that the authorities were building on pre-war practice—forcible committals by police and health offices had already become prevalent.[18] However, in addition to the established emphasis on security that empowered the police and health offices, two new factors played a significant role in committals from 1941 to 1945: first, the changed situation brought about by the war and the Brandt Campaign, and, second, the war-specific reasoning articulated by members of patients' social milieu. Together, these three aspects helped ensure that committal-related rationales broke through their previous limitations and took on a more radical form. In addition, against the background of the Nazi murder of the sick, compulsory committals must be considered a particularly extreme form of exclusion.[19]

In what follows, I seek to illuminate which actors were involved in committals on the grounds of "danger to public safety" (*Gefahr für die öffentliche Sicherheit*) under wartime conditions and to what extent patients' families had any room for maneuver. This question is linked to the issue of who the forcibly committed patients were and what reasons were given for their committal. I shed light on three groups of patients in succession whose forcible committals had war-specific characteristics. First, soldiers. The focus here is on committals to the asylums within the "Reich" examined in this book, a limited perspective since I look neither at military hospitals nor asylums near the front. I then scrutinize committals of elderly individuals. This group occupied a social position completely different from that of soldiers. The elderly were a non-combatant and non-working segment of the population to whom no immediate "utility" was attributed.[20] Lastly, I turn to forcible committals of women, which lay in the field of tension between sexuality, capacity for work, and class affiliation. Women accounted for the vast majority of wartime compulsory committals by police and health offices—in marked contrast to the gender ratio of postwar forcible committals.

Soldier committals at the front and "home front"

One group of patients directly linked to the war and subject to strict committal regulations were soldiers.[21] War-injured servicemen played a role in committals on the "home front" in two senses. First, they were quartered in psychiatric facilities, as parts of the clinics and asylums were repurposed as special or military hospitals. This outside use of asylum premises as reserve hospitals for non-mentally ill patients affected all the institutions dealt with in this book, especially the Land Sanatorium in Marburg, which had already developed a focus on military psychiatry during World War I and expanded it from 1938 onward. The sanatorium eventually contained more beds for soldiers than civilians.[22]

Second, soldiers themselves formed a specific group of psychiatric patients, prompting the Wehrmacht and the asylums to enter into agreements regulating their committal.[23] These accords reflected the course of the war. Originally, the plan was to send soldiers to sanatorium-nursing homes in their respective military districts[24] but toward the end of the war, this ceased to be viable, and new agreements were made as the front moved across the map. A special agreement was concluded with Untergöltzsch, for example, as late as March 1945, which provided for the admission of soldiers who were supposed to be sent to sanatorium-nursing homes rendered out of bounds as the front drew nearer.[25]

The sample taken for the present book includes only soldiers suffering from brain injuries and those who were diagnosed in a field hospital with somatically induced psychoses, such as schizophrenia,[26] but no so-called *Kriegszitterer* of the kind familiar from World War I. It is difficult to assess how representative the sample is in this regard[27] but the findings appear consistent with the development of military psychiatry from World War I onward. As a "lesson" from World War I, in which numerous *Kriegszitterer* appeared for the first time, this branch of psychiatry had embraced the view that the best cure for mentally damaged soldiers was combat fire.[28] Ailments were always to be treated close to the front, so that there was no prospect of returning home that might have encouraged subterfuge.[29] From 1943 onward, soldiers whom doctors judged unfit for combat could also be sent to a concentration camp.[30] In light of this, it is unsurprising that the sample contains only cases in which physicians explicitly mentioned that there was no connection between front-line deployment and the soldier's illness.[31] The evidence thus indicates that the "insights" of military psychiatry were reflected in practice.

If it did take place, the committal of soldiers was subject to special rules and was carried out by the Wehrmacht itself: "The patients were effectively treated as the property of the German Wehrmacht. They were admitted to an 'insane asylum' because the army's regular facilities were poorly suited to treating their symptoms. They were not allowed to leave this institution until their condition was deemed improved 'in consultation with the military doctor' and as soon as the legal provisions (sterilization) permitted."[32] This is a reference to the 1933 law on hereditarily ill offspring, which stipulated that soldiers diagnosed with schizophrenia had to be sterilized.

Against this background, it is noteworthy that there was a third way of dealing with soldiers classified as exhibiting mental abnormalities.

If their ailments were accepted as endogenous conditions, such as schizo-phrenia or MDI, rather than suspected of being undesirable reactions to front-line service, soldiers were not always committed to an asylum in line with official policy.[33] Some were sent home. In the sample, such soldiers only appear if they were in fact subsequently admitted to an institution by a different route. Again, it is an open question how often this happened. However, given the rigid approach to mentally ill soldiers, it is astonishing that such cases occurred at all. It may be that these irregular discharges were related to difficulties in organizing a place in an asylum in the Reich, which could take months. Furthermore, the asylums on the "home front" sometimes refused to admit soldiers because it was not entirely clear who would bear the costs. At other times, the relevant asylum had been closed, while other institutions declared certain cases outside their jurisdiction.[34] One example is that of Dietrich K., who was diagnosed with schizophrenia. The report on his discharge by the medical officer at the Eglfing-Haar Reserve Hospital states:

> This is an endogenous disease, which is not causally but is temporally related to military service. Once the procedure for military discharge is underway and the patient no longer requires hospitalization, he will be discharged to the 4th Schiffstammabteilung Wilhelmshafen [a naval unit] on October 5, 1942.[35]

The medical officer explicitly stressed that this was not a psychological reaction to the war. According to the regulations, Dietrich K. should only have been discharged to a sanatorium-nursing home in his military district, and it is not clear from the file why this did not happen. Six months later, he was forcibly committed from his home village on the initiative of his wife, who stated that he was beating her and wrecking their home.[36] Once again, it is apparent that committals could occur not only because a medical institution had established the presence of mental abnormalities, but also on the initiative of relatives.

This case also makes it clear that committals in wartime and under National Socialism did not necessarily have to be Nazism- or war-specific. Coalitions of (often female) family members and doctors against violent (often male) patients are neither particular to wartime situations, nor to the German case, nor even to the twentieth century. Similar committals are found not only in the postwar period, but also in the nineteenth century.[37]

The committal of soldiers in ways that sometimes departed from the prescribed norms shows in itself that even compulsory committals cannot be grasped solely in the light of rules and institutional actors. Families and the social environment remained important even during the war, and doctors at the front also had room for maneuver at times, although they operated in a highly regimented domain. In what follows, I scrutinize the power relations of different groups of actors with reference to two large groups of patients who were often forcibly committed: the elderly and women, the latter often in connection with sexuality. Due to the much larger source basis, we are in a better position to discern discrete patterns of reasoning with regard to these two groups than in the case of soldiers.

The elderly as a threat: the radicalization of committal practices by institutions and the social milieu

Even before the war, old people were treated from a highly utilitarian perspective in the newly emerging research on old age (*Altersforschung*) expedited by the Nazi regime for ideological reasons. One key question pursued by this research was how older people could be retained as part of the "workers' front" for as long as possible.[38] In addition, as the war progressed and old people's homes were increasingly transformed into substitute hospitals, the elderly were transferred to psychiatric asylums in ever greater numbers.[39] Cases are known in which large groups of elderly people were sent to sanatorium-nursing homes following the closure of an old people's home.[40] At the same time, especially in the last two years of the war, rumors circulated about poorer care for the elderly and their murder.[41] In addition to shedding light on these changes, the individual psychiatric case files provide insights into the treatment of the elderly in everyday wartime life, about which little is known.[42] In what follows, I analyze committals of elderly people "on grounds of danger to the public" (*auf Grund von Gemeingefährlichkeit*) in order to illuminate their position within their social environment and in medical establishments. We can distinguish four variants of the committal pathway typical of the elderly.[43]

First, they were transferred from old people's or nursing homes (*Altersheime* and *Pflegeheime*) to state sanatorium-nursing homes. There were major regional differences here.[44] Before their committal to Untergöltzsch, 10.7 percent of patients were in an old people's home and 7.1 percent in a nursing home.[45] In Munich and the surrounding area, meanwhile, no one was admitted from old people's homes.[46] However, this does not mean that no elderly people were committed to Eglfing-Haar. Its in-house statistics show that, compared to the postwar period, neither a conspicuously small nor a particularly large number of old people were admitted. What was special was the wartime-specific evocation of danger to others.[47] Furthermore, the medical records demonstrate that the sanatorium-nursing home serving Munich and the surrounding area often functioned as an alternative to an old people's home during the war, because from 1941 onward several municipal facilities of the latter type were converted into "auxiliary hospitals" (*Hilfskrankenhäuser*). The residents of the old people's homes were mainly sent to the religious institution of Schönbrunn, not to Eglfing-Haar.[48] New placements in old people's homes, meanwhile, which were difficult or impossible to arrange, were replaced by admissions to the latter.

In addition, older patients were often transferred from surgical departments to sanatorium-nursing homes after operations. This was legitimized—and here we have the second variant—either with reference to the increasing overburdening of hospitals or—third—to relatives' refusal to let their elderly family members return home. In contrast to the findings on independent physicians in Chapter 2, there is no evidence that hospitals committed significantly fewer patients during the war than in the postwar period,[49] which is bound up with the fact that they formed part of the medical arm of the war machine: they were constantly being called upon to free up beds for injured soldiers. Arguments centered on overburdening mostly referred to instances in which patients were perceived as disruptive on the ward and there were no relatives nearby. In these cases, the procedure in itself is not specifically "Nazi" in character, because similar steps were often taken, for example, after 1945 in connection with refugee flows from the former eastern territories, and also in later periods. However, this procedure was legitimized with reference to the war and was facilitated by the fact that old people in hospitals were generally regarded as a "waste of resources."[50]

However, referrals from hospitals to psychiatric facilities cannot be explained solely with reference to practical wartime constraints. Patients were not necessarily transferred to such institutions to free up beds but were also discharged to their families under certain circumstances. For a comprehensive understanding of the overall committal constellation, it is important not to overestimate hospitals as actors or to underestimate the role of the social environment. This is illustrated by the story of Lina V., who was admitted to Eglfing-Haar in December 1940 with a diagnosis of senile dementia.[51] Previously, her brother had arranged for her to be admitted to the Munich university psychiatric clinic. Her medical record there notes with regard to her transfer to the Eglfing-Haar Sanatorium-Nursing Home:

> Request was made for placement in an old people's home. Patient was continent during clinic stay. Residence in the old people's home is possible in our opinion despite occasional states of confusion. Patient is to remain at Eglfing-Haar until the application, which is ongoing, has been completed. Brother also wants patient transferred to Eglfing[52] due to low costs.[53]

Lina V.'s placement in the sanatorium-nursing home was thus an interim solution expedited by the authorities and her brother. The asylum had to admit the woman because she was considered a "threat to public safety" (*Gefährdung der öffentlichen Sicherheit*). A constellation in which hospital doctors and relatives cooperated was a regular occurrence, not only at Eglfing-Haar but also at Untergöltzsch and Marburg, with the patient's social milieu often backing such compulsory committals.[54] Lina V's committal shows that her brother was relatively indifferent to where she was placed. Originally, he had taken his sister to the Munich university clinic. Whether the initiative for this came from him or from an independent physician cannot be inferred from the file. The doctors there did not consider placement in a psychiatric facility necessary but were nonetheless willing to refer the patient to one. At the same time, it is clear that the brother did not want to take his sister home, because this option—the most uncomplicated as well as the most economical one for the hospital physicians—finds no mention in the university clinic file. Still, this does not mean that this possibility might not have been discussed between the hospital physicians and her brother. However, if her brother rejected this and both he and the hospital doctors wished to arrange for temporary committal instead, it would not have been expedient to mention other less expensive possibilities in the referral. The file sheds no light on the brother's possible motives.[55]

The example of Lina V. illustrates that even in wartime there was room for maneuver both for the hospital as an institution and for the patient's social environment, even if an individual was forcibly committed to an asylum. Lina V.'s brother made a quite willful decision, and while it is possible that the hospital doctors put this option to him, he at least appropriated it.

Some relatives who had lived for years at home with a family member exhibiting psychological abnormalities refused to take them back, even after surgically indicated hospitalization. This was the case, for example, for 69-year-old Meta C., who was committed to Eglfing-Haar in September 1942 "as a danger to the public" (*wegen Gemeingefährlichkeit*).[56] The senior medical officer justified this as follows in his expert report:

> C. had already been at the Stralsund Sanatorium-Nursing Home from 1928 to 1930, after which she lived with her brother for years. In May or June 1942 she was taken to Pasing Hospital due to an ulcerated leg, from which she was transferred to the university clinic as she was exhibiting psychological abnormalities. This was a manic disorder resulting from cerebral sclerosis. [...] Her relatives refuse to take the patient in. She must therefore be placed in a closed institution because she is a danger to the public.[57]

Why the relatives refused to care for the woman at home is unclear in this case, but their decisive role is plainly apparent. University psychiatric clinics acted as a crossroads when it came to the question of whether or not someone was to be placed in a sanatorium-nursing home on a long-term basis. This was a far from automatic matter. From a medical point of view, most patients at a university clinic were able to return home even after a lengthy stay if their relatives took them in. At times—albeit rarely—relatives even took their elderly family members out of an asylum against medical advice. For example, 76-year-old Ina. M. was taken home by her nephew at his own risk from the Marburg Land Sanatorium, where she had been staying following an attempted suicide in July 1941.[58]

These exemplary accounts of referral from a hospital to Eglfing-Haar demonstrate that committals cannot be traced via institutions alone. Even forcible committals could be a process of negotiation in which different interests competed with each other and whose outcome depended on the conduct of those in the social environment of the committed. A sole focus on institutions, meanwhile, obscures our view of the relationship between patients and members of their immediate social setting under the conditions of World War II.

In many cases, committals were initiated by health offices together with family members or patients' social milieu. In this context, patient files often include the argument that still spry elderly people who showed slight signs of senility posed a danger at home if not supervised. They might, for example, leave the house without being properly dressed, disturb the neighbors by telling confused stories, fail to observe the blackout during bombing raids, or hinder speedy entry into the air-raid shelter.[59] Two points in particular were repeatedly cited: failure to comply with blackout regulations and letting ration cards expire. Both aspects coincided in the committal of 72-year-old Lydia K. Her guardian requested that she be committed because "she is quite unaware of the blackout regulations, and certainly does not observe them."[60] He also stressed that she was incapable of leading her life independently: "She is unable to take care of her own affairs; she lets ration cards expire!"[61]

The argument from danger was frequently made in direct connection with wartime conditions. I am not arguing here that members of the patient's social milieu instrumentalized the asylum in pursuit of their own interests—this is an open question. It can be shown, however, that the concept of danger to others (*Fremdgefährdung*) vis-à-vis the elderly was very broadly defined and included merely potential safety risks. In 1940, for example, a landlord wrote to the Chemnitz Health Office:[62]

To Chemnitz Welfare Office
  Mitte 6/4552
  I hereby inform you that Mr. [N.], who has been residing in my property as a boarder and is currently in hospital, cannot move back into the room I had rented out to him. I ask you to make arrangements for his placement in an old people's home or care home (*Fürsorgeanstalt*). Mr. [N.] is likely no longer in full possession of his faculties as a result of his old age, which is especially noticeable in his very careless handling of fire and naked flames. He lights his room with a kerosene lamp and sometimes cooks on an alcohol stove. Then there is the great uncleanliness [...].
  Since there is now a great risk that the vermin will spread within the building, and there is a risk of fire due to his handling of kerosene and flames, the residents of the house have lodged complaints with me on a number of occasions, especially since there are small children in the building—and I am forced to terminate Mr. [N.]'s tenancy with immediate effect.

Heil Hitler![63]

The health office accepted this line of argument and Mr. N. was committed directly from the hospital to the Zschadraß Sanatorium-Nursing home. The reference to his handling of kerosene was regarded as sufficient circumstantial evidence that he might cause a fire to break out, while vermin in the old man's quarters could plausibly be presented as a danger to children in other rooms in the building.

Cases in which—fourth—the police picked up people on the street in a confused state also reveal the interplay, characteristic of the committal of the elderly, between medical laypersons and the executive authorities, such as the police and the health office. In May 1943, for example, Alfred S. stopped a policeman in Munich and called his attention to the fact that a "mentally disturbed" (*geistesgestört*) old man was disrupting traffic. According to his medical records, the 70-year-old man claimed that he was looking for his former place of work. The police officer then took him to the health office. There, the public health officer certified that he needed to be placed in a closed institution as a "danger to public safety" (*Gefahr für die öffentliche Sicherheit*). He did not receive a preliminary diagnosis. On the basis of the certificate issued by the health office, he was first taken to the Munich university psychiatric clinic but was immediately referred on to Eglfing-Haar.[64] This rapid onward referral featuring several medical waystations in one day emerges as a specific feature of forcible police committals and is otherwise almost entirely absent from the medical records. It was also common, for example, in police compulsory committals of women suffering from STDs. In the case of the old man above, the ground had already been laid by the police officer's concurrence with the passerby's assessment and his decision to take him to the health office. The fact that the man arrived at Eglfing-Haar without a preliminary diagnosis points in the same direction. It indicates that this was a committal resulting solely from the assessment of the old man as disruptive. To be committed without a preliminary diagnosis was unusual, even compared to other police committals. For example, women with venereal diseases, another group often committed by the police, received a diagnosis despite the rapid committal process.

The rationales for the committal of old people, in which they were described as a "danger to the public" with reference to the war, reveal a tendency to exclude this group from wartime society. The key factor here is that the elderly could plausibly be portrayed as a danger to their own families as well as to the "national body" (*Volkskörper*) as a whole, regardless of whether this danger was taken seriously or was a purely instrumental assertion.[65] In any case, the argument from danger proved strong enough to make admission happen. Hospitals and health offices played a major role in this. At the same time, however, we can clearly discern an impetus "from below," since the social environment—and sometimes even completely uninvolved third parties—tolerated or initiated many of these committals. In both cases, committals sometimes took place without backing from asylum doctors. It was not uncommon for this category of physician to note in the patient's file that this was not a psychiatric admission but in fact a case for an old people's home. At other times, asylum doctors noted that the best solution would be to return the patient to their family. This was not necessarily due to any special thoughtfulness on the part of the doctors but was likely a result of the fact that the admission of old people as "cases not amenable to cure" (*Verwahrungsfälle*) ran counter to the asylums' orientation toward efficient medical care and psychiatric treatment as intended by the doctors.[66] Maria O., for example, ended up at Eglfing-Haar contrary to the asylum doctors' assessment. She was committed with a certificate from the health office as a "danger to herself and the public" (*selbst- und gemeingefährlich*) because she was suffering from a "mental illness (senile dementia)."[67] She remained there, although the doctors did not consider a stay in the asylum necessary, because her family was unwilling to take her home until a place in an old people's home had been found. The family favored Eglfing-Haar as a residential option because of its lower costs.[68] Maria O., however, never made it to an old people's home, dying like many others at Eglfing-Haar.

The limits of what could be said and done, of what was tolerated, were congruent with the specific circumstances of the time. It was legitimate for families and hospital doctors to devote their time and energy to matters that were considered more important than caring for elderly citizens: the war, gainful employment, and young families.[69] Yet it was still possible for relatives to decide otherwise and to bring their elderly relatives back home, as, for example, in the case mentioned above at the Marburg Land Sanatorium. At other times, actors proceeded in clear alignment with these shifts in the sayable and the new opportunity structures. The decision to place elderly people in sanatorium-nursing homes could be rationalized, especially during the war, as inevitable and ultimately as serving the "national good" (*Volkswohl*) and "security."[70] This was not without consequences. Due to the poor supply situation, old people often died far earlier than they might have between 1941 and 1945, even if they were described as spry and having a clear sense of time and place (*zeitlich und örtlich gut orientiert*) when they entered a psychiatric institution and were perhaps only waiting for a place in an old people's home.

In sum, along with the conversion of many homes for the elderly into substitute hospitals, the widespread use of the argument from safety or security facilitated the de-differentiation of asylums.[71] The distinction between the mentally ill and the elderly, which had been engendered by the professionalization of psychiatry, was blurred to some extent during World War II.[72] This leveling out—though not necessarily intended by all the involved parties—was impelled as much by health offices, hospitals, and relatives as by central agencies (through the Brandt Campaign and the like).[73] It was not primarily the doing of asylum doctors, who had no interest in their institutions becoming catch-all quartering facilities, which undermined their aspiration to run cost-efficient institutions.

Security, sexuality, and work: committals of "asocial female psychopaths"

Overall, women accounted for the vast majority of forcible committals by police and health offices during the war period, as evident at both Untergöltzsch and Eglfing-Haar. At Untergöltzsch, two-thirds of those forcibly committed between 1941 and the end of the war were women.[74] For the postwar period, statistical data based on the sample collected for Untergöltzsch/Rodewisch is not meaningful, as forcible committals make up such a small proportion of patients that a further breakdown would tell us nothing.[75] A different picture pertains when it comes to the Bavarian asylum, where more data is available thanks to its yearbooks. There were more committals of women than men at Eglfing-Haar in the years 1941–1945, likely due to war-induced changes in population structure on the "home front." But even considering the higher number of women committed overall, their share of forcible committals was disproportionately high. Women accounted for about one-fifth more of the total number of committals. Among those admitted "as a threat to public safety" (*wegen Gefahr für die öffentliche Sicherheit*), however, there were about twice as many women as men. In 1949, forcible committals broke down more or less equally by gender, after which the trend reversed.[76] By the following year, twice as many men as women were committed by the police.[77] Even compared to forensic committals, which were three to four times more likely to involve men than women throughout the entire period investigated in this book, the number of non-judicial forcible committals of women during the war years was high. While forensic committals were broken down by crime in the Bavarian annual reports, this is not the case for compulsory committals by the police. What we can say is that many forcibly committed women were declared "asocial." In his research on the persecution of so-called "asocials" during the Nazi era, Wolfgang Ayaß has found that before the war began, the focus was on the arrest of male "vagabonds," while from 1940 onward, the emphasis shifted markedly to "prostitutes."[78] This did not necessarily involve sexual services for payment, but could simply mean women who were accused of frequently changing sexual partners.[79] "Asocials" were sometimes placed in asylums, but they were mostly sent to workhouses and concentration camps or barracked in so-called "asocial colonies" in the cities.[80] The high number of forcibly committed women must, therefore, be viewed against the background of the various internment options. Here, gender-specific differences in the nature of persecution soon become apparent.

Reviewing medical records from the wartime period, it is striking that when it comes to women's committals, the topics of safety, sexuality, and ability or willingness to work were often intertwined at the argumentational level. This applies both to the reasoning typical of the social environment and especially to police measures. As with the elderly, it was common for members of the social environment to get in touch with the health office and for admissions to take place as a result. In April 1944, for example,

Mrs. K. phoned the Munich Health Office to report that her neighbor Minna W. was paranoid and constantly disturbing the domestic peace. This had been preceded by years of disputes about everyday issues such as noise and cleanliness.[81] In addition to such scenarios, however, there were committals in which the police apprehended women and initiated their forcible committal. This section is devoted primarily to cases of this kind in order to shed light on the full range of compulsory committals during the war. Committals of old people shine a light on one end of the spectrum of possibilities, at which mainly relatives and the social environment could often exert influence. In some instances of forcible committal, however, institutional actors occupied the key position. This applied, for example, to the compulsory committal of women with venereal diseases.

Four aspects of the forcible committal of women—of both a gender-specific and more general nature—will be elaborated in what follows. Many compulsory committals were clearly gendered and most of these also had a class-specific component. Once again, the broad interpretation of the concepts of safety and danger plays a key role here. Ultimately, the forcible committal of women with sexually transmitted diseases points to a vacuum of responsibility at the institutional level in Nazi wartime society.

Even before the Nazi era, it was common practice to force women to undergo inpatient treatment for venereal diseases. This fits the entrenched interpretative paradigm, which focused exclusively on women as carriers of such diseases.[82] From 1933 onward, however, the preventive detention of women with venereal diseases was also possible.[83] Committals to psychiatric institutions were a step beyond the compulsory inpatient treatment in a dermatological clinic that was common in Weimar:[84] the "solution" to the risk of infection was not to treat the disease but to detain the carrier. Police committals to sanatorium-nursing homes were even more consequential than those to skin clinics, since these placements were of indefinite duration. During World War II, against the backdrop of the murder of the sick, they were also potentially lethal.

A typical example of the forcible placement of women with venereal diseases is the committal of 31-year-old Sina N. from Munich in 1941.[85] The Health Police (*Gesundheitspolizei*) initiated this step with the following statement:

She was dismissed from the special school (*Hilfsschule*) due to educational incapacity. She can perform only the most modest forms of domestic work; she is incapable of shopping. In 1939 she was rendered infertile. For some time, she has been roaming the streets seeking male company. She has already been arrested twice by the police after taking to the streets of Munich in search of men. On each occasion, she was diagnosed with a venereal disease (gonorrhea). Admonitions are fruitless. The feeble-minded N. is unable to see the public danger that her behavior represents and is incapable of mending her ways. She is a proven source of infection for venereal diseases. It must be feared that she will continue to spread venereal diseases. Her detention in a closed institution pursuant to Art. 80/II of the Police Criminal Code is thus imperative.

From her medical record at the Munich university psychiatric clinic, a copy of which is attached to the file at Eglfing-Haar, it emerges that the police apprehended this woman while she was talking to a man on the street. She herself stated that she had a steady partner and had been approached by the man. Nevertheless, Sina N. was committed with the diagnosis of "feeble-minded [*debil*], asocial psychopath," as typical of such cases. The associated procedure, in which the ability to work—here referenced in the statement that Sina N. was capable only of the simplest forms of housework—and sexuality were implicitly intertwined, fit ideological tropes that ascribed to so-called "asocials" a particularly pronounced sex drive.[86]

While this argumentative link between sexuality and work was ubiquitous,[87] the diagnosis of "feeble-minded, asocial psychopath" highlights class-specific differences. Among lower-class women, "work-shyness," sexuality, and venereal disease had formed an interlaced thematic complex since the days of the German Empire. Prostitution was subsequently debated as part of the "psychopath problem."[88] The linking of the themes of security, work, and venereal disease in officially initiated forcible committals is illustrated in a particularly incisive way by the committal of 24-year-old Fredericke W. in 1940. The health office committed her to Untergöltzsch with an initial diagnosis of "psychopathy" and the following explanation:[89]

Arrested during a hotel inspection, she was taken to the Polyclinic for Skin and Venereal Diseases (Poliklinik für Haut- und Geschlechtskranke), found not to be ill, and admitted to the Catholic Girls' Home in Leipzig, where she exhibited abnormal behavior after a few days, complained of headaches, failed to go to work, and had to 'think a lot.' She became impudent and told lies at her workplace, was therefore dismissed without notice, and again failed to turn up at a new job after a few days; sitting by the oven in the home dressed to go out, she made no move, and said nothing.

Made a somewhat dreamy impression on examination, was quite standoffish, and gave no explanation for her behavior.[90]

Although the suspicion of STDs was not confirmed, the woman, having come to the attention of the Health Police, remained in their sights. The only reason for her committal was now the statement that she had failed to show up for work on several occasions. Her complaints of headaches were investigated no further, and no other organic disease was found. It is not uncommon to find cases in the records of the psychiatric facilities considered in this sample in which patients who failed to show up for work "only" due to complaints such as headaches attracted the attention of company physicians or the Health Police. In such cases, both women and men could be committed to an asylum with a diagnosis of "psychopathy." In practice, this term functioned virtually as a medical synonym for "asocial,"[91] though often people were classified more unambiguously as "asocial psychopaths."

Who was responsible for persecuting "female psychopaths" and how exactly they should be dealt with remained a matter of some dispute—a finding that fits with the well-established notion that the Nazi state, with its polycratic structures, was characterized by overlapping competencies. Researchers have underlined that these structures led to competition and thus ultimately helped make the state's draconian measures more efficient.[92] When it comes to Munich, however, which is of particular importance to the present book, Annemone Christians paints a somewhat more nuanced picture, demonstrating that the necessary processes of negotiation could sometimes diminish efficiency.[93] Much the same can be said of wartime committal practices. It is beyond doubt that the jurisdictional spread between different institutions led to increased persecution of women who had been declared "asocial." Sometimes, however, none of the institutions involved, which became increasingly overburdened as the war wore on, were willing to assume responsibility and shuffled women with STDs back and forth between them. In February 1945, for example, Lisa L. was committed to the Untergöltzsch Sanatorium-Nursing Home on the same argumentative basis as Sina N.[94] The Glauchau Health Office stated:

> She [L.] is subnormal (*minderbegabt*) and an unstable psychopath who sleeps around. She poses a risk, especially to members of the armed forces, as she demonstrably engages in sexual intercourse in spite of her illness. I therefore consider detention necessary in order to remedy a state of affairs that is contrary to police regulations.[95]

The explicit reference here to the risk of infecting soldiers crops up frequently and was intended to reinforce the urgency of the situation. Nevertheless, the asylum immediately discharged her as cured and noted:

> Should Mrs. L. take to sleeping around again, police measures would no doubt be appropriate, but not committal to a sanatorium-nursing home. This has also been communicated to the mayor responsible for the Glauchau Municipal Welfare Office."[96]

The sanatorium-nursing home condemned the woman for "sleeping around" (*herumtreiben*) and expressed support for official intervention, but refused to accept responsibility for this. Thus, although in such cases the patient was at the mercy of various institutions, it sometimes took a long time for them to be admitted to an asylum because none of the establishments or agencies involved accepted responsibility. This is indicative of a kind of negative competition or jurisdictional vacuum at the institutional level, especially during the war. The shunting of people back and forth between institutions that declared themselves not responsible was already evident in the above-mentioned case of Lina V., the elderly woman who was committed from a surgical ward to the Eglfing-Haar Sanatorium-Nursing Home, although the doctors saw no real medical need for this. The forcible committal of old people from hospitals, meanwhile, makes it clear that asylums usually had to back down amid the struggle to reject responsibility. This is because old people admitted from hospitals could not simply be discharged. Someone or some establishment had to be found to take them in, whether relatives or an old people's home. The compulsory committal ultimately took place because no one was willing to do so. Hospitals had the option of passing on responsibility to the asylum by means of such a committal. The asylum itself, however, could refer patients no further—in these cases, it was the final stop on their institutional journey.

The argumentative interweaving of "prostitution," suspicion of the spread of venereal diseases, and the ability to work shows that the committal of women with STDs had a class-specific component. If they were middle-class, doctors treated them quite differently. For example, in 1944, 33-year-old Katharina L., a mother of four whose husband worked as a civil servant (*Reichsangestellter*), was admitted to the Greifswald university psychiatric clinic. During her stay there, her husband wrote to the clinic from the front, making inquiries and sending money.[97] The diagnosis was "progressive paralysis," a condition caused by the venereal disease of syphilis. Nevertheless, in contrast to the other cases we have looked at, her committal was not based on coercion. When the clinicians questioned Katharina L. about STDs, she herself confirmed her infection. She stated that she had been an outpatient at the skin clinic but had discontinued the treatment "because she felt healthy."[98] This was contradicted by the statements of the "duty-year girl" (*Pflichtjahrmädchen*),[99] which the so-called objective anamnesis reproduces as follows:

> ... When not crying, she was constantly wandering around the room rubbing her hands together. About eight days ago, the patient ceased to perform household tasks and instructed the duty-girl to do so. She could not go on. The children were taken in by relatives, while the youngest child and the patient were taken care of by the duty-year girl ...[100]

Although the woman was neglecting her household and children and had discontinued treatment for her venereal disease, she was not admitted to a sanatorium-nursing home, let alone forcibly committed to one. Instead, the doctors recommended that Katharina L. be permitted a recuperative stay at the Leba health resort.[101]

Even in the course of committals not related to STDs, sexuality frequently played a key role in connection with the ability to work. Adele S. is a prime example. This case also brings out once again the importance of class affiliation and relatives' engagement to the course of a committal. In this instance, such involvement even led to the doctors subsequently rendering the committal "invisible."

Adele S. came from a wealthy family that owned a large amount of land. Although she lived in Berlin, she was committed by the police to Bethel in January 1942.[102] Normally, a police committal would have seen her taken to a state-run institution near her place of residence. However, her brother had advocated for her to be admitted to the Bodelschwingh Asylums—further evidence that even in the case of a forcible committal during the Nazi era, no institutional automatism came into play that prevented relatives or the social milieu from taking action.

The reason given for this admission by the police was that she was hounding a senior high-school teacher (*Studienrat*) who had been drafted into the Wehrmacht, accusing him of having raped her. Whether this was true cannot be verified. However, it is clear from the medical records that the doctors never considered the possibility that the woman might actually have been raped. At the same time, they failed to make a diagnosis because they found no abnormalities other than the alleged "bogus rape claim." The patient and her family were therefore asked about any problems in her past, as typical of case histories. The patient herself and her relatives foregrounded the fact that she had done poorly at school as a child and had later been "lazy," showing little desire to work, and changing jobs several times as a result. Her brothers saw the allegedly invented rape as directly connected with their sister's attitude to work, of which they took a highly negative view. They stated that, given this mentality, they were not surprised that she had invented "such a story." One of her brothers surmised that her frequent change of jobs could be explained by her sexual debauchery.[103]

The administrative file in this case contains numerous letters from various family members and the public health officers involved in the committal. The patient had a half-brother, for example, who informed the attending physician at Bethel that the other side of the family suffered from hereditary diseases, information the doctors followed up on.[104] While this claim of hereditary disorders was still being investigated, the other branch of the family sought her immediate release from Bethel. A sister-in-law wrote several times to the pastor there, assuring him that her family would take care of things and ensure that the patient stayed away from the teacher.[105]

Bethel, however, initially ruled out discharge categorically due to the extant "danger to the public." Officially, a patient committed by the police could in any case only be discharged with the approval of the relevant police authority. However, about a week after the Bethel doctors had ruled out her discharge, they allowed the patient to leave anyway. In the context of her release, her last place of residence was given not as the Bethel Asylums, as would have been formally correct, but as the district of Gadderbaum. The pastor explained to the brother who took Adele S. in that the reference to this locale was intended to avoid difficulties in registering her in the brother's place of residence.[106] Contrary to the officially prescribed procedure, this temporary committal was no longer immediately apparent in the patient's papers. It had, as it were, been erased from her personal history. This erasure as well as the authorizing of her discharge were the result of the patient's brother's engagement. He had personally approached the public health officer, who then wrote to Bethel that in his opinion there was no reason why the patient could not be discharged immediately.[107] Due to their social position, the family had considerable room for maneuver and asserted their influence with the authorities. This case exemplifies relatives' potential to lobby for a family member to remain in an asylum or to be released quickly, even in the case of a police forcible committal.

Interpretation: compulsory committals during the war

During World War II, police officers and public health officers were central actors in committals at the institutional level. Hospital physicians also played an important role. Asylum doctors, conversely, had little influence, while judges were the deciding factor only in the rare cases of forensic committals. Yet even in the case of forcible placements, there was often some room for maneuver for relatives and members of the patient's social milieu, as the committals of soldiers and especially the elderly reveal. This scope for action took various forms and could be used both to the benefit and detriment of the patient.[108] As the examples considered above demonstrate, room for maneuver potentially depended on the social position of the committed and their family, as well as on their gender and age.

However, there were also cases in which people were entirely at the mercy of institutions, while their social environment was not involved in the committal at all. We might recall Sina N. from Munich, who was forcibly committed by the police "due to the risk" that she would spread venereal diseases. Despite agreeing on the "inferiority" of their clientele, in such cases, the various institutions sometimes sought to foist responsibility onto each other. For those affected, this jurisdictional vacuum could enable them to evade both police and psychiatrists. Alternatively, they might end up in the institution least able to decline responsibility, namely, a psychiatric facility.

Capacity for work/utility and sexuality served as the most important building blocks in the argumentative construction of a security risk. Age, class, and gender aspects were fused together here. These elements, however, were not related to each other in rigid fashion but were interdependent. We can only understand their concrete manifestations if we consider the scope of action enjoyed by the actor in a given case. The practice of exclusion, then, was not based on objective criteria. While, for example, the danger posed by women with STDs was a common theme in the course of committals, other elements could come into play and significantly influence how these women were dealt with. In particular, the attribution to the patient of a capacity for work and usefulness to the "community," as well as the social status of their family, ruptured the exclusionary pattern of presenting women with venereal diseases as a threat. The argument from usefulness also played a role in the committal of the elderly.

The extension of the argument from danger and its anchoring in everyday life by means of the topics of work, sexuality, and age made a mockery of the promise that the individual was safe and sound within the "National Community." Exclusion and committal to an asylum, with its potentially lethal outcome, could be triggered in many different ways and often fell back on the powerful argument of "endangering public safety." The effectiveness and applicability of exclusionary practices, including committals, can be explained by the fact that they could build on well-known patterns and criteria of exclusion. Arguments based on age, sexuality, and gender emerge as characteristic of the wartime period not because of their subject matter, but only because they were put forward in ever more radical ways. Thus, psychiatric ailments of old age such as dementia and Alzheimer's disease were a classic field of activity for psychiatrists and neurologists. Similarly, the focus on women in combating venereal diseases was certainly not typical only of wartime. However, the issue was tackled in an increasingly radical way: from compulsory treatment at skin clinics in the Weimar Republic through the possibility of forcible committal to psychiatric facilities to the persecution of women declared "prostitutes" during the war. The connection between "incapacity for work" and sexuality was not a new topic either. It was already an established feature of discourses on "the underclass" and so-called "asocials."[109] During the war, however, this argumentative paradigm was extended to female patients from affluent backgrounds, as in the committal of Adele S. Yet such committals were negotiable to a much greater extent than in cases involving lower-class patients and could be mitigated by social capital. Hence, it was not particular themes that were specific to the practice of forcible committal during World War II, but rather the expansion and radicalization of exclusion in association with established "problem areas." Processes of hierarchization were informed by the themes of capacity for work and performance (*Leistungsfähigkeit*), sexual behavior, gender, and age. Here, a process of radicalization of a social utilitarian hue is evident not only on the part of the police and medical institutions, but also clearly among the general population as well.[110] This more radical practice of compulsory committal on all sides by means of the—potentially infinitely expandible—concept of danger is congruent with the hypotheses of Birthe Kundrus, who has argued that a permanent, potentially ever-expanding wartime practice of exclusion would have led to the self-destruction of the National Community had the conflict not ended.[111]

Forcible committal practices during World War II thus had two defining features: the radicalization of established patterns of exclusion and the active and broad participation of a variety of actors both at the institutional level and within the social microcosm.

Unregulated spaces: the new power of doctors and relatives in the GDR

Police committals in the FRG and the GDR differed from those in the Nazi era both in their number and in the rationales given for them. In both states, forcible committals by the police and health offices decreased significantly, not exceeding 10 percent.[112] In contrast to the wartime period, the police carried out committals in the 1950s mostly on the grounds that patients—now mostly men—were extremely violent. We might think here first and foremost of cases of domestic violence, as described in the context of Walther M.'s regular committals to the LHA Marburg. Neighbors or the family called the police, who then took Walther M. to the psychiatric facility.[113] Second, the police continued to apprehend people who were considered to be acting in a violent or destructive way in public. Frank A., for example, was taken to Rodewisch by the police in 1953 after smashing a shop window.[114] Police committals that operated with an extreme concept of danger, as typical of those involving women with STDs or declared "unwilling to work" during the war, did not exist in either East or West Germany in the 1950s. Below, I first examine how the police were marginalized in the committal process in the postwar period. I then explore how committals involving coercion proceeded when not carried out by the police, first in East Germany and then, in the next section, in the FRG. A new legal regulation on compulsory committals by the police and health offices was not enacted in the GDR until 1968. What did this mean for forcible committals in early East Germany at the level of rules and practice?

The regulation of forcible committal in the GDR

Both in the Soviet occupation zone and in the GDR, decrees, guidelines, and advice on committal were issued. The rules on compulsory committal have already been researched in detail by Sabine Hanrath and I will merely summarize them briefly here before scrutinizing changes in practice.[115]

The Decree on the Institutional Care of the Mentally Ill (*Verordnung über die Anstaltspflege von Geisteskranken*), issued in 1946, contained a significant innovation when it came to compulsory committal on grounds of danger. This was now to be carried out without the involvement of the police and instead on the basis of a judicial order and medical criteria. This, however, was changed again as early as 1948. In general, committals were now to be initiated by means of a medical certificate, but in the case of danger to the public, the police regained their powers. In contrast to the Nazi period, when the asylums had had to accept committals by the police, the final decision now rested with the asylum's medical director even in the case of committals on grounds of public danger.[116] This significantly strengthened the asylum physicians' position compared to the Nazi era. In 1959, Guidelines on the Placement of Mentally Ill and Mentally Deviant Persons in Psychiatric Hospitals and Nursing Facilities (*Hinweis auf die Unterbringung psychisch kranker und psychisch Abwegiger in Krankenanstalten und Pflegeeinrichtungen*) issued by the Minister of Health and the Prosecutor General (Generalstaatsanwalt) then ordained that the PVG of 1931 would remain in force temporarily. However, the district medical officer (*Kreisarzt*)[117] was now to be responsible for compulsory committal and was to cooperate closely with the police (Volkspolizei) and the Public Prosecutor's Office (Staatsanwaltschaft).[118] All in all, this meant that forcible committals by the police were again permitted in exceptional cases from 1948 onward, while the position of the asylum physicians was considerably strengthened, and public health officers remained important.

It has already been mentioned that the number of compulsory committals initiated and carried out by the executive branch, in other words the police and the health offices, had already decreased significantly before the founding of the state in 1949. This remained the case until 1963. While 25 percent of the committals to Untergöltzsch during the war were forcible committals by the authorities, this only applied to a maximum of 10 percent of later committals to that asylum.[119] Does this mean that fewer patients were in the Rodewisch and Großschweidnitz asylums against their will in the early GDR? This may partly explain the decline; overall, however, the discrepancy in the figures is mainly due to the fact that forcible placements proceeded quite differently. The term "compulsory committal" (*Zwangseinweisung*) always referred to committals imposed by the authorities, not to other forms of coercion, such as that exercised by relatives. In 1959, for example, the medical director of the Rodewisch Specialist Hospital, Dr. Walther, in a statement requested by the Ministry of Health on the newly composed draft Guidelines on the Placement of Mentally Ill and Mentally Deviant persons in Psychiatric Hospitals and Nursing Facilities, declared that:

> As hitherto, it must be possible for any licensed physician to commit a mentally ill person by providing the appropriate certificate. It has so far been the next of kin that have given their consent to the committal of patients who are not incapacitated, and the same applies to the required consent to treatment. This existing procedure should be sanctioned by law.
>
> Forcible committals would then be limited to the small number of cases in which relatives with a poor level of understanding wish to prevent a committal or prematurely terminate one that has already taken place (at their own risk). One would also have to add those patients who have no relatives.[120]

Hence, at Rodewisch and—the statement suggests—apparently other institutions as well, patients were admitted against their will, provided that their relatives agreed.[121] Officially, however, these were not forcible committals. Relatives thus occupied a recognized position of power in early East Germany, even if this was not legitimized by law. Although we can clearly observe a change in the practice of compulsory committal compared to the

Nazi period here, the true rupture is far less evident in relatives' stronger position than in the loss of power suffered by the police and public health officers. As shown above, relatives often had room for maneuver in the event of compulsory committal during the war and could initiate them, consent to them, or impede them. In the GDR, the falling away of the executive organs placed family members in an even more decisive position. A twofold shift in power also took place within the medical profession. First, the asylum directors' authority was considerably enhanced. They had the final say over admission decisions, whereas in the Nazi era they had no choice but to admit patients in the event of forcible committal. Second, while a medical certificate was sufficient for compulsory committal even under the PVG of 1931, in practice the vast majority of such committals up to 1945 were handled by the health office. Committals via the latter had already decreased considerably in the Soviet occupation zone and remained at a low level. This indicates that other physicians played a more important role in these non-official committals carried out against the will of the persons concerned.

How many such committals ultimately took place is not clear. When it comes to Rodewisch, in a statement for the Ministry of Health in 1959, Dr. Fabian, the medical director, gave a figure of 90 percent of current patients.[122] Thus, the decision to commit patients to Rodewisch almost always rested with relatives and physicians. In practice, the standard that was being established here—that in case of doubt the family and the asylum physicians should be the responsible parties—potentially extended to all committals. Conversely, the notion that the patient themself should sign the declaration of voluntariness was abandoned. Instead, their relatives rose to become the physicians' primary negotiating partner. This was not a new practice: it was de facto already family members who chiefly negotiated with physicians. But now this familiar procedure underwent massive expansion. Whether this applies to the same extent to all asylums in the GDR cannot be determined on the basis of the sources used in this study, but it seems likely. The committal decision ultimately rested with the asylum director, so differences in practice are possible. But in view of psychiatrists' ongoing struggle for official recognition of their decisions, made in consultation with the family—including with respect to official compulsory committals[123]—there is good reason to assume that practices in Rodewisch were typical of committal decisions in East Germany as a whole.

Hence, a feature of signal importance that the "Third Reich" and the GDR had in common is that patients in both systems lacked an advocate when they were committed against their will. In East Germany, responsibility and decision making lay mainly with the patient's social milieu and with doctors. But local authority institutions also played a role on many occasions. An unofficial negotiation process in a law-free space thus compensated for an insufficiently regulated procedure. Unlike in the Nazi dictatorship, then, there was no large-scale intervention by the executive branch in the case of imposed committals in the GDR.[124] The state and its executive organs had much less interest than in the Nazi era in influencing the practice of committal and intervening in this particular way in the everyday lives of its citizens. Equally, though, until 1968, there was no restructuring of compulsory committal through the involvement of the judicial branch. Who required institutional-ization was decided by families and physicians. This finding does not dovetail straightforwardly with common historiographical interpretations of the SED dictatorship, which assume that while purposeful (*eigensinnig*) action was possible in East Germany, it must always be understood in relation to dictatorial rule. Ultimately, the prevailing opinion has been that even the spheres of everyday life, some of which could be shaped through purposeful action, were infiltrated by representatives of the regime.[125] On this view, no area of life is conceivable without reference to the dictatorship. Yet this concept captures the practice of committal only partially.

It is true that the vacuum of rules that existed until 1968 meant that negotiation between families, the social environment, and doctors was per-missible "within the limits of the basic structure" of the dictatorship, as en-visaged in Lindenberger's concept of the "dictatorship of limits" (*Diktatur der Grenzen*).[126] Yet there was no need for purposeful action vis-à-vis the dic-tatorship, since there was simply no point of contact with it. Families' negotiation of committals took place with psychiatrists, the vast majority of whom did not support the new state in the 1950s.[127] Contrary to common perceptions of the GDR, then, the practice of committals had no direct connection to the level of rule. There are two reasons for this. First, psy-chiatrists saw themselves as the opponents of any political intervention in the practice of committals.[128] Second, the committal event was in no way a predictable one that could be straightforwardly regulated through the orga-nized political penetration of society. It did not take place within any of the numerous prescribed political structures, such as youth or women's organi-zations, trade unions, or enterprise brigades (*Betriebsbrigaden*). Political infiltration from below by representatives of state power was, therefore, not possible. The concept of the "dictatorship of limits"—and to an even greater extent that of a *durchherrschte Gesellschaft*,[129] a society governed to the point of saturation, which was often used in the past—is rooted in the extremely high degree of organization of East German society, right down to the lowest levels. With the help of this concept, it can for example be shown to impressive effect that the "self-organized" working class and its brigades—while indeed acting in a purposeful way—could be subverted by re-presentatives of power. Psychiatric committals, however, took place on a level not accessible through this form of organization.[130] In many cases, therefore, the practice of committal was not characterized by the inter-weaving of "state power, the practice of domination [*Herrschaftspraxis*] and a fragmented society"[131] as imagined in the notion of a "dictatorship of limits."[132] Committal decisions certainly entailed an interplay of institutions including clinics, asylums, and polyclinics, as well as the social microcosm. Yet in individual cases, committals against the patient's will were often driven chiefly by families or the immediate social milieu, such as neighbors or landlords. This "necessity" was then pursued quite straightforwardly in collaboration with a medical profession that was fighting against the political control and regulation of its activities.[133] This did not require fundamentally new arrangements: a form of committal that had to some extent been practiced previously—but that was in any case favored—managed to become broadly established thanks to the legal vacuum.

Ultimately, committal practices saw various actors appropriate an unregulated space in which social microcosms and state institutions came into contact. In the context of committal practices and "successful" self-regulation, the existence of this space does not call into question the theoretical concepts explaining the connections between dictatorship and everyday life *per se*. It does raise doubts about their reach. In the practice of committal, the interaction between state and social microcosm was often merely indirect in nature, even in the context of compulsory committals. The kind of questions generally raised in light of the field of tension between dictatorship and purposeful conduct relate to people's burning need to come to terms with the dictatorship in whatever way. In the first instance, these questions do not arise with respect to the practice of committal.[134] This does not mean that we cannot examine committal in the early GDR with a view to possible impacts of the socialist regime, let alone that we are dealing here with a space free of domination or a niche far removed from politics. That would be going too far. The way people dealt with political-ideological control or the consequences of economic reconstruction are plainly apparent in rationales for committal. Yet this did not entail direct control of the mechanisms for entry into psychiatric institutions, but, for instance, ideological rhetoric of a more general nature, which was implicitly referenced in reasoning about committals. What we can discern in committal practices, then, are the indirect but potentially profound consequences of SED rule. For example, committal rationales shed instructive light on the ways people dealt with egalitarianism as a guiding socialist norm[135] and the role played by work in the construction of a healthy self within the "workers' and peasants' state."[136]

Standards and decisions: the coalition of practice encompassing asylum physicians and families

The following three examples illustrate how civil committals against the patient's will functioned in East Germany. These cases represent common family constellations when it comes to civil committals that were decided over the patient's head. In the first example, the patient's sister initiated the committal. The second case involves a woman whose parents were involved in the committal decision. I then turn to the case of an elderly man whose son expedited his committal. In the first example, the negotiation took place solely between family members and physicians, much as in the committals of Karin F. and Albin H. considered in Chapter 2. In the other two committals, various other parties sought to assert their interests. Even in these cases, though, it is evident that relatives' interests and physicians' assessments were ultimately decisive.

The committals of Walpurga R., admitted to Großschweidnitz nine times between 1947 and 1956, were typical.[137] In most cases, her sister, who lived with her, initiated the 46-year-old woman's admission. Walpurga R. received various diagnoses, such as "reactive depression," "endogenous depression," and "schizophrenia."[138] However, the decisive factor in the sister's decision to pay a visit to the doctors—regardless of the exact medical classification—was situations that she described as having become unbearable and beyond what she could fairly be expected to cope with. When she was committed in 1947, Walpurga R., according to her sister, refused to eat for fear that she might be poisoned.[139] In 1953, her sister stated that she could hardly communicate with her because she was hearing voices.[140] The patient only ever remained in the asylum for a few weeks at a time, until doctors and her sister agreed that Walpurga R.'s symptoms had subsided to the extent that she could live with her sibling again.

In the case of Petra Sch., who was committed several times in the early 1950s and suffered from epilepsy, her family, landlord, and home munici- pality, as well as the asylum doctors, were all involved, each with their dif- fering concerns, during her third committal in 1951. Petra Sch. was admitted to Untergöltzsch with an acute epileptic seizure after a doctor had given her a sedative injection.[141] The patient's mother argued against a lengthy stay in the asylum, writing to obtain a leave of absence that might serve as a trial for discharge. The leave of absence was granted and Petra Sch. was released into her mother's care.[142] Immediately after this, the asylum received a letter from the local council arguing vehemently that the patient required institu- tionalization. The letter briefly recapitulated the circumstances of the com- mittal before emphasizing that it was not in the interest of the committing physician, the municipality, or the owner of the building in which Ms. Sch. lived that she be discharged:

> The committal of [Petra Sch.] took place at the instigation of the physician Dr. Nier, who has, however, been on vacation for several weeks. The admission forms will be sent to you as soon as he returns.
>
> Further, the social committee of the municipality of Raum also dealt in detail once again with the case of [Sch.] at its last meeting, as there was a request from the building owner whose property [Sch.] lived in, in which he asked that [Sch.] not be lodged in his building again after her return, since she had already broken windows, etc.
>
> Since [Sch.'s] condition is unlikely to improve in the near future, and the seizures recur regularly, we ask you not to grant her leave after a few weeks, let alone discharge her, since we have also had difficulties with the doctor, who is no longer willing to give [Sch.] a sedative injection in the event of a seizure due to the risks involved.
>
> We ask for your understanding and look forward to your reply.[143]

The local council, the owner of the building, and the doctor cited pragmatic reasons for long-term institutionalization, which related exclusively to disruptions to the smooth running of community life. The director of the asylum took a different view in her letter of reply while adopting a mediating stance between the interests of mother and community:

The above-named has behaved in a calm, orderly, and inconspicuous way during the last few weeks of her stay here, so the request of the patient's mother was granted and Miss [Sch.] was given a trial leave of absence in her mother's household on September 6, 1951.

Your letter of August 31, 1951 had not yet reached me at that time.

From the medical point of view, it is legitimate to give a patient whose condition has improved considerably a trial leave of absence, especially if the relatives have given assurances of diligent care and supervision—as in this case.

If there are any concerns in this regard on your part after the domestic situation has been reviewed, a request will be made for the patient's immediate return.[144]

The medical arguments made by the doctor played no role in the reasoning of the municipal council. Yet she in no way rejected its alternative point of view, but conceded the possibility of readmission should the patient's family fail to ensure that Miss Sch. cease to cause disturbances. The doctor thus reflected multifunctionality that typified psychiatric institutions in all three political systems and that I addressed at various points in the previous chapter.[145] It is remarkable that the views of the patient herself, who was committed without even an admission form—a failure to comply even with procedures for a civil committal—are not mentioned at all in the medical record. If the asylum doctor was seeking to mediate between all serious parties, the patient was obviously not considered one of them. Four traits typify the course of committals that were formally not compulsory but in which a patient who was not incapacitated was deprived of any role in the decision. First, it was ultimately asylum physicians and relatives who decided on prolonged institutionalization. Second, other parties attempted to exert influence. This could be significant—after all, in this example, it was the actions of a local physician that led to the admission in the first place—but was not usually decisive in determining whether an individual should remain in an asylum. Third, the patient had little—and in this case, no—involvement in the decision. Fourth, the reasoning of local authorities tended to be purely pragmatic in character, as in this case, which is reminiscent of the rationales put forward in the Nazi era. But these pragmatic arguments were more pivotal in wartime than they were in the 1950s GDR. In the latter, however, they had excellent prospects of prevailing if they came from relatives. The medical assessment of a patient's state of health, as in this example, became more important again in the postwar period, as did the apposite placement of relatives, especially elderly ones.

The de-differentiation of old people's homes and sanatorium-nursing homes persisted during the occupation. In Untergöltzsch, an entire old people's home was incorporated into the sanatorium-nursing home as late as 1947. As a result, the individual case files contain no medical history, exploration, or diagnosis. Instead, they merely identify the reason for the patient's stay in general terms: "Transferred as a result of the integration of the Obergöltzsch Old People's Home into the nursing department of the Untergöltzsch Land Asylum."[146] Immediately after the war, meanwhile, many confused old people fleeing from the former eastern territories became separated from their families and were placed in asylums.[147] During the war, and then in the FRG and GDR, no clear distinction was made between those for whom an old people's home was an appropriate option and those who desperately needed care in an asylum. In wartime, the asylum was in case of doubt the last stop in a series of onward referrals of elderly people, whereas in the GDR the boundary between asylum and old people's home was permeable in both directions. The East German asylums' lack of capacity meant that in the 1950s there were people who, in the opinion of doctors and relatives, should have been in a sanatorium-nursing home, but who ended up in an old people's home. Here we find a line of reasoning diametrically opposed to that so prevalent in wartime, when it was regularly argued that an individual should be admitted to an asylum because there were no places in old people's homes. This can be seen in the medical records at Greifswald: university psychiatric hospitals often played a decisive role among medical institutions when it came to determining where an individual would be placed. For example, 63-year-old Lothar Z., who had been cared for by his wife and son for years but no longer recognized them in 1952—nor did he know who he himself was—was taken by his family to the Greifswald university psychiatric clinic.[148] His file notes: "After consultation with his relatives—since a transfer to a sanatorium-nursing home is not possible due to overcrowding—the patient is to be placed in a home for the elderly that is under medical supervision."[149]

By the time of the Soviet occupation zone, the files had already ceased to show evidence of committals of old people suffering only a minor degree of impairment that were initiated by their families on the grounds that they represented a "security risk" (*Gefahr für die Sicherheit*). The lack of space and the food situation in the asylums during this period were, however, even worse than during the war. It is thus possible that such attempts at committal continued to be made but cannot be traced because they were unsuccessful. Due to the desperate situation of psychiatric facilities in the immediate postwar years, it is impossible to determine whether the way lay people dealt with the elderly had already changed.

By the 1950s, meanwhile, the way the elderly were treated by their relatives had certainly changed, while older patterns persisted among the committing institutions. This became apparent in the course of reviewing almost 400 medical records from Greifswald, Rodewisch, and Großschweidnitz for the postwar period. Elderly people were regularly committed to all three institutions. But while the social milieu continued to initiate committals in which the argument from safety played a decisive role, the rationales put forward here were different in quality than during the war. They no longer referred to potential safety risks of an indirect nature, such as the spread of vermin through lack of cleanliness. Rationales relating to wartime conditions naturally ceased to appear, such as fears that the elderly would be unable to maintain blackouts. Typical now were references to an acute hazard and its potential recurrence. The aforementioned committal of a 62-year-old widow to Rodewisch who had thrown her grandson out of a window is a striking example of this.[150]

This shift in approach is also evident in relatives' protests against the committal of old people by the authorities, which continued to use asylums for old-age care. In 1955, for example, 65-year-old Martin K. was committed to Rodewisch.[151] Living with his son and his family and perceiving himself as a burden on them, he had contacted the Karl-Marx-Stadt Welfare Center (*Betreuungsstelle*) himself requesting a place in an old people's home. Instead, he was sent to the Untergöltzsch Sanatorium-Nursing Home via the Welfare Service for the Psychiatrically and Mentally Ill (*Fürsorge für psychiatrische und Nervenkranke*). The family then wrote several times to the senior staff at Untergöltzsch stating that it was beyond their comprehension that he had ended up in a psychiatric facility: he was old and ill, but completely "normal."[152] The conflation of geriatric and psychiatric care was no longer so straightforwardly accepted.

Judicial compulsory committal: new regulations and their implementation in the FRG

In West Germany, in contrast to the GDR, new legal regulations on forcible committals had already come into force in the 1950s. What were the effects of—and what resistance was there to—this restructuring of the practice of committal by the democratic state? Since placement regulations were essentially a matter for the federal states or *Länder*, my discussion of the FRG begins with an examination of the new regulations and their acceptance in Bavaria, Hesse, and North Rhine-Westphalia, the locations of the three West German psychiatric institutions whose medical records I analyze in the present book.[153] They cannot be considered representative of West Germany as a whole. In fact, given the differences that emerge below between these three federal states, it seems likely that there were major regional differences in responses to the new committal laws. After exploring this topic, the next section sheds light on the practice of committal decisions.

New regulations and their acceptance

On a societal level, Cornelia Brink has shown that the postwar public discourse on psychiatric facilities in the FRG was characterized by a fear of inappropriate committals, while the purpose of such institutions was questioned in the press and patients were portrayed as somewhat eccentric victims.[154] The mandatory involvement of a local court prior to forcible placement, meanwhile, was intended to prevent arbitrary committals. How did the implementation of the new rules proceed in practice?

Figures on compulsory committals and what they tell us

The introduction of judicial placement, which will be explained in more detail below, broadened the spectrum of procedures. While forcible committals during the war years were mainly carried out without a judicial order on the grounds of danger to the public, new modes of committal now came into play. But even after the introduction of the new placement laws, police committals continued to be made to Eglfing-Haar and Marburg. At the latter, 10 percent of all admissions from 1955 to 1963 were judicial committals,[155] while nearly 7 percent were carried out by the police.[156] At Eglfing-Haar, many official forcible committals occurred even in the 1950s, on a scale comparable to the war years, though now judicial committals greatly outnumbered those made by the police. After the introduction of the Bavarian Detaining Act of 1952, which I elucidate in more detail below, judicial committals accounted for about a quarter of all admissions.[157] The larger number of forcible committals to Eglfing-Haar compared to Marburg, meanwhile, was due mainly to the two asylums' differing orientations, with the LHA being intended for shorter stays.

In the early FRG, a total of about 3–6 percent of patients were assessed by psychiatrists as a danger to the public, but the number of forced committals was significantly higher.[158] There are no official statistics for the 1950s and 1960s, but "[t]he Psychiatry Inquiry found that the rate of compulsory committals in the *Länder* in 1974 ranged from 6.4 percent of all committals in Baden-Württemberg to 49.1 percent in Hesse."[159] These figures, though, are of limited use. Not only are the numbers for the period under study in this book highly uncertain, but the surveys that do exist do not always capture the same legal realities. Forcible or compulsory committal (*Zwangseinweisung*) was not always understood in the same way in the 1950s. In Hesse, for example, committals of incapacitated patients were considered to be compulsory committals for a time, but this did not apply in Bavaria or North Rhine-Westphalia. The limitations of purely quantitative surveys are clearly evident here. In what follows, I first examine the new legal regulations and the debate on who ought to be responsible for compulsory committals, before addressing the implementation of the new order.

New regulations on compulsory committals in Bavaria, Hesse, and North Rhine-Westphalia

In 1949, the adoption of the constitution or Basic Law (*Grundgesetz* or GG) kicked off a debate in the FRG on forcible placement, which, according to

Art. 104 of the GG, required a court order.[160] This meant that the regulations set out in the PVG of 1931 on "committal on grounds of danger" (*Gefahreneinweisung*) no longer conformed to the Basic Law, since the PVG allowed for forcible committal without the involvement of a court. After a lengthy debate on the deprivation of liberty, the Federal Law on the Judicial Process in Cases of Deprivation of Liberty (*Bundesgesetz über das gerichtliche Verfahren bei Freiheitsentziehung*) was therefore passed in 1956.[161] In that debate, physicians had taken a stand against the involvement of courts in compulsory committals. "The presumed relationship of trust between physician, patient, and relatives became an argument against judicial involvement."[162] The medical profession thus favored a regulation that would have legally enshrined a procedure similar to that in the GDR. But despite the rapid reconstruction of their power structures, physicians ultimately had to accept a regulation that restricted their official scope of action with respect to committal practice.[163]

In addition, however, Land law continued to apply when it came to the deprivation of the liberty of the "mentally ill" (*Geisteskranke*).[164] The laws for Bavaria and Hesse were passed as early as 1952 and were very similar with respect to the material preconditions for "placement in case of danger" (*Unterbringung bei Gefahr*).[165] In both cases, the law referred to danger to others and danger to self.[166] These laws differed, however, with regard to the concept of danger. In Bavaria, the placement merely had to be necessary for reasons of public safety and order.[167] In Hesse, the danger involved had to be considerable and not otherwise avertable,[168] a state of affairs that is legally much more difficult to prove than risks to security and order.[169] The legislation in North Rhine-Westphalia was even more restrictive. It contained a specific section on the preconditions for placement, which read: "The placement of mentally ill (*geisteskrank*), feeble-minded (*geistesschwach*) or addicted (*suchtkrank*) persons is permissible only if and as long as there is a present danger to public safety or order as a result of their behavior toward themselves or others that cannot be averted in any other way."[170] The phrase "present danger" (*gegenwärtige Gefahr*) possesses enormous significance if we consider previous practice during the war, when individuals were regularly committed due to *potential* dangers, as in the committals of women with STDs or the elderly described earlier. In contrast to the Bavarian terminology, which left a good deal of latitude that could potentially be used to the detriment of the persons concerned, North Rhine-Westphalia took a more restrictive approach.

The differences become more apparent still if we subject the Code of Criminal Procedure (*Strafprozessordnung* or StPO) to comparative examination. Its Sec. 126a regulated "temporary placement to avert a threat" to public safety. This was applied if there was reason to believe that the defendant, first, would be classified as of unsound mind or of diminished mental capacity (*vermindert zurechnungsfähig*), second, posed a threat in the interim, and, third, it was likely that preventive detention would be imposed.[171] In Bavaria, the defendant could then be held until they were shown not to represent a danger.[172] Moreover, this type of placement was once again the responsibility of the police rather than the court.[173] In Hesse, meanwhile, only one-day police detention was possible, and the subsequent asylum placement (of a maximum of two months) had to be ordered by a judge.[174] In North Rhine-Westphalia, there was no possibility at all of temporary placement to avert a threat. In accordance with Art. 104 of the Basic Law, the police were only allowed to commit people for one day. After that, the forcibly committed person had to be released or placed in an institution on a long-term basis through a court order.[175] There were, therefore, considerable differences in the new rules on placement in the different federal states.

Resistance to the new regulations on forcible committal

Conversely, immediately after the introduction of the Basic Law, all the federal states were united by uncertainty about how to proceed with respect to the practice of police committals. In May 1950, the German County Association (Deutscher Landkreistag) thus wrote to the Federal Minister of the Interior to clarify the implications of the aforementioned Art. 104 of the Basic Law:

> The German County Association is receiving a growing number of inquiries as to whether the powers of the administrative authorities, laid down in former laws, to forcibly place unruly individuals harmful to national health or society [*widerspenstige Volksgesundheits- oder Sozialschädlinge*] (such as asocial tuberculosis sufferers, lunatics, and asocials) in asylum houses [*Asylierungshäuser*], lunatic asylums [*Irrenanstalten*], or workhouses, are compatible with Art. 104 of the Basic Law.
>
> The German County Association has so far taken the view that administrative staff should in the first instance adopt the position that the existing regulations do not contradict Art. 104. It remains to be seen whether further legal declarations will be made on Art. 104.[176]

We can thus observe a general tendency to perpetuate entrenched police committal practices. Still, major regional differences are discernible during this period of legal uncertainty.

The Bavarian legislation was built on regional welfare regulations and practices that gave greater weight to security issues than to individual liberty.[177] Even before the Bavarian Detaining Act was passed, it was already clear that the authorities were striving to maintain their regional "welfare tradition" and circumvent the Americans' attempts to reorganize the field of committal "on grounds of danger to the public" (Art. 80, Para. II, PolStGB). On March 9, 1949, the Bavarian State Ministry of the Interior ordered[178] an end to committal by the police; only judicial committal was to be permitted in relevant cases. This was complied with. In 1949, only 48 people were forcibly committed by the police to the Eglfing-Haar Sanatorium-Nursing Home. This was a significant decrease, though we should bear in mind that forcible committals without judicial intervention had undoubtedly declined before then. In 1946, 461 out of 660 patients had still been admitted under Art. 80/II PStGB; in 1948, the figure was 245 out of 1,564. In 1949, this had dropped to just 48 out of a total of 1,638 admissions.[179] At the same time, however, attempts were made to get round this regulation. The Health Department of the Bavarian State Ministry of the Interior wrote to the Bavarian State Ministry of Justice in response to the order of March 9, 1949, stating that all police committals must cease. It argued that in the interest of public safety the new procedure could not be put into practice, and made a proposal as to how, in its opinion, it might best be circumvented. The Health Department contended that courts far too often rejected temporary placement to avert a threat to public safety,[180] calling the judges' assessment fundamentally into question and making the case for an extraordinarily broad interpretation of the concept of danger:

With respect to the unpredictability of a mentally ill person who constitutes a danger to the public, as a rule, an objective criminal threat to public safety is to be regarded as given. In his unpredictable behavior lies a constant threat—to the persons around him in terms of acts of violence and to the property of others in the form of damage and destruction. [...] Urgent grounds for the assumption that a person has committed a punishable act in a state of unsoundness of mind can be assumed to exist if the mentally ill person has threatened to attack those in proximity to him in a fit of rage.[181]

The Ministry of the Interior now inquired as to whether the Ministry of Justice might urge the courts to much more frequently order placements out of consideration for public safety. The Interior Ministry argued that the American military government had shifted responsibility from the police to the judicial authorities, "which must fulfill this obligation in the interest of the general public."[182] If the courts "do not believe they can justify" placements on grounds of danger,[183] an application should be made for expedited incapacitation, which should include a request for the newly incapacitated person's placement.[184] Here, then, the Bavarian Health Department portrayed any deviation from its comprehensive definition of safety as a neglect of judicial responsibility to the public. Instead of accepting the new more liberal-democratic regulations, those in positions of authority sought to identify legal sleights of hand that would render them inoperative.[185]

While the Bavarian Ministry of the Interior was unwilling to accept the new regulations, in Hesse protection for the freedom of the individual was for a time interpreted as broadly as possible. In 1955, in the *Staatsanzeigen f. d. Land Hessen*[186] (the official gazette for the state of Hesse), the Hessian

Minister of the Interior retracted his interpretation of Art. 104 of the Basic Law, which was geared toward liberal-democratic ideals, because it clashed with the decision of the Federal Supreme Court, which took a less far-reaching view:

Under No. 1, 2, Para. 2, of the First Implementing Decree on the Deprivation of Liberty Act, I have taken the position, with respect to the voluntary nature of placement, that even in the case of persons who are legally incompetent or of limited legal competence, their own volition and not that of a legal representative (holder of parental authority or legal guardian [*Vormund* or *Pfleger*]) is in principle paramount, and that the only exception to this applies to persons under fourteen years of age.

This interpretation was based, first, on § 15, Para. 2 and § 22 of the Deprivation of Liberty Act [The Hesse Deprivation of Liberty Act (*Freiheitsentziehungsgesetz*) of 1952]. It was rooted, second, in the legal opinion that Art. 104, Para. 2, Sent. 1 of the Basic Law extends to any deprivation of liberty, that is, not only to measures by holders of public authority, but also to deprivations of liberty by the holder of parental authority or the legal guardian.[187]

However, the Federal Supreme Court ruled that the involvement of the courts applied only to the deprivation of liberty "by holders of public authority."[188] In the early 1950s, however, this had still been subject to debate. In 1954, for example, in the context of discussions on the specific form to be taken by the new Deprivation of Liberty Act, the Bundesrat proposed that legal guardians no longer be allowed to carry out committals to closed institutions without a decision by the guardianship court (*Vormundschaftsgericht*). The federal government rejected this.[189]

This affected a fair number of the "adult" patients considered in this study. In addition to incapacitated persons, those not yet of age must also be considered here.[190] This is because, in terms of psychiatric practice, people were usually admitted to adult wards from the age of sixteen, depending on their physical development. Beginning in 1960, even committals with the consent of the legal guardian required a judicial decision.[191] Views on the legal change proposed in 1954, which did not take place, are nevertheless interesting with respect to committal practices, since those expressing them argued in light of experience with compulsory committals. Ernst Lösch, an administrative judge in Düsseldorf, made two points regarding judicial placement of underage or incapacitated persons. First, he argued in favor of judicial decisions to prevent abuse of committals arising from legal guardians pursuing their own interests. Second, he justified his call for this judicial role with reference to the fact that, in his experience, legal guardians often failed to arrange for appropriate placement "because they balk at a burden of responsibility resting solely on their shoulders."[192] The opposing camp made the inverse argument: there were no known cases of abuse and legal guardians might be avoiding committals because they did not wish to involve the court.[193] What is remarkable about both arguments is the central importance they attached to the behavior and decisions of relatives. The priorities at play here went well beyond protecting incapacitated or underage persons from abuse, which was not even deemed necessary by all those involved in the debate.

In general, unofficial compulsory committals reflect asymmetrical power relationships in families. This applies not only to children's dependence on their parents, but often, reversing the generational relationship, to a parent's dementia: older family members affected by this condition could also be incapacitated. In these cases, a relative usually became their guardian. I examine both constellations in what follows.

Informal preliminary decisions by families and physicians

Practice in the FRG deviated from the legal norm, placing greater power in the hands of physicians: "With remarkable openness and great satisfaction, Medical Officer of Health [*Medizinalrat*] Schulze could report to his colleagues in 1956 how legal norms and committal practice had diverged: 'Due to our passive resistance, the average, civil admission procedure continued to function as before. We relied on our old admission regulations and made our report. And then, gratifyingly enough, it became increasingly apparent that the public prosecutor's offices were coming to see things our way.'"[194] In every instance recorded in the sample taken for this book, the local courts did in fact concur with the doctors' opinion. But how exactly did this work in specific cases, and what role did patients and relatives play? What happened prior to the physician's report to the courts?

I seek to exemplify this here with reference to the committal of patient Miranda L., whom we met in the last chapter. In 1952, she was admitted[195] to the LHA Marburg for the third time. A certificate authorizing this had been provided by an independent physician. After summing up her previous committals, he wrote:

> Now the relatives are complaining about new bouts of restlessness, along with constant talking and complaining. The only person who might care for her now is her aged mother, but she is afraid of the patient in her states of agitation. All the other residents of the farm are busy working in the fields and can only step in temporarily to care for her. The relatives therefore wish to place the patient in an asylum. [...]"[196]

The Wolfhagen District Health Office, in the shape of the public health officer, gave this certificate its seal of approval a day later. The last sentence of his letter reads: "The Wolfhagen District Court has been notified." This was, therefore, officially a juridical committal. In reality, however, the admission had long since taken place. The retrospective obtaining of a judicial order was common in the early FRG.[197] As this case shows, such belated authorization by a judge was not only an emergency solution for patients who were an acute danger to themselves or their environment: according to her relatives, Miranda L.'s committal was essentially a matter of ensuring her supervision. The relatives' decision depended both on structural circumstances, such as the demands on the entire family in the shape of agricultural work, and on the specific family situation, such as the fact that the mother was afraid of her daughter and therefore could not look after her. There is no mention of danger in the admission records. At most, it is inherent in the supervision problem, though it is not discussed explicitly. This kind of compulsory committal was not unusual, with several similar cases at the LHA appearing in the sample. Furthermore, the documentation of the committal itself indicates that this was not a special case requiring explanation. In the medical certificate for the admission, the committing physician merely echoed the supervision problem, without adding, for example, that he discerned an acute danger to the patient or her milieu as a result. It is impossible to say whether the notification provided by the public health officer was any different, since it is not attached to the medical record. But at least in the communication between the committing independent physician and the admitting institution, there was no need to explicitly evoke a threatening scenario in order for the institution to admit the patient prior to the judge's decision. Although the judge had jurisdiction, this case shows how significant the decisions of relatives and the independent physician remained. The problem of supervision once again became the pragmatic legitimation of committal.

At least at the LHA Marburg, then, the relatives were decisive actors even in the case of judicial compulsory committals. Presumably, this was not unique to this facility. Such negotiation of forcible committals had already been practiced in cases of police committals both to Eglfing-Haar and the LHA Marburg. This may well have been an entrenched *modus vivendi* maintained by doctors, relatives, and asylums that was now perpetuated in West Germany, with the courts as new actors. In principle, it was always possible for judges to decide against a committal. In the sample taken for this book, however, this never occurred.[198] Plainly, if we seek a deeper understanding of the processes that brought people into an asylum, we need to look at more than just the rules on forcible committal.

Miranda L. was committed from a domestic setting. As in wartime and in the GDR, however, committals from hospitals were common in the FRG as well. This included those against the patient's will, such as the committal of 66-year-old Ludwig M. to the LHA Marburg. Much as in East Germany in the 1950s, the individual case files show that even in the early FRG relatives no longer participated in the committals of older family members in the same way as during the war. As in the GDR, the extremely broad "argument from danger" ceased to appear, and there are many instances of relatives reacting indignantly to committals to a psychiatric institution. In 1953, Ludwig M.

was committed to the LHA from the surgical department of the Marburg university psychiatric clinic.[199] The certificate states:

As agreed by telephone, I am transferring (patient)

He is suffering from acute urinary retention due to a prostate adenoma. Acute state of confusion this evening, tore out his catheter and wishes to walk home. There is an urgent danger that he will harm himself. He stated that he wishes to throw himself in front of a car.

There is also an urgent danger that he will cause damage in the room housing new post-operative patients. While dressing, he fell several times against the bed of a patient who underwent surgery four days ago.

Since there is just one night nurse for the entire clinic, the patient cannot be kept here.[200]

This man was "discharged to his home" two days later "after the symptomatic psychosis had abated, in an orderly condition. Is being collected by his relatives, who are complaining that he was transferred from the surgical ward to this asylum."[201]

Summary: practices of compulsory committal in comparative perspective

At the formal level, the pathways of forcible committal differed greatly in all three systems. While in the Nazi era, they were the responsibility of the police and in the FRG they required a judge's order, in the GDR there was no new legal regulation until 1968. Within West Germany, it is also important to note the regional differences in the implementation of judicial authority.

The routes to committal were directly bound up with the actors involved and their room for maneuver. Although the police were a much more important and powerful actor in compulsory committals in the "Third Reich" than they were later, they did not disappear completely from committal practices in either successor state. In addition to judicial compulsory committal in the FRG, the justice system was decisive in forensic committals under § 42b StGB in all three systems.

Even in the case of judicial and police committals, however, a medical report was required. Doctors thus played an important role in all three systems in every type of committal, whether it involved coercion or not. Yet a sometimes profound shift occurred with respect to which physicians and health care institutions carried out committals. During the war, the public health officers in the health offices were tremendously important. In the GDR, asylum physicians held a much greater position of power than under National Socialism or in the FRG. In the latter, independent physicians were particularly relevant. In all three systems, hospitals functioned as key institutions with respect to both civil and compulsory committals.

Relatives too consistently played a decisive role. Once again, however, we have to be alert to the nuances involved. Even during the war, relatives were not always powerless in the face of forcible committals. On the contrary, they were sometimes able to initiate them themselves, consent to them, or try to prevent them—but not always. Particularly in the case of committals initiated by the police, this depended largely on the position of the patient and their family in society. Lower-class women who had been declared "asocial" were at the mercy of the system if committed due to a venereal disease. But the wartime period also featured the shifting of patients back and forth between institutions in a way that affected both "asocials" and the elderly. In this process, patients sometimes fell through a jurisdictional gap, which could potentially empower their relatives. State authorities were much less involved in committal negotiations in the GDR than in Nazi Germany. The two dictatorial systems differed significantly in this regard. Nowhere were relatives in such a powerful position vis-à-vis sick family members as in East Germany: due to the lack of legal regulations, committals against the patient's will were negotiated by family members and physicians. This negotiation of committals remote from power cannot be accurately grasped with the explanatory models established in the research that conceptualize the SED state as a "dictatorship of limits," let alone as a *durchherrschte Gesellschaft*.[202] It is true that in West Germany, too, despite judicial regulation, relatives were often in a key position with respect to forcible committals, but not to the same extent as in the GDR.

Patients' potential to negotiate their fate was much more limited during the war than in the early GDR or FRG and in all three systems, their position was directly related to that of their relatives. In the context of formal compulsory committals, the patient was the object of negotiations rather than party to them. In the Nazi period, those subject to committal were usually powerless within the police placement process, although this was not necessarily true of their relatives. In East Germany, informal committals against the patient's will made them particularly dependent on their relatives and on physicians. Unlike police committals, however, these cases did not require official authorization of discharge by the authorities. Thus, depending on the constellation at play in a specific case, patients in the GDR were more likely to be in a position to end their asylum stay more rapidly than during the Nazi era. In West Germany, on the other hand, the involvement of the courts in the formal compulsory committal procedure was supposed to give the patient the opportunity to at least express their views to an independent authority. The extent to which this procedure altered patients' position in practice, however, varied greatly. Judges' decisions commonly depended heavily on the two medical opinions that had to be obtained for every judicial compulsory committal in the FRG. These medical opinions, in turn, typically involved intensive questioning of the relatives. In reality, under certain circumstances, an individual could already find themselves in an institution before the judge had made their decision. In all three systems, pragmatic concerns could play a role in committals, be it the interest of a municipality or relatives. But this is especially true of the wartime period, with the danger-based arguments made by both relatives and institutions prominent in this regard. Furthermore, as we saw in the previous chapter, families often tried to avoid state institutions, or patients sought to evade inpatient admissions. What all these points have in common is that committal to an asylum during World War II had little to do with the treatment of illness.

Notes

1 LHA Marburg, Patient file sign. 16K10740F, Statements by mother-in-law, March 15, 1946, LWV Hesse 16.
2 Ibid.
3 Ibid., Statements by the patient, March 15, 1946.
4 On preventive detention, see Schewe, Jörg, *Die Geschichte der Sicherungsverwahrung. Entstehung, Entwicklung und Reform* (Dissertation, Kiel 1999).
5 HPA Eglfing-Haar, Annual Report 1942, AB Upper Bavaria, EH, 7; HPA Eglfing-Haar, Annual Report 1943, AB Upper Bavaria, EH, 8.
6 HPA Eglfing-Haar, Annual Report 1956, AB Upper Bavaria, EH, table 8; for details on the new regulations on forcible committal in the FRG, see the section "Judicial compulsory committal: new regulations and their implementation in the FRG" in this chapter.
7 KA Großschweidnitz, Re: Composition of the Contingent of the Sick 1956, BAB, DQ1/20523; KA Rodewisch, Re: Composition of the Contingent of the Sick 1956, BAB, DQ1/20523. For a text that shows that preventive detention was not abused by the GDR regime as in the Soviet Union, see Süß, *Politisch mißbraucht*.
8 Forcible committals were also possible at Greifswald and Marburg. However, both were geared toward short stays with the aim of rapid recovery, diagnosis, or assessment.
9 See Appendix: Statistical Analysis of the Committal Pathway (categories "health office" and "police"): T12, T27, T40, and T52.
10 HPA Eglfing-Haar, Annual Report 1941, Table: Movement of Patients, AB Upper Bavaria, EH; HPA Eglfing-Haar, Annual Report 1942, Table: Movement of Patients, AB Upper Bavaria, EH; HPA Eglfing-Haar, Annual Report 1943, Table: Movement of Patients, AB Upper Bavaria, EH; HPA Eglfing-Haar, Annual Report 1944/45, Table: Movement of Patients, AB Upper Bavaria, EH; HPA Eglfing-Haar, Annual Report 1946, Table: Movement of Patients, AB Upper Bavaria, EH; HPA Eglfing-Haar, Annual Report 1947, Table: Movement of Patients, AB Upper Bavaria, EH; HPA Eglfing-Haar, Annual Report 1948, Table: Movement of Patients, AB Upper Bavaria, EH; HPA Eglfing-Haar, Annual Report 1949, Table: Movement of Patients, AB Upper Bavaria, EH. On the connection with the new legislation in the FRG and legal uncertainty during the occupation and in the early FRG, as well as on how informative figures on forcible committals are, see the section "Figures on compulsory committals and what they tell us" in this chapter.
11 HPA Eglfing-Haar, Annual Report 1953–59, Table: Movement of Patients, AB Upper Bavaria, EH.
12 Herbert, *Best*, 163ff.; Wagner, *Kriminalisten*, 56ff.
13 See Götz Aly on the possibility of releasing patients earmarked for murder at their relatives' request when they were already in the intermediate institutions en route to the killing centers (*Tötungsanstalten*): Aly, *Belasteten*, 39 and 281.

14 As mentioned in chapter 1, the "Law for the Unification of the Health System" of 1935 established health offices throughout the country. See Süß, "Volkskörper," 36. During World War II, the Health Police was mostly subordinate to the health offices but also formed a subunit of the police at times. In Munich, the Health Police was only integrated into the Municipal Health Office in 1941, having previously been part of the Munich Police Headquarters. See *Münchener Gemeindezeitung*, April 24, 1941, Copy, StdA Munich, 117. On the structure of the Munich Health Office during the war, see Christians, *Amtsgewalt*, 54.
15 Brink, *Grenzen*, 259.
16 See Appendix: Statistical Analysis of the Committal Pathway (categories "health office" and "police"): T11–15.
17 Director HPA Eglfing-Haar, Re: Statement on direct admissions, September 23, 1939, AB Upper Bavaria, EH 604.
18 On the police as an actor in the field of psychiatry during the Nazi era, see Brink, *Grenzen*, 259ff.
19 On the need to evaluate health policy inclusion and exclusion, a phenomenon not originally "Nazi" in character, differently in the context of National Socialism, see Thießen, Malte, "Medizingeschichte in der Erweiterung. Perspektiven für eine Sozial- und Kulturgeschichte der Moderne," AfS 53, 2013, 562.
20 On the demand that old people work as long as possible in order to be useful to the "community," see Möckel, Benjamin, "'Mit 70 Jahren hat kein Mensch das Recht, sich alt zu fühlen.'—Altersdiskurse und Bilder des Alters in der NS-Sozialpolitik," *Österreichische Zeitschrift für Geschichtswissenschaften* 22, 2013, 112–134.
21 Müller, Roland, "Militärpsychiatrie im Zweiten Weltkrieg. Die Reservelazarette III und IV in der Landesheilanstalt," in Peter Sandner et al. (eds.), *Heilbar und nützlich. Ziele und Wege der Psychiatrie in Marburg an der Lahn* (Marburg 2001), 307.
22 Grundmann, Kornelia, "Vom Kaiserreich über die Weimarer Zeit bis zum Nationalsozialismus: Die Landesheilanstalt zur Zeit von Prof. Dr. Jahrmärker (1914–1937)," in Peter Sandner et al. (eds.), *Heilbar und nützlich. Ziele und Wege der Psychiatrie in Marburg an der Lahn* (Marburg 2001), 253.
23 On Marburg, see Müller, "Militärpsychiatrie." Eglfing-Haar also entered into an agreement on the admission of soldiers. In August 1938, a contract was concluded to this end between the "Corps physician, VII Army Corps (local army physician [Wehrkreisarzt]) and the district municipality as proprietor of the Upper Bavarian Sanatorium-Nursing Home of Eglfing-Haar," which provided for the admission of psychiatrically ill servicemen. See Contract between VII AK and HPA Eglfing-Haar, August 23, 1938, AB Upper Bavaria, EH 604.
24 Berger, Georg, *Die Beratenden Psychiater des deutschen Heeres während des Zweiten Weltkrieges* (Freiburg 1997), 145.
25 Special agreement between HPA Untergöltzsch and Reserve Hospital 706/15, March 22, 1945, Copy, HPA Untergöltzsch, Patient file sign. 9683, SächSta Chemnitz, 32810.
26 HPA Untergöltzsch, Patient file sign. 9704, Medical record, Tapian Field Hospital, November 9, 1944, SächSta Chemnitz, 32810.
27 To reach more substantial conclusions about this topic one would have to examine systematically a large number of medical records of committed soldiers.
28 Quinkert et al., "Einleitung," 20.
29 Goltermann, *Gesellschaft*, 167.
30 Ibid., 183.
31 See for example HPA Untergöltzsch, Patient file sign. 8704, Report by Medical Officer, Eglfing-Haar Reserve Hospital, October 5, 1942, SächSta Chemnitz, 32810.

32 Müller, "Militärpsychiatrie," 306.
33 In these cases, the procedure for discharge from military service provided for mandatory discharge to a sanatorium-nursing home. See Berger, *Beratenden Psychiater*, 145.
34 Ibid., 145 f.
35 HPA Untergöltzsch, Patient file sign. 8704, Report by medical officer, Eglfing-Haar Reserve Hospital, October 5, 1942, SächSta Chemnitz, 32810.
36 Ibid., Medical certificate, June 5, 1943. In the sample taken for this book, there are only four comparable cases in which the patient was discharged from military service due to endogenous psychosis but was then committed by relatives on the "home front."
37 Gründler, *Armut und Wahnsinn*, 119ff.
38 Möckel, "Altersdiskurse," 119ff; Schwoch, Rebecka, "'... leider muss ich feststellen, dass man mich hier abgestellt hat.' Alte Menschen in den Wittenauer Heilstätten 1945 und 1946," in Thomas Beddies and Andrea Dörris (eds.), *Die Patienten der Wittenauer Heilstätten in Berlin 1919–1960* (Husum 1999), 462–498; Hahn, Susanne, "Pflegebedürftige alte Menschen im Nationalsozialismus," in Christoph Kopke (ed.), *Medizin und Verbrechen. Festschrift zum 60. Geburtstag von Walter Wuttke* (Ulm 2001), 131.
39 Süß, "Volkskörper," 297ff.
40 On Sachsen, see Hahn, "Pflegebedürftige," 132. On the closure of municipal old people's homes in Munich in 1941, see Christians, *Amtsgewalt*, 278ff.
41 See the evaluation of SD reports in: Aly *Belasteten*, 259ff.
42 Süß, "Volkskörper," 297.
43 The extent to which these war-specific patterns of justification were at the same time Nazi-specific would have to be explored by comparing them to the practice of committal in other wartime societies. Dietmar Süß's comparison of Germany and England at war suggests that the exclusion of older people, as traced in what follows, was indeed specific to National Socialist wartime society. He concludes that race-, class-, and gender-based conflicts were present to a far greater degree than in England. His account, however, addresses generational conflicts only very peripherally. Süß, Dietmar, *Tod aus der Luft. Kriegsgesellschaft und Luftkrieg in Deutschland und England* (Munich 2011), 331 and 346 f.
44 Overall, there were major regional differences between 1941 and 1945. Both the transfers and the decentralized murder of the sick depended on local and regional decision-makers. See Süß, "Volkskörper," 320ff. and 340ff.
45 Appendix: Statistical Analysis of the Committal Pathway: T7.
46 Ibid: T8.
47 Admissions by age were divided into four groups: 16–30, 31–45, 46–60, and over 60. In the 1946–49 period, the over-60 category was the second largest, and between 1941 and 1945 it was the third largest, but also accounted for between 15 and 20 percent of new arrivals. See HPA Eglfing-Haar, Annual Report 1941, Table: Movement of Patients, AB Upper Bavaria, EH; HPA Eglfing-Haar, Annual Report 1942, Table: Movement of Patients, AB Upper Bavaria, EH; HPA Eglfing-Haar, Annual Report 1943, Table: Movement of Patients, AB Upper Bavaria, EH; HPA Eglfing-Haar, Annual Report 1944/45, Table: Movement of Patients, AB Upper Bavaria, EH; HPA Eglfing-Haar, Annual Report 1946, Table: Movement of Patients, AB Upper Bavaria, EH; HPA Eglfing-Haar, Annual Report 1947, Table: Movement of Patients, AB Upper Bavaria, EH; HPA Eglfing-Haar, Annual Report 1948, Table: Movement of Patients, AB Upper Bavaria, EH; HPA Eglfing-Haar, Annual Report 1949, Table: Movement of Patients, AB Upper Bavaria, EH.
48 See Christians, *Amtsgewalt*, 278ff.

49 At Untergöltzsch/Rodewisch, for example, 14 percent of committals were by non-psychiatric hospitals during the war; the figure was 10 percent between the end of the war and 1949, and 25 percent between 1950 and 1955. At Großschweidnitz, 17 percent of committals were referrals from a hospital between 1956 and 1963. For figures on all the institutions considered in this book, see Appendix: Statistical Analysis of the Committal Pathway: T11–15, T26–30, T39–42, and T51–54.

50 For example, in early 1944, the deputy medical officer in Leipzig reported to the Saxon Ministry of the Interior 111 nursing cases "that were clogging up the hospitals." Quoted in Hahn, "Pflegebedürftige," 136.

51 HPA Eglfing-Haar, Patient file sign. 6212, AB Upper Bavaria, EH.

52 Ibid., PsychN Munich, Entry in medical record, December 18, 1940, Copy.

53 The daily rate for sanatorium-nursing homes was lower than that for hospitals throughout the period studied in this book.

54 In this context, it should be noted that non-action is also the result of a decision with consequences. See Reemtsma, Jan Philipp, "Über den Begriff 'Handlungsspielräume,'" *Mittelweg* 36, 3, 2004, 6.

55 It is, therefore, impossible to judge to what extent these might have been morally questionable.

56 HPA Eglfing-Haar, Patient file sign. 6528, AB Upper Bavaria, EH.

57 Ibid., Letter, September 15, 1942.

58 LHA Marburg, Patient file prov. sign. 9903 F, LWV Hesse, 16.

59 On blackouts and getting to the air-raid shelter, see for example HPA Eglfing-Haar, Patient file sign. 2933, AB Upper Bavaria, EH; HPA Eglfing-Haar, Patient file sign. 778, AB Upper Bavaria, EH.

60 KA Rodewisch, Patient file sign. 1737, Letter from guardian, July 13, 1944, SächSta Chemnitz, 32810.

61 Ibid.

62 HPA Untergöltzsch, Patient file sign. 10857, SächSta Chemnitz, 32810.

63 HPA Untergöltzsch, Patient file sign. 10857, Letter [n. d., late 1940] SächSta Chemnitz, 32810.

64 HPA Eglfing-Haar, Patient file sign. 4988, Entry, May 25, 1943, AB Upper Bavaria, EH.

65 Generally, whether those making the argument from danger believed it or were making a purely strategic move cannot be determined in light of the available sources.

66 On Eglfing-Haar director Pfannmüller's interest in short clinic stays and efficient use of the asylums in connection with patients' labor, see, for example, Aly, *Belasteten*, 197.

67 HPA Eglfing-Haar, Patient file sign. 6212, Certificate issued by Health Office, December 6, 1940, Copy, AB Upper Bavaria, EH.

68 Ibid., Entry, December 18, 1940.

69 For a general account of young families and armament workers as "winners of the war" in contrast to older people, see Süß, "Volkskörper," 292ff.

70 As a parallel to this, on the way wartime necessities shaped the health system, see ibid., 41 and 275ff.

71 Paradoxically, there were still talks at the official level in the summer of 1944 about a planned division of sanatorium-nursing homes into "quartering" institutions and sanatoriums. Ibid., 309.

72 On the professionalization of psychiatry in Germany, see esp. Kaufmann, *Aufklärung*; Engstrom, *Psychiatry*; Lengwiler, "Sozialtechnologie"; on the outsourcing of old age in the Weimar Republic from families to institutions, see Schwoch, "Alte Menschen," 464ff.

73 The Brandt Campaign mainly served to create special hospitals for the treatment of injured soldiers and "national comrades" (*Volksgenossen*), by requiring, for example, old people's homes and psychiatric facilities to make some of their beds available. Although this campaign was probably not an attempt to continue the murder of the sick, it did much to worsen patients' lot in the asylums. On the Brandt Campaign, see for example Süß, "Volkskörper," 76ff.

74 Appendix: Further Statistical Analyses: T56.

75 On the reasons for the decrease in forcible committals, see the section "Unregulated spaces: the new power of doctors and relatives in the GDR" in this chapter.

76 HPA Eglfing-Haar, Annual Report 1941, AB Upper Bavaria, EH, 7; HPA Eglfing-Haar, Annual Report 1942, AB Upper Bavaria, EH, 7; HPA Eglfing-Haar, Annual Report 1943, AB Upper Bavaria, EH, 8; HPA Eglfing-Haar, Annual Report 1944/45, AB Upper Bavaria, EH, 8; HPA Eglfing-Haar, Annual Report 1946, AB Upper Bavaria, EH, 8; HPA Eglfing-Haar, Annual Report 1947, AB Upper Bavaria, EH, 8; HPA Eglfing-Haar, Annual Report 1948, AB Upper Bavaria, EH, 7; HPA Eglfing-Haar, Annual Report 1949, AB Upper Bavaria, EH, 8.

77 Throughout the 1950s, it remained the case that men were committed "on grounds of danger" about twice as often as women. However, new rules on compulsory committal came into force in Bavaria in 1952.

78 Ayaß, *"Asoziale,"* 186ff.

79 Ibid., 187.

80 Ibid., 136.

81 HPA Eglfing-Haar, Patient file sign. EH 10389, Entry, April 2, 1944, AB Upper Bavaria, EH. The reasoning of the social milieu in such cases is analyzed in chapter 5 in the section "At the threshold: work and institutionalization, 1941–1963."

82 See for example Lindner, "Traditionen," 222; Steinbacher, Sybille, *Wie der Sex nach Deutschland kam. Der Kampf um Sittlichkeit und Anstand in der frühen Bundesrepublik* (Munich 2011), 86.

83 Lindner, *Gesundheitspolitik*, 298.

84 On compulsory treatment and the reporting of venereal diseases before and after the Nazi era, see Lindner, "Traditionen," 222ff.

85 HPA Eglfing-Haar, Patient file sign. 6250, AB Upper Bavaria, EH (original emphasis).

86 Eberle, *Sozial-Asozial*, 212.

87 As in the demand for sterilization of so-called "asocials" due to the excessive sexual activity and degeneracy attributed to them. See for example the speech by the head of the Office of Racial Policy (Rassenpolitisches Amt), Dr. Walter Groß, at a rally organized by that institution's Oberdonau branch in Linz on March 14, 1940, reprinted in Ayaß, *Gemeinschaftsfremde*, 242–244.

88 Althammer, Beate, "Pathologische Vagabunden. Psychiatrische Grenzziehungen um 1900," GG 3, 2013, 307.

89 HPA Untergöltzsch, Patient file sign. 1851, SächSta Chemnitz, 32810.

90 Ibid., Health Office certificate, March 1940.

91 Götz Aly contends that the two words were used to mean the same thing: Aly, *Belasteten*, 217.

92 On the municipal level, which is particularly relevant in the present book, see Gotto, Bernhard, *Nationalsozialistische Kommunalpolitik. Administrative Normalität und Systemstabilisierung durch die Augsburger Stadtverwaltung 1933–1945* (Munich 2009).

93 See Christians' account of the establishment of a "central assembly point for currently ill people" in Munich: Christians, *Amtsgewalt*, 59ff.

94 HPA Untergöltzsch, Patient file sign. 1423, SächSta Chemnitz, 32810.

95 Ibid., Entry, March 16. 1945.

96 Ibid., Letter, March 17, 1945.

97 PsychN Greifswald, Patient file prov. sign. 1944/871, UA Greifswald, PsychN.

98 Ibid., Entry, April 17, 1944.

99 A girl or unmarried woman below the age of twenty-five enlisted in the Nazis' so-called Duty Year program, who was required to work for a nominal fee for a family with a large number of children or in an agricultural enterprise.

100 Ibid., Entry, March 20, 1944.

101 Ibid., Doctor's letter, May 2, 1944.

102 vBS Bethel, Patient file sign. 32/41, HAB, Patient files Mahamain I.

103 Ibid., Entries, January and February 1942.

104 Ibid., Letter, August 15, 1942 to Public Health Officer, Tecklenburg State Health Office.

105 Ibid., Letter (n.d.).

106 Ibid., Letter, August 28, 1942.

107 Ibid., Letter, August 10, 1942.

108 Lüdtke, Alf, "'Fehlgreifen in der Wahl der Mittel.' Optionen im Alltag militärischen Handelns," *Mittelweg* 36, 12, 2003, no. 1, 61–75.

109 Ayaß, *"Asoziale,"* 13.

110 Dietmar Süß identified a similar phenomenon in discussions of access to bunkers, which included calls for working people to be given priority over mothers. Süß, *Tod*, 347.

111 Kundrus, Birthe, "Der Holocaust. Die 'Volksgemeinschaft' als Verb-rechensgemeinschaft?" in Hans-Ulrich Thamer and Simone Erpel (eds.), *Hitler und die Deutschen. Volksgemeinschaft und Verbrechen* (Berlin 2010), 135.

112 Appendix: Statistical Analysis of the Committal Pathway (categories "health office" and "police"): T11–15, T26–30, T39–42, and T51–54. On the relationship between civil and forcible committals, see also section 1 in the previous chapter.

113 LHA Marburg, Patient file sign. K10563M, LWV Hesse, 16.

114 KA Rodewisch, Patient file sign. 5451, Letter from Dr. K. to father of patient, December 10, 1953, SächSta Chemnitz, 32810.

115 Hanrath, *Euthanasie und Psychiatriereform*, 351ff.

116 Ibid., 360 f.

117 The administrative reform of 1952 created two types of local area physician (*Bezirksarzt* and *Kreisarzt*). See ibid., 355.

118 Ibid., 363.

119 Appendix: Statistical Analysis of the Committal Pathway (categories "health office" and "Police"): T12, T27, T40, and T52.

120 KA Rodewisch, Letter to MfG, August 25, 1959, BAB, DQ1/22108, fol. 2.

121 This is true of the Großschweidnitz asylum, which is also examined in this book.

122 KA Rodewisch, Letter to MfG, August 25, 1959, BAB, DQ1/22108, fol. 3.

123 On the establishment in law of physicians' demands, see Hanrath, *Euthanasie und Psychiatriereform*, 360ff.

124 This is not to say that there was no such intervention at all, nor that there were no individual cases of political abuse. On the discussion of political abuse of psychiatric institutions following the publication of Sonja Süß's work, see Weinberger, Friedrich, "Schizophrenie ohne Symptome? Zum systematischen Mißbrauch der Psychiatrie in der DDR," *Zeitschrift des Forschungsverbundes SED-Staat* 25, 2009, 120–132. However, none of the cases cited in the latter

publication occurred during the period investigated in this book; Süß, *Politisch mißbraucht.*

125 See for example Lindenberger, "Herrschaft"; Sabrow, Martin, "Sozialismus als Sinnwelt. Diktatorische Herrschaft in kulturhistorischer Perspektive," *Potsdamer Bulletin für Zeithistorische Studien* 40/41, 2007, 14ff; Lindenberger, Thomas, "In den Grenzen der Diktatur. Die DDR als Gegenstand von 'Gesellschaftsgeschichte,'" in Rainer Eppelmann et al. (eds.), *Bilanz und Perspektiven der DDR-Forschung* (Paderborn 2003), 239–245.

126 See Lindenberger, "Herrschaft." The space between these limits, however, is surprisingly large and relates to an important issue of security that had already come under the jurisdiction of the executive. In principle, moreover, compulsory committal was a sphere accessible to the state. Yet until 1968 the state made little or no effort to impose its will on this realm and even in the new regulations on compulsory committal physicians continued to play the pivotal role, as Sabine Hanrath has shown. See Hanrath, *Euthanasie und Psychiatriereform*, 359ff.

127 Hanrath explains the vacuum of rules, which was not filled by state intervention and made this room for maneuver possible, with reference to the strong position of psychiatrists, who were able to assert their interests in the GDR to a greater degree than in the FRG. Hanrath does not explain the regulatory vacuum *per se*—beyond reconstructing the long-running struggle between physicians and politicians. See ibid.

128 Ibid.

129 Kocka, "Gesellschaft"; Lüdtke, "Helden," 188.

130 The practice of committal suggests that areas of life not amenable to structuring and organization cannot be fully captured by the interpretive models established in the research.

131 Lindenberger, "Diktatur der Grenzen," 244.

132 Indirectly, the practice of committals was shaped by GDR-specific framework conditions, as shown in the previous chapter, such as the institution of the polyclinic and the transfer of authority over asylums to the district level, along with the systematic underfunding this entailed.

133 Hanrath, *Euthanasie und Psychiatriereform*, 359.

134 Such questions have been raised with respect to many aspects of the GDR since the 1990s, such as collectivization and the allocation of land to so-called "new farmers" (*Neubauer*), work experiences in state-owned enterprises, and young people's confrontations with the SED state. Bauerkämper, Arnd, *Ländliche Gesellschaft in der kommunistischen Diktatur. Zwangsmodernisierung und Tradition in Brandenburg 1945–1963* (Cologne 2002); Wierling, Dorothee, *Geboren im Jahr Eins. Der Geburtsjahrgang 1949—Versuch einer Kollektivbiographie* (Berlin 2002); Lüdtke, "People." These studies were initially inspired by the disputes between Sigrid Meuschel and Ralph Jessen: Meuschel, Sigrid, "Überlegungen zu einer Herrschafts- und Gesellschaftsgeschichte der DDR," GG 1, 1993, 5–14; Jessen, Ralph, "Die Gesellschaft im Staatssozialismus. Probleme einer Sozialgeschichte der DDR," GG 1, 1995, 96–110; for a retrospective summary, see Lindenberger, "Diktatur der Grenzen."

135 On the significance of egalitarianism to everyday worlds of meaning under socialism, see Sabrow, "Sozialismus," 18.

136 See Chapter 5, "Work and Performance."

137 KA Großschweidnitz, Patient file sign. 2741, HSta Dresden, 10822.

138 Ibid., Medical record entries relating to admissions in 1947, 1949, and 1953.

139 Ibid., Entry in the medical record, May 6, 1947.

140 Ibid., Entry, August 2, 1953.

141 KA Rodewisch, Patient file sign. 4833, Letter from Local Council, August 31, 1951, SächSta Chemnitz, 32810.
142 Ibid., Letter from head of department, September 19, 1951.
143 Ibid., Letter from Local Council, August 31, 1951.
144 Ibid., Letter from head of department, September 19, 1951.
145 On physicians' awareness of this multifunctionality and their self-reflection on their role, see the following chapter, "Disease and Diagnostics."
146 See for example KA Rodewisch, Patient file sign. 5174, Entry, August 1, 1947, SächSta Chemnitz, 32810.
147 For more detail, see Chapter 2, Section 2, "Committal practices in a 'society in a state of collapse' (*Zusammenbruchgesellschaft*) (1945–1949)."
148 Patient file prov. sign. 1952/1312, Entry, May 23, 1952, UA Greifswald, PsychN.
149 Ibid.
150 KA Rodewisch, Patient file sign. 4772, Entry, September 15, 1953, SächSta Chemnitz, 32810.
151 KA Rodewisch, Patient file sign. 10157, Entry, April 2, 1955, SächSta Chemnitz, 32810.
152 Ibid., Letter from son, March 4, 1955.
153 North Rhine-Westphalia is not the focus here, as the asylum examined in that state in the present book is confessional in character, which means it was not responsible for state care. Forcible committals by the authorities to that facility were, therefore, few and far between.
154 Brink, *Grenzen*, 376ff.
155 This 10 percent includes both preventive detention committals and judicial committals under the new Placement Act.
156 Appendix: Statistical Analysis of the Committal Pathway: T53.
157 At the same time, a comparatively much smaller proportion of patients was committed under Sec. 81 and Sec. 126 of the Code of Criminal Procedure. See HPA Eglfing-Haar, Annual Report 1941, Table: Movement of Patients, AB Upper Bavaria, EH; HPA Eglfing-Haar, Annual Report 1942, Table: Movement of Patients, AB Upper Bavaria, EH; HPA Eglfing-Haar, Annual Report 1943, Table: Movement of Patients, AB Upper Bavaria, EH; HPA Eglfing-Haar, Annual Report 1944/45, Table: Movement of Patients, AB Upper Bavaria.
158 Brink, *Grenzen*, 385 and 401.
159 Ibid., 401.
160 See http://www.bundestag.de/bundestag/aufgaben/rechtsgrundlagen/grundgesetz/gg_09.html (accessed November 14, 2013).
161 Neither the antecedent discussions nor the law itself referred specifically to placement in psychiatric institutions. The federal law met the demand for the involvement of a judge made in Art. 104 of the Basic Law.
162 Brink, *Grenzen*, 389.
163 Hanrath, *Euthanasie und Psychiatriereform*, 269 f.
164 Brink, *Grenzen*, 390.
165 The 1952 laws were the first at *Länder* level, the last of which came into force in 1958.
166 Baumann, Jürgen, *Unterbringungsrecht und systematischer und synoptischer Kommentar zu den Unterbringungsgesetzen der Länder* (Tübingen 1966), 216–220.
167 Ibid., 216.
168 Ibid., 218.
169 Voßkuhle, Andreas, "Der Gefahrenbegriff im Polizei- und Ordnungsrecht," *Juristische Schulung* 10, 2007, 908–910.
170 Baumann, *Unterbringungsrecht*, 219.
171 Ibid., 193.

172 Ibid., 109.
173 Ibid., 110.
174 Ibid., 114.
175 Scholars disagree, however, on whether this ultimately had more advantages or disadvantages in practice for those subject to placement. It is possible that long-term placements were quickly ordered to avoid having to discharge an individual again immediately. Ibid., 116.
176 German County Association, Letter to BMI, Re: Isolation of infected persons and placement of the mentally ill—implementation of Art. 104 GG, 1949–1955, BAK, B 142/1017, 21.
177 On Bavarian welfare practice, see Eberle, "Sozial-Asozial"; Stockdreher, "Heil- und Pflegeanstalt," 344ff.
178 SMI, Order, March 9, 1949, BayHStA, Minn. 80911, 1.
179 HPA Eglfing-Haar, Annual Report 1941, Table: Movement of Patients, AB Upper Bavaria, EH; HPA Eglfing-Haar, Annual Report 1942, Table: Movement of Patients, AB Upper Bavaria, EH; HPA Eglfing-Haar, Annual Report 1943, Table: Movement of Patients, AB Upper Bavaria, EH; HPA Eglfing-Haar, Annual Report 1944/45, Table: Movement of Patients, AB Upper Bavaria, EH; HPA Eglfing-Haar, Annual Report 1946, Table: Movement of Patients, AB Upper Bavaria, EH; HPA Eglfing-Haar, Annual Report 1947, Table: Movement of Patients, AB Upper Bavaria, EH; HPA Eglfing-Haar, Annual Report 1948, Table: Movement of Patients, AB Upper Bavaria, EH; HPA Eglfing-Haar, Annual Report 1949, Table: Movement of Patients, AB Upper Bavaria, EH.
180 The reference here is to committals under Sec. 126a of the Code of Criminal Procedure.
181 SMI, Order, March 9, 1949, BayHStA, Minn. 80911, 2.
182 Ibid., 3.
183 Ibid.
184 This was possible through a combination of § 646 (2) ZPO and § 656 ZPO; see ibid. The combination of incapacitation and committal thus became, on the whole, a more frequently used mode of committal in the FRG. See Brink, *Grenzen*, 398.
185 After the new Bavarian Detaining Act, which regulated judicial placement, came into force, Eglfing-Haar's annual reports show a marked increase in forcible committals from 1953 onward. 387 judicial committals were already carried out in 1953—and this does not include forensic committals. This is a significant increase from the low point of compulsory committals in 1949, when the debate on this practice began. In that year, a total of 48 persons were forcibly committed. HPA Eglfing-Haar, Annual reports 1949 to 1953, Table: Movement of Patients, AB Upper Bavaria, EH.
186 Hesse MdI, *Staatsanzeigen für das Land Hessen* 45, November 5, 1955, BAK, B 106/36773.
187 Ibid.
188 Ibid.
189 *Deutsches Verwaltungsblatt*, vol. 69, no. 20, October 15, 1954, BAK, B 106/36773, 663ff.
190 The committal of incapacitated patients was the responsibility of the guardian in all three systems. For a long time, however, these cases were not treated as compulsory committals in any of the three systems, since these were understood to mean compulsory committals by the authorities. In the period up to 1963, this changed only in the FRG. See *Deutsches Verwaltungsblatt*, vol. 69, no. 20, October 15, 1954, BAK, B 106/36773, 663ff. On the GDR, see 7th Decree on Committal, Admission and Discharge at Psychiatric Hospitals and Nursing

Facilities, BAB DQ1/6486; on the Nazi period, see Lange, Johannes, *Kurz gefasstes Lehrbuch der Psychiatrie* (Leipzig 1936), 257.
191 Brink, *Grenzen*, 399.
192 *Deutsches Verwaltungsblatt*, vol. 69, no. 20, October 15, 1954, BAK, B 106/36773, 663ff.
193 Ibid.
194 Brink, *Grenzen*, 396.
195 LHA Marburg, Patient file sign. K12962F, LWV Hesse, 16.
196 Ibid., Admission, April 10, 1952.
197 In such cases, the court order was sometimes obtained by telephone.
198 Compulsory committals were carried out by a number of different district courts, so we are dealing here with the practices of more than one court. However, it is possible that there were regional differences that would become visible only through evaluation of medical records in other parts of the FRG.
199 LHA Marburg, Patient file sign. K12091M, LWV Hesse, 16.
200 Ibid., Referral, June 3, 1953.
201 Ibid., Entry, June 5, 1953.
202 See for example Lindenberger, "Diktatur der Grenzen"; on the older model of the *durchherrschte Gesellschaft*, see Kocka, "Gesellschaft," and Lüdtke, "Helden," 188.

4 Disease and diagnostics

Medical aspects of committal

It was by no means only (mental) illnesses that were negotiated at the threshold of the asylum. Still, across political systems, committal remained tied to attributions of illness. It is true that during the Nazi era, one of the key grounds for committal was clearly distinguished from illness in the shape of "endangerment."[1] Yet all those committed received a diagnosis once in the asylum or clinic, if not before. In the case of Martina R., admitted to the Marburg Land Sanatorium in March 1946 after a fit of rage, the diagnosis was "reactive depression."[2] The asylum thus added specificity to the findings of the committing physician, who had diagnosed a "depressive mood disorder" (*depressiver Verstimmungszustand*).[3] This difference between the diagnosis underpinning committal and that provided in the asylum itself is typical. The doctor's certificate essentially described the condition, while the asylum physicians added the adjective "reactive" and thus a cause: Martina R. was suffering from a depression triggered by external circumstances. The obverse diagnosis would be "endogenous depression," with endogenous illnesses being conceptualized as somatic and fated to occur. The extent to which Martina R.'s symptoms were assessed as reactive is illustrated by the summary of her illness on the day of discharge:

> This was a reactive depression in connection with her lying-in [postpartum confinement], triggered by burdensome situational problems and complicated by constant tensions with her husband's family (mother-in-law, daughter-in-law).[4]

Two key aspects emerge in this description. First, depression is associated with a gender-specific physical event, namely, childbirth and "lying-in" (*Wochenbett*). This was often the case for female patients. Second, the description incorporated elements of the patient's narrative. Family problems, which both the patient and her mother-in-law had mentioned at the asylum, served as evidence of the medical assessment. Such congruence was by no means always present; the interpretations of illness put forward by physicians and laypersons could differ fundamentally. From the laypersons' point of view, asylum committals could in fact revolve around aspects far

DOI: 10.4324/9781032716237-5

removed from illness, such as threats to self and others or pragmatic considerations. But while the attribution of illness was not always the decisive
criterion for committal, it was ultimately a necessary one. The distinction
between illness and health, then, was pivotal in the practice of committal, but
as such it only arose—and can only be understood—in direct connection with
other factors entailed in constructions of the need for institutionalization.[5]
There could be a substantial temporal gap between the attribution of illness
by laypersons and that of the need for institutionalization by both laypersons
and physicians. A fundamental commonality in lay and medical conceptions
of illness, which may seem trivial at first glance, is that both psychiatrists
and patients, along with the latter's families, not only attributed illness but
classified it in specific ways. Physicians assigned a diagnosis to the patient that
was in accordance with a broader schema of syndromes.[6] Laypersons classified diseases in terms of life paths and life contexts. These two classifications
came into contact in committal practice: they became intertwined, were
partially congruent, coexisted, and were (or were not) subject to discussion.
From the point of committal onward, they formed a nexus that constituted
the admission. The attribution of illness within the committal process, then,
was multi-layered in terms of both time and content. I approach it in this
chapter by first scrutinizing physicians and then laypersons.[7]

During the war, however, the boundary between disease and health
and the assignment of specific diseases occupied a subordinate position in
committal practice in a dual sense. Overall, with the onset of World War II,
"the procurement and securing of medical resources and disease control
superseded 'hereditary and racial cultivation' as the [health system's]
core task."[8] There were also fewer theoretical psychiatric debates during the
war. The journal *Der Nervenarzt* was in fact discontinued in 1943. But even in
decisions on clinic and asylum stays, the issues of diagnosis and treatment
played only a very marginal role in the interaction between physicians and
laypersons—and were even less significant to the police. Diagnostic classifications remained of great importance chiefly when the patient was committed
for a sterilization evaluation.[9] During the war, then, the distinction between
sick and healthy was of little relevance to the vast majority of committals that
were not for evaluation. To put it differently, this distinction was mainly
significant to attempts to avoid asylum stays. It was a distinction that was
subverted in several ways. First, it was undermined by patients' and their
relatives' knowledge of the murder of the sick. As shown in Chapter 2, those
whose illnesses featured in a propaganda film might decide not to stay in an
inpatient facility despite an urgent need for treatment.

Second, the patient's decision to stay in such a facility was usually based on
safety considerations. Here we might recall the case, described in Chapter 2,
of Herbert M.,[10] who was firmly convinced that he would kill himself or his
family if not in an asylum. Relatives too were focused on issues of "safety,"
the limits of the tolerable,[11] and protecting the patient. They tended to
foreground either the option of placing the patient in a private institution, as

evidenced by the unofficial requests for admission to Bethel, or purely pragmatic concerns of broad scope. The latter might revolve around the supervision of elderly relatives under conditions of aerial bombardment, the need for protection from a violent husband, or a homeowner's desire to get a tenant out of their property.

Third, the committing institutions too were primarily concerned with "endangerment" or solving war-related problems of space: women with venereal diseases were committed prophylactically as a "danger" to the "national body," while hospitals used their beds for sick people who were considered useful to the "National Community," such as soldiers.

In both the GDR and the FRG, in contrast to the wartime period, the category of "illness" represented a much-discussed topic both in the psychiatric journals that were beginning to reappear and in the communication between physicians and laypersons with respect to committal decisions. We can thus discern a highly instructive disparity in the use of clinics and asylums in World War II and in the postwar period.

The role of the psychiatrist

By probing the position of the psychiatrist and examining theoretical aspects of diagnostics and diagnostic qualification we can begin to approach physicians as individuals involved in the practice of committal. In journal articles, they reflected on, explained, and legitimized their professional self-image and addressed their relationship with their patients. The field of medical practice encompasses explaining, alleviating, ameliorating or curing illnesses, ordering/classifying them, and making prognoses. When it comes to psychiatry as a field of medical action and knowledge, two special attributes should be borne in mind. First, the young discipline of psychiatry's sometimes heady hopes of healing were shelved as the twentieth century progressed.[12] Second, and directly related to the first point from the physicians' point of view, by the end of the period examined in this book, namely, the 1940s and 1950s, no causes had been found for many psychiatric illnesses. They could not be treated in a targeted, sustained way, let alone cured, because it was not possible to address the cause. Against this background, psychiatrists were left with only two areas of activity: first, alleviation/amelioration/care, and second, the classification and description of clinical pictures, in other words nosology. Under National Socialism, the field of alleviation/amelioration/care was perverted by the murder of patients in the asylums.[13] Since all practices from treatment to murder took place after admission, I do not consider them in this chapter. But the other remaining field of psychiatry, nosology, is directly linked to committal practices. The *sine qua non* for entering an asylum, the attribution of illness, was officially legitimized by the medical diagnosis,[14] with patients receiving this diagnosis in the clinic or asylum at the latest. In most cases, though, this was preceded by a diagnosis provided by the committing physician, and not infrequently several physicians, potentially with differing specialties. Diagnoses can be read as a genuine medical contribution to committals. Committal certificates, on the other hand, often reflect to a greater extent than diagnoses the interaction between the committing physician and the patient's family or the sick person themself. The case of Miranda L.'s committals to the LHA Marburg in the previous chapter comes to mind here, with the committing physician referring to the reasons for committal identified by the family in the certificate.[15]

In what follows, I first ask whether, and if so how and why, the diagnostic classifications used in the event of committal to psychiatric institutions changed (or remained the same) after 1945 and were (or were not) subject to discussion. Here, I focus first on disease names and the diagnostic systems used in the asylum or clinic in general, before going to examine the concept of schizophrenia[16] in more detail. After analyzing theoretical concepts, I turn to the negotiation of diagnoses between various physicians in practice. My goal is to trace the psychiatric debate on a practicable diagnostic system. I do not aim to present the various diagnostic systems and proposals in detail or to analyze and evaluate their content. Instead, I scrutinize when and why diagnostic classifications became subject to discussion in the GDR and FRG as well as whether, and if so how and to what end, local, national, "global," "socialist," or "American" standpoints were invoked and evaluated. Finally, I analyze how psychiatrists and neurologists presented themselves as experts within the debate on the practical application of diagnostic systems.

The relationship between doctor and patient

I turn now to the interaction between physician and patient. My first step here is to evaluate contemporary textbooks' guidance on the psychiatrist's first contact with the patient and instructions on taking their history. I then seek to reconstruct the perspective of the committed and their relatives on the basis of ego-documents. Here, I focus on patients with the psychiatric diagnosis of schizophrenia and the neurological diagnosis of multiple sclerosis. Since the theoretical debate on diagnostics and psychiatrists' self-placement only becomes comprehensible in contradistinction to neurology, it makes sense to consider a neurological diagnosis as well. Schizophrenia and MS seem like excellent candidates in this regard due to three shared traits. Both disorders were first distinguished diagnostically from diseases of old age, schizophrenia from Alzheimer's disease, and MS from Parkinson's disease. Their essential characteristic was thus that symptoms otherwise observed in older people appeared in younger people and resisted classification. This classificatory problem persisted until well into the period under investigation in this book as neither a cause nor treatment options was identified for either diagnosis. Furthermore, both conditions were considered common in their associated medical specialisms.[17] They thus provide us with a useful means of illuminating how physicians and laypersons dealt with "uncertain" diagnoses and limited treatment options.

The psychiatrist as expert: diagnostic classifications and the clinical picture of schizophrenia in the Nazi era and early FRG

The Würzburg Key as a diagnostic scheme in the "Third Reich"

Caesuras in the political sphere and in the history of psychiatry do not necessarily coincide. When it comes to periodization in the history of psychiatry, Benoît Majerus and Volker Hess correctly summarize that "political caesuras do not necessarily fit in with the 'landmarks' in scientific and medical development. To understand mental illness, its treatment and society's contact with it, surely much more decisive developments, given their significance, are: the invention of psychoanalysis around 1900, the advent of biological psychiatry with the formation of neurosciences; the introduction of convulsive shock therapy and the development of new diagnostics in the 1920s and 1930s that produced graphs and images; the psychopharmacological 'revolution' in the mid-1950s; and the de-institutionalization of psychiatry since the 1970s and 1980s."[18] In line with this, asylums changed significantly as a result of the murder of the sick and the Brandt Campaign during World War II, but psychiatric diagnostic classifications did not. The asylums worked with the same diagnostic key as before, and it was not subject to major discussion. Hence, this section only briefly recapitulates the state of affairs during the Nazi period and then focuses on the question of continuities and ruptures in the postwar period. By looking at changes in the latter era, it nevertheless reveals a connection with the Nazi period. In what follows, I explore in detail where we might identify continuities and discontinuities and how we might locate and explain them within the field of tension engendered by the various caesuras in the history of society and medicine. Classification is to the fore here in a dual sense, namely, with respect to both diagnostic classifications and practical diagnostics, which were interconnected in the theoretical debate.

With the exception of the Greifswald University Psychiatric Clinic, all the institutions studied in this book based their diagnoses during World War II on the so-called Würzburg Key.[19] This had been developed, tested, and then recommended for general use by the German Psychiatric Association (Deutscher Verein für Psychiatrie) between 1930 and 1932.[20] Although this recommendation was not binding, this was undoubtedly the definitive classification scheme, which reflected the prevailing medical theories. While the dissemination of this classification system from 1933 onward coincided with the beginning of Nazi rule, it had been developed in advance of it. The scheme comprised 21 numbers,[21] with the organic syndromes occupying 1–15. The larger number of somatic diagnoses reflects the view that these conditions constituted diseases, in other words, the core field of medicine. Only two numbers, 16 and 17, were reserved for psychiatric borderline conditions. The distinction between clinical pictures interpreted as organic and other kinds was fundamental to the understanding of psychiatric conditions: "organic" encompassed all ailments with clearly localizable causes, such as sequelae of meningitis, poisoning, or venereal diseases. Also included were diseases for which a somatic cause was postulated but had (as the discipline saw it) "not yet" been found. These were the so-called "endogenous" psychoses, manic-depressive insanity (number 15), and schizophrenia (number 14). When it came to diseases conceived as organic, including endogenous psychoses, the focus was on the course of the disease.[22]

Fundamentally differentiated from these were "reactive" forms of "abnormal" behavior. These too were divided into two categories: "psychopathic personalities" (number 16) and "abnormal reactions" (number 17). Neither was typically ascribed pathological significance during the Nazi or postwar periods and they were distinguished by their "content" rather than their "form." In his 1936 *Lehrbuch der Geisteskrankheiten* ("Textbook of Mental Illnesses"), Oswald Bumke[23] (1877–1950) described this fundamental distinction within psychiatry. On "organic mental illness," he summarized: "In all these cases, then, the orientation toward the brain is the only possible basis for all scientific work."[24] He distinguished people suffering from "organic" diseases from those

> who appear to us—in a positive or negative sense or even in both—unusual, in other words who are brilliant, notable, gifted or, at the other end of the spectrum, antisocial [*gesellschaftswidrig*] and unfit for life [*lebensuntüchtig*]. (...) These cases [are] connected with health by fluid transitions and they regularly feature a good many quite normal characterstics alongside the unusual ones. These inherited psychophysiological predispositions we call psychopathies (...).[25]

Hence, while it was thought possible for a "normal" person to put themself in the shoes of "psychopaths" on the basis of "fluid transitions," in other words, the content of their thoughts was basically comprehensible, this did not apply to organic mental illnesses; the prevailing view was that the latter could not be described in terms of their content, but only in light of their progression.[26] Psychotherapeutic approaches were thus ruled out *per se* as a means of treating schizophrenia, for example.[27] This shows that the classification and basic understanding of psychiatric diseases were directly related to prognoses and forms of treatment.

The classification and understanding of widely recognized psychiatric disorders were based solely on the postulate that they had somatic underpinnings. Thus, Kurt Kolle[28] (1898–1975) stated in his textbook that while the exact physical basis was known, for example, in the case of paralysis or cerebral arteriosclerosis, "with regard to the overwhelming majority even of those mental illnesses that are undoubtedly contingent upon physical factors, the cause and preconditions are still shrouded in complete darkness."[29] These included the two psychoses of manic-depressive insanity (*Manisch Depressives Irrsein* or MDI) and schizophrenia.[30] Yet Kolle optimistically opined that psychiatry was set fair to become a full-fledged medical discipline in the future.[31] His comparison brings out the sore spot in the self-image of psychiatry, namely, its uncertain status within the field of medicine. This was bound up with psychiatry's unusual emergence as a medical subdiscipline.[32] In his textbook, Kolle went on to explain that modes of knowledge proper to the "humanities"[33] had the same significance in psychiatric diagnostics as chemistry, for example, did in the rest of medicine.[34] But he emphasized that this was only a preliminary state of affairs before psychiatry developed into a more somatic discipline.[35]

The way psychiatrists classified their own profession in connection with their practical diagnostic activity allows us greater insight into their self-image as practicing physicians. This self-image can be traced in more detail for the postwar period, as debates about the use of diagnostic systems and practical diagnostics arose in both successor states—whereas during World War II diagnostic classifications were not a topic of discussion. I seek to show how the presentation, legitimization, and contextualization of diagnostic classifications were related to psychiatrists' self-concepts in the context of both their medical milieu and the political-social situation.[36]

Practice, tradition, and local knowledge: the diagnostics debate in the FRG

In West Germany, the Würzburg Key was replaced as a classificatory system in 1967 by the International Statistical Classification of Diseases and Related Health Problems (ICD) drawn up by the World Health Organization (WHO).[37] Diagnostic classifications had, however, already been discussed and modified locally. Between 1947, when *Der Nervenarzt* appeared for the first time since 1943, and 1963, five articles appeared whose sole subject was a comprehensive diagnostic scheme. One was published in 1948, two in 1959, and two in 1963. It can be assumed that the spate of articles from 1959 onward is no coincidence but was indirectly related to a debate, also gaining momentum in 1959, on an internationally uniform classification of psychiatric diseases. In 1959, British psychiatrist Erwin Stengel (1902–1973) wrote a 60-page paper on the "Classification of Mental Disorders" for the expert committee of the WHO, which was published in the *Bulletin of the World Health Organization* the same year.[38] The core demand set out in this paper, in which Stengel compared numerous national classification systems—including, among many others, the Würzburg Key—was for the use of a standard international scheme. But none of the four articles subsequently published in *Der Nervarzt* referred to this. This means that it is merely an assumption that the topic arose in the FRG as a result of the international debate.[39] What is clear is that, if this was the case, in *Der Nervenarzt* it merely prompted consideration of the issue but did not engender the broad reception or discussion of Stengel's or the WHO's proposals. The problems and suggestions in all five articles moved between the two cornerstones of local and national knowledge.

Five points connect these texts and are instructive with regard to the self-conception and external description of the disciplines of psychiatry and neurology: the significance of local knowledge, the relationship between neurology and psychiatry, the importance of practice and the individual psychiatrist to the discipline of psychiatry, the crucial role of schizophrenia as a clinical picture in overarching diagnostic classifications, and the issue of the relationship between tradition and reform.

None of the five authors referred to international discussions. In fact, four of them took as their starting point a diagnostic system road-tested in their own clinic and proposed its general use. The approach of Richard Jung (1911–1986),[40] a well-known neurologist at the Freiburg University Psychiatric Clinic, who published a proposal for a "neurological-psychiatric diagnostic scheme" in *Der Nervenarzt* in 1948, is exemplary.[41] Unlike psychiatry, in which the Würzburg Key had been used since the early 1930s, neurology did not have a recognized diagnostic system even in the 1950s. Jung lamented this state of affairs and suggested that the system that had proved its value in his clinic should be used generally.[42] He made two main arguments. First, he emphasized its proven practical applicability. His second point was also bound up with this claim: he proposed a common diagnostic system for psychiatric and neurological disorders on the basis that they were treated together in university psychiatric clinics and sanatorium-nursing homes and partly overlapped. The scheme he proposed was an expanded version of the Würzburg Key, into which he incorporated the neurological diseases by adding new numbers (22–50).[43]

In addition to Jung's scheme, another proposal for a new or modified diagnostic system came from a neurologist. Werner Scheid (1909–1987), director of the Cologne university clinic, published the article "Aufbau der Diagnose und Differentialdiagnose in der Neurologie" ("Structure of the diagnosis and differential diagnosis in neurology") in 1959.[44] Much like Jung, he emphasized the nosological and diagnostic acuity and reliability of neurology through a negative comparison with psychiatry:

Psychiatry today is still comparable to a building complex that is partly completed but with important and quite centrally located sections no more than bare brickwork that is accessible only by invisible staircases and is merely provisionally compartmentalized. Wherever psychiatry *has to delineate disease entities on the basis of psychopathological criteria* alone there will be *differing nosological systems,* one of which may be more appealing, clearly structured, or convenient in the context of everyday work than the other. [...] The sister discipline of psychiatry, *neurology*, is *more complete* in this respect. Its diagnoses in no way differ fundamentally from those of, for example, internal medicine, of which neurology is of course a direct offshoot.[45]

The two neurologists thus emphasized the locally bounded nature of psychiatric diagnostic classifications and diagnostic practices. On this view, the diagnoses made in the process of committal to psychiatric institutions depended more on local tradition than in the case of admissions to other kinds of medical facility. Scheid attributed the problematic search for a nosological schema in psychiatry to the fact that this field, unlike neurology, was not a full-fledged, in his words "complete," medical subdiscipline. Its attempts at diagnostic classification, he contended, were open to attack because the disease entities to be classified were themselves controversial. Psychopathological criteria, he believed, were a vaguely defined, makeshift means of constructing clinical pictures. Both Scheid and Jung elaborated on this point in detail. Referring to his own classification system of neurological disorders, Jung suggested categorizing them in light of etiological aspects, in other words their causes.[46] Only if this was not possible should topographical[47] and then symptomatological-descriptive aspects be used for purposes of classification.[48] Scheid articulated a more nuanced view of this problem, concluding that a combination of etiologic and morphologic elements could generate the clearest and most practicable clinical pictures.[49] Thus, for both of them etiology was decisive and they used it to distinguish neurological from psychiatric syndromes in accordance with the two disciplines' potential for diagnostic classification. The causes of many psychiatric diseases were in fact disputed or completely unknown. This applied, for example, to schizophrenia and manic-depressive insanity. In his publication, Scheid underlined that the problem of diagnosis was not theoretical but had consequences for psychiatric practice in the negative sense and for neurological practice in the positive sense:

> With a side glance at our sister science, psychiatry, it can be stated to our relief that the same or at least similar-sounding neurological diagnoses are made everywhere. Furthermore, apart from understandable errors, the individual case will essentially receive the same diagnostic evaluation wherever neurological diagnostics is an established practice. What constitutes a brain tumor or a tabes [dorsalis][50] does not depend on the attitude of the diagnostician.[51]

As mentioned above, psychiatrists classified diseases according to "descriptive-symptomatological criteria,"[52] which highlight the role of the psychiatrist as person in the diagnostic process, an outsize one from the neurologists' point of view. This is emphasized again in the above statement that in neurology the diagnosis does not "depend on the attitude of the diagnostician." At the same time, Scheid underscored that diagnoses often varied greatly because of the special role of the psychiatrist. The idea here was that the psychiatric patient was particularly dependent on an individual physician and on local tradition when it came to the admission diagnosis. For the neurologists Scheid and Jung, it was central to scientifically based diagnoses that they turned out the same everywhere, regardless of the treating physician. Here they were operating within a scientific paradigm that had held sway since the middle of the nineteenth century and whose guiding principle was objectivity without regard for the person involved.[53]

The denigration of psychiatry as a non-somatic and inexact discipline that did not proceed in a medical-scientific way was already familiar to psychiatrists from the preceding decades.[54] Articles published in *Der Nervenarzt* reveal a specific way of dealing with these accusations, namely, by making absolutely no attempt to dispel them. Instead, their authors emphasized psychiatrists' ability to deal with the impossibility of scientific diagnosis as their special form of expert capital. In 1959, the director of the Göttingen University Psychiatric Clinic, Klaus Conrad (1905–1961), a psychiatrist by trade, wrote an article entitled "Das Problem der 'nosologischen Einheit' in der Psychiatrie" ("The problem of 'nosological uniformity' in psychiatry"),[55] which highlighted the difference between "expertise" (*Kennerschaft*) and "science" (*Wissenschaft*).[56] He explained that science is characterized by a "valid theory of causes," whereas expertise is a preliminary stage of science, with psychiatry being an example of this stage.[57] Conrad cited mineralogy as a science and art history as a case of expertise. In mineralogy, he contended, every object can be clearly assigned to a category by measuring certain properties, whereas art history essentially entails a subjective approach.[58] Unlike the articles by the two neurologists, however, this paper valorized psychiatrists' ability to compensate for scientific imprecision as a special skill. It described psychiatric diagnosis as an individual capacity: "Only in light of the coexistence of different symptoms, their successive occurrence, data on the individual and family history, and a wealth of other additional determining factors do we construct the diagnosis."[59]

As in the other two articles by psychiatrists, Conrad used the clinical picture of schizophrenia to illustrate his arguments.[60] The role of the psychiatrist as a person and his or her personal judgment was in fact mentioned in many articles on schizophrenia. In a 1960 paper entitled "Zur Diagnose der Schizophrenie" ("On the diagnosis of schizophrenia"), Giessen-based psychiatrist Richard Kraemer explicitly addressed Conrad's article.[61] Kraemer agreed with his division between science and expertise and his clear classification of psychiatry as a form of the latter. His article, however, reads like a plea against Conrad's concomitant concession that there simply was no sure criterion for diagnosing schizophrenia. Kraemer interpreted the individual physician's expertise, which Conrad too emphasized positively, even more broadly, namely, as a guarantee of reliable diagnosis in practical contexts.[62] Kraemer stated that diagnostic problems hardly ever occurred and that no one would claim "that it is not generally quite possible to distinguish between psychoses and neuroses—merely through expertise. [...] The essential point probably lies in the conception of expertise. Is it not the wellspring of science?"[63] He argued that expertise too features criteria "that are not to be scoffed at."[64] To back this up, he cited Karl Jaspers (1883–1969):[65]

"In his recent Wiesbaden lecture, Jaspers stated that biological insight is by no means exhausted by scientific methods. The method of *Verstehen*-based insight (which foregrounded emotional engagement, particularly empathy, and detailed descriptions), he stated, is a valid means of making sense of things."[66] This reference to Karl Jaspers reflected the prevailing psychiatric doctrine of the 1950s, which took its lead from Kurt Schneider (1887–1967),[67] who in turn drew heavily[68] on Jaspers.[69]

Kraemer went on to elaborate on the potential of *Verstehen*-based insight in the diagnosis of schizophrenic disorders. His focus was on the intuitive recognition of those suffering from schizophrenia, which he called the "praecox feeling"[70:]

> Diagnosis by expertise is closely related to that by intuition—by a feeling (*Gefühl*), or better a sense (*Gespür*). Petrilowitsch[71] has explained that intuition's borders with science can be fluid. Rümke[72] refers to the praecox feeling and what he means by this is a widely recognized experience, though one with which we are familiar more from lectures and observation room [*Wachsaal*] practice, and far less from textbooks. To mention something of this kind scientifically perhaps seemed not quite serious. Yet coming up against a brick wall, that odd, typical, enduring experience of lack of access, of unbridgeable distance, of strangeness, is familiar to every psychiatrist.[73]

According to Kraemer, the diagnostic technique of intuition was rooted in the fact that people suffering from schizophrenia differed from other people in a fundamental way, such that a "healthy person" immediately viewed them as alien. The idea here was that rather than entailing interpersonal relationships and potentially taking a variety of forms, relations between those suffering from schizophrenia or other "mentally ill"[74] people and the healthy were characterized by the impossibility of relationship. As previously indicated, Kraemer's views were certainly in line with the psychiatric mainstream. The term "praecox feeling," introduced by Rümke, built on older descriptions of encounters with people suffering from schizophrenia. In 1925, for example, Kurt Schneider, a particularly widely received author in the postwar period, referred to an "atmosphere" that "envelops one" upon meeting a schizophrenic.[75]

Psychiatrists did not acquire this alleged ability to intuitively diagnose schizophrenia through scientific reading or from textbooks. Kraemer described a form of learning through oral transmission, in lectures, and through practical experience in the observation room. As presented in his article, this is a phenomenon well captured by the term "tacit knowledge" coined by Polanyi.[76] I use that term here—following Harry Collins—to mean "knowledge or abilities that can be passed between scientists by personal contact but cannot be, or have not been, set out or passed on in formulae, diagrams, or verbal descriptions and instructions for action."[77] Practice and daily interaction were considered crucial. Kraemer highlighted the "praecox feeling" to make the diagnosing psychiatrist appear not only equal to the scientist in light of their expertise, but also to stylize psychiatry as a more challenging field than more "scientific" disciplines, such as neurology. On this view, successful psychiatrists were not just implementing specialist knowledge that could be looked up in a book: his article underlined that their diagnostic activity depended on "aptitudes and endowments."[78] Here, the focus was on the individual psychiatrist as a particularly gifted figure. The origin of diagnostic ability was discerned not in learnable scientific knowledge, methods, and practices, but in the nature of the physician. Kraemer thus laments that the pursuit of scientification is leading to a loss of true "experts" among the new generation of psychiatrists: "Often, it is the seasoning of expertise that is just what modern diagnostics lacks; it is characterized by a loss of self-confidence and self-reliance—there are fewer experts than there used to be—and there is always a risk that, rather than prompting efforts to offset it, this loss will turn into the abandonment [of expertise]."[79]

In four steps, I will now locate—and interpret—the styling of the psychiatrist as expert within the contemporary historical context. I begin by briefly introducing the two concepts of scientific self-presentation and knowledge acquisition common in the mid-twentieth century, namely, "scientific objectivity" and "trained judgment" (*geschultes Urteil*). I then argue that the portrayal of the expert cannot be explained solely in light of the scientific status of psychiatry, because in many ways it had yet to achieve that status. Building on this insight, I show that "expertise" shares similarities with the concept of "trained judgment" but differs from it in essential ways. Finally, I probe the function of this specific representation of a medical subdiscipline in terms of its position and remit within society.

In her article "On Scientific Observation," Lorraine Daston points out that the scientist as a person and their intuition always play a role in scientific knowledge acquisition. But whether intuition is viewed positively within a given field and the scientific community or is even discussed depends on long-term trends. While intuition was still regarded as crucial in the early modern period, this changed appreciably with the introduction of measurement methods. From the mid-nineteenth century onward, the ideal of objectivity meant that science should be as detached as possible from individual characteristics.[80] In the monograph *Objectivity* by Daston and Peter Galison, we learn that the ideal of objectivity was deposed though not supplanted entirely by that of trained judgment from the mid-twentieth century onward.[81] Trained judgment is characterized by the "necessity of seeing scientifically through an interpretative eye" and thus represents a vital complement to mechanical procedures.[82]

By emphasizing expertise, Conrad and Kraemer classified psychiatry as pre-scientific, contending that it lacked objective methods. Yet contrary to the claims made in their articles, objectification and measurement had played a role in psychiatry since its professionalization in the final third of the nineteenth century, though they did not supplant non-objectifiable empirical knowledge. Eric Engstrom points out that psychiatric knowledge in asylums, and in the clinics established much later, is based on observation, but on differing kinds of observation. He describes the psychiatric knowledge of the nineteenth century as "essentially empirical, experiential, and asylum-based."[83] Departing from the asylums' practices, university clinics legitimized their observations by adopting methods from somatic medicine. Kraepelin in particular introduced psychophysical measurements redolent of natural scientific precision in their quantification and visualization.[84] Yet the establishment of university psychiatric clinics failed to facilitate the identification of causes or potential cures, so it was of signal importance to psychiatry as a profession that it promote its representatives as experts in the diagnosis and classification of "mental illnesses." In the German Empire, their expertise in attributing and classifying mental disorders was indispensable to the assessment of unsoundness of mind and, above all, played a key role within the new social security system.[85] But as evident in enduring disputes over the training of psychiatrists in university psychiatric clinics and/or asylums, the experiential knowledge gained in asylums remained important as well.[86] In the 1930s, psychiatry underwent another phase of technization, which saw the introduction, for example, of shock therapy.[87]

Psychiatry, then, featured a variety of approaches, some of which were avowedly intuitive and some of which entailed the attempt to achieve objectivity. Nevertheless, in the 1950s, psychiatrists responded to frequent accusations that psychiatry was not an exact science not with reference to measurement, quantification, or technical treatment methods but by styling themselves as "experts" rather than scientists.[88]

A brief look at neurology demonstrates that presenting oneself as an expert was not the only viable way of dealing with uncertain diagnoses. Neurologists portrayed themselves in an entirely different way in their articles. This is not, as asserted in Jung's and Scheid's articles, because neurology was devoid of diagnostic problems and produced the same diagnoses everywhere. In fact, almost every issue of the *Der Nervenarzt* contained one article and sometimes several articles on trigeminal neuralgia[89] or multiple sclerosis, a deluge of texts reflecting the fact that neither a cause nor a successful treatment method could be found for either neurological phenomenon, both of which were considered difficult to diagnose. Thus, for psychiatry and neurology, the point of departure was similar, even if there were fewer "uncertain" disease entities in the latter. Significant to the two disciplines' self-image is the fact that neurologists and psychiatrists had pursued a completely different approach to diagnostic uncertainty. In their articles in *Der Nervenarzt*, psychiatrists not only admitted that many clinical pictures could not be diagnosed scientifically but also presented this as a hurdle that the discipline had managed to overcome. Meanwhile, the much-discussed conditions of trigeminal neuralgia and MS played no role in neurologists' general reflections on diagnostics. The longstanding search for a diagnosis for MS, for example, was not addressed at all in the more general neurology articles. Neurology presented itself as a medical science in no way different from any other branch of natural science.[90]

Yet going by the narrative in the psychiatrists' articles discussed above, their expertise was not trained judgment in the true sense of the term, but rather an emotion- and character-based form of judgment. Kraemer explicitly underscored that experience played only a very minor role: "Experience is required only to a limited extent and tends to add little. There is no appreciable development. The feeling arises anew each time and with the same force. The youngest assistant and the oldest senior [psychiatrist] are equally subject to it. There is no assimilation. It is a fact."[91] This exemplifies a self-understanding that was much more widespread in the nineteenth century, according to which the psychiatrist's character played a key role in treatment. According to this venerable conception, one could gain access to the sick by empathizing with them. The person's psychological and emotional experience was imagined as regulated by an "inner core," and it was the strength of the asylum directors' "inner core" that supposedly allowed them to "educate" the sick.[92] Kraemer's intuition is evidently not the same construct. While the nineteenth-century asylum director's strength of character enabled him to empathize with the sick, this empathizing was impossible due to schizophrenic patients' allegedly "alien" character (*Wesensfremdheit*).[93] This impossibility of empathy was in fact seen as an aid to diagnosis. Yet central to both constructs is the personality of the psychiatrist.

We can thus observe tremendous continuity in psychiatrists' self-portrayal as experts. Certain argumentative tropes of the 1940s and 1950s bear a structural resemblance to the traditional self-perceptions of the previous century but had a quite different thrust. Major socio-historical caesuras do little to explain this change. More important are conceptions of illness and their social classification, which remained relevant across these caesuras. Key examples here are, first and foremost, Griesinger's conception of "mental illnesses" as "brain diseases" and, in the case of schizophrenia, Kraepelin's conception of dementia praecox as an endogenous psychosis. Griesinger worked with the idea of a so-called unitary psychosis (*Einheitspsychose*), while Kraepelin differentiated between psychoses, but both assumed a lasting somatic change and their thinking thus clearly differed from earlier conceptions.[94] Psychoses were now considered somatic states, rather than mental states with which one could empathize. In addition, the notion of a "degenerate underclass" and the concept of "psychopathy" were taking root. While "psychopathies" were considered comprehensible, empathy was no longer appropriate from the point when late nineteenth-century psychiatry increasingly began to imagine the "underclass" as a threat.[95] With the establishment of the notion of pension neurosis (*Rentenneurose*) in the 1920s, "psychopathies" were now interpreted merely as cases of misbehavior that required correction.[96] Instead of understanding, the emphasis now was on signposting clear boundaries in order to cure the patient of their desire-based representations (*Begehrvorstellungen*). It was thus impossible to empathize with somatic diseases, while empathy with the psychiatric borderline states known as "psychopathies" was possible but undesirable.

How might we explain the fact that in the 1950s psychiatry strategically foregrounded expertise to counter accusations that the field lacked scientific precision? This proactive approach to diagnostic challenges becomes understandable if we consider the interplay of several factors. Structurally, psychiatry could build on the paradigm of self-portrayal established since its founding phase by emphasizing character and talent. At the same time, this self-representation was consonant with its role in society: this was not the desperate strategy of a discipline still in its founding phase. As we have seen, by now psychiatry enjoyed sweeping interpretive sovereignty over major societal "problems." Ultimately, psychiatrists' diagnostic practices faced no fundamental challenge. They formed the accepted basis for cost-intensive inpatient stays, the granting of pensions, and for establishing unsoundness of mind. As we will see in the remainder of this chapter, moreover, when legitimizing their diagnoses psychiatrists also fell back on practices that, in contrast to their valorization as "experts," were typical of the paradigm of scientific objectivity. It is thus fair to say that intuition-based practice was understood as a form of capital specific to psychiatry.

"Expertise" was a capacity that was also attributed to lay people, at least to some extent. Here, the difference from "trained judgment" comes to the fore. Whereas specific experiential knowledge and training are necessary to the latter—without eliminating the level of intuition—the attribution of psychiatric deviations was based on a feelings-centered appraisal that every "healthy" person was ultimately capable of producing.[97] Expertise thus constituted a basis for the attribution of "mental illness" and for institutionalization common to both psychiatrists and lay people. This perspective harmonized with the fact that clinics and asylums were often dependent on committal decisions made within the patient's social milieu. The major role played by the relatives of those committed in the "Third Reich," FRG, and GDR, emphasized on a number of occasions throughout this book, shows that committals were impossible without an assessment that was—to a certain degree at least—shared by laypersons and medical experts.[98] This was all the more crucial in view of the many different schools of thought on the causes of various psychiatric illnesses. Expertise represented a shared benchmark, an anchor in society.

The construction of expertise, which lay people also possessed in a rudimentary sense, dovetailed with ideas of community that stood in continuity with the Nazi era.[99] Expertise functioned as a means of inclusion and exclusion and facilitated the identification of "the other" within the community. In the case of the "praecox" feeling, a community of healthy people was imagined whose members possessed the ability to recognize non-healthy "schizophrenics." This was a fundamental distinction that, it was believed, was prior to any form of social differentiation—exhibiting parallels with the organic notion of the *Volksgemeinschaft* as a "natural" community.[100] Psychiatrists' self-interpretation as experts is congruent with the picture of the 1950s drawn by Ulrich Herbert, who highlights the widespread critique of the "subordination of the great individual to the masses, to the dictates of bureaucracy, rationalization, and civilization."[101] Expertise as an individual, intuitive achievement beyond rationally justifiable or even describable procedures fits neatly with this picture.

As shown in Chapter 3, "Danger and Security," however, social differentiation as well as gender-specific attributions played an important role in the practice of committals during World War II. The same point is demonstrated in the present chapter, in the section "The relationship between doctor and patient," for the postwar period. References to intuitive "expertise" had a dual role here. They concealed the non-medical aspects inherent in the identification of "mental illness" by attributing to medical laypersons too the ability to sense it. At the same time, in practice this notion of expertise also enabled the negotiation of non-medical issues, as regularly occurred at the threshold of the asylum. This kind of professional attribution of illness, that is, legitimized the powerful role of individual psychiatrists. Free of the justificatory constraints typical of an objectified, discipline-specific epistemic order, they could address the widely varying gender-, class-, and context-specific concerns expressed by lay people. I will discuss the justification of differing diagnoses in more detail in the next section.

Psychiatrists' proactive approach to diagnostic difficulties—in addition to building on traditional self-conceptions and on their practical role—gave psychiatry a singular status. The ability to deal with and classify illnesses that could not be entirely grasped by science was a quality that distinguished psychiatry from other medical subdisciplines. The classification of that which resisted "objective" ascription was a niche successfully occupied by psychiatry in the second half of the twentieth century, a period characterized by scientification in the sense of the embrace of an objectively comprehensible order that imposed meaning on reality.[102] This argumentative strategy worked because it was deployed in a context in which objectivity was accepted as a scientific paradigm. Only against this background could expertise be stylized as an exceptional ability. Yet the emphasis on intuitive judgment was far from outlandish. Scientists' presenting themselves as experts who supplemented objective procedures with trained judgment was an ever more common feature of the mid-twentieth century. Though not every interpretation portrayed expertise as a form of such experience-based judgment, the individual person was always highlighted as crucially important—and here we can see common ground with the idea of trained judgment and a fundamental difference from the paradigm of "objectivity."[103]

Self-representation as an expert echoed older forms of psychiatric self-understanding. In the following, I scrutinize continuities and changes in this regard by taking a closer look at schizophrenia as an individual syndrome.

Continuities and ruptures in diagnoses of schizophrenia in the FRG

The end of World War II did not mark a turning point in debates on the clinical picture of schizophrenia. In the 1950s, discussion of the causes of the disease adhered to the same basic premises that had held sway in the 1940s, the prevailing assumption being that schizophrenia was a heritable somatic disorder. Within this framework, opinions differed as to which forms of schizophrenia were inherited and with what degree of probability.[104] While the hypothesis that schizophrenia was a metabolic disorder was discussed and tested in the 1940s, this ceased to be considered in the late 1950s. Periodic upsurges in somatic explanations influenced the topics that psychiatrists researched and published on. For example, in light of the metabolic hypothesis, cerebrospinal fluid studies were carried out on schizophrenics[105] and the results were published in *Der Nervenarzt*.[106] Consonant with the basic assumption that schizophrenia was an organic disease, successful cases of somatic treatment were published and discussed, with shock therapy being the most common example of this.[107]

The debate on causes was thus subject to continuous change, which essentially reflected medical-technical innovations and did not, in the first instance, mirror the demise of the "Third Reich." This dovetails with the statement made by Hess and Majerus, quoted at the start of this section, that periodization issues in the history of psychiatry do not necessarily coincide with those in general history.[108] Indeed, articles on schizophrenia did not change significantly until the mid-1950s—in direct connection with the introduction of psychotropic drugs. These drugs, however, were not simply presented, discussed, and evaluated as a new treatment method, but helped stake out a new discursive spectrum. The debate on classification systems in the FRG had oscillated between a focus on those tried out at the local level and the aspiration to adopt a uniform psychiatric and neurological schema. From the second half of the 1950s onward, however, articles on schizophrenia also referred to the views of American researchers, which had generally been dismissed in the early 1950s.[109] Psychiatry thus exhibited an attitude toward the United States that ranged between outright hostility and occasional expressions of interest, one that has been identified as typical of West German society as a whole in the 1950s.[110]

During that decade in the United States, one school of thought interpreted schizophrenia psychoanalytically as a disease caused by family circumstances. The roots of this perspective lay chiefly in the work of psychiatrist Adolf Meyer (1866–1950) and that of psychoanalyst Harry Stack Sullivan (1892–1949).[111] Meyer adduced biological and psychological elements in his explanations and emphasized the importance of schizophrenic patients' life course. In sum, he interpreted the condition as an attempt to escape from an everyday life with which the future patient could no longer cope.[112] Inspired by this, Sullivan construed schizophrenia as an interpersonal event, and his focus was on the patient's family. It is significant to the practice of committal, in which the family was usually involved, whether and if so how psychiatrists related the family to the illness and its course. In both North America and Switzerland, the use of psychotherapy to treat schizophrenia was directly linked with psychoanalytic explanations.[113]

The majority of German psychiatrists rejected the views of Meyer and Sullivan out of hand, consonant with the institutional division between psychiatry and psychology in the 1950s.[114] Yet during the second half of that decade, in some cases psychotherapy was embraced as a fruitful form of treatment for schizophrenia despite the ongoing assumption that it was a somatic disorder. This was closely bound up with the potential for treatment with psychotropic drugs. The growing number of articles on the use of these drugs to treat schizophrenia repeatedly underlined that this approach opened up potential for psychotherapeutic methods.[115] Thanks to these new drugs, one did not have to share the premises of American psychoanalysts in order to consider psychotherapy for schizophrenics.

The more far-reaching psychoanalytic ideas at large within American psychiatry were also received. After the Second International Congress of Psychiatry in Zurich in 1957, which focused on schizophrenia, an increasing number of articles on the latter appeared in *Der Nervenarzt*. As mentioned above, all relevant articles in that publication explained the difficulties of psychiatric diagnosis and nosology with reference to the example of schizophrenia. This was not a specifically German trend. Manfred Bleuler (1903–1994), son of Eugen Bleuler (1857–1939), well known for his research on schizophrenia,[116] began his opening address at the Second International Congress of Psychiatry by highlighting the deep disagreement among psychiatrists: "Our congress is not only a daring venture because of the difficulty and importance of the issue at hand. It is daring above all because the nature of schizophrenia is more controversial today than ever before. Every researcher now assesses it in his own way."[117] The cause and treatment of schizophrenia were, he claimed, the key bones of contention.[118] While the search for an appropriate classification system in *Der Nervenarzt* did not refer to international debates until 1963—the international schema was only introduced in 1967—a few articles on schizophrenia did consider the ideas of scholars abroad. The majority of articles, however, failed to discuss such ideas. The prevailing view was that a person was born with a predisposition for schizophrenia, and social factors were not addressed—either as trigger or cause.[119]

The basic distinction between endogenous and reactive psychoses was widely accepted among West German psychiatrists, with most of them following Kurt Schneider (1887–1967) in this regard.[120] On this view, the types of psychosis differed in that endogenous psychoses were characterized by their form and "psychopathies" by their content. In the case of endogenous psychoses—and schizophrenia's placement within this category was undisputed—this meant that the course of the disease was decisive.[121] According to Schneider, who followed Jaspers here, somatically induced psychoses were not amenable to *Verstehen* or understanding. The approaches of Meyer and Sullivan, which were widespread in the United States, thus ran counter to the prevailing conception of schizophrenia and the basic classification of psychiatric abnormalities in West Germany. The use of psychotherapy in combination with psychotropic drugs, conversely, did not represent the same kind of challenge, since it had a completely different meaning and status in the FRG than, for example, in Sullivan's approach.[122]

However, between 1961 and 1963, American research was considered sporadically in *Der Nervenarzt* beyond the topics of psychotropic drugs and psychotherapy. Lutz Rosenkötter, for example, went so far as to describe schizophrenia not as a somatic disease but as a developmental one. This is no great surprise given that Rosenkötter himself was a psychoanalyst. In an attempt to prove his claim, he referred not only to well-known American psychiatrists and psychoanalysts, but also to the stress research carried out by the Canadian Hans Selye (1907–1982).[123] He thus considered both psychological and somatic symptoms, but reversed the causality typically assumed in the FRG. He wrote: "Since Selye's studies on adaptation syndrome, we know that this may well entail somatic reactions to psychological stress rather than psychosis inevitably being the consequence of somatosis."[124] Tellingly, Selye's research on stress garnered little attention in Germany.[125] In his article, Rosenkötter focused on patients' families, and not in the usual way. Most of the time, families were discussed in connection with genetic factors or as suffering due to their relatives' disorders. Rosenkötter's paper, meanwhile, addressed dysfunctional families as potentially causing the illness of a family member.[126] Another article heaped praise on American research. But the author, Helm Stierlin (b. 1926), had himself lived and practiced in the United States since 1957.[127] In addition to these articles, several other essays appeared in *Der Nervenarzt* that highlighted the role of the family in explaining schizophrenia and thus addressed psychotherapy beyond the context of psychotropic drugs. Their authors were all based in Switzerland,[128] where research on schizophrenia was strongly influenced by Eugen Bleuler, a champion of a social-psychological explanatory approach and, therefore, also an advocate of psychological treatment methods.[129] *Der Nervenarzt* certainly provided space for discussions of differing international research findings, but this space went unused by German psychiatrists.

To sum up, we can identify a variety of forms of intellectual transfer in the early FRG. American and Swiss concepts were published in *Der Nervenarzt*, but West German psychiatrists barely addressed them in their publications. Some incorporated psychotherapy as a treatment method while retaining their fundamentally somatic perspective.[130] The lack of discussion of social-psychological explanatory approaches and treatment methods can be read as an example of boundary marking, of negative transfer. Given the focus on schizophrenia at the Second International Congress of Psychiatry, we can assume that the contrasting conclusions reached by different researchers were generally known. The incorporation of psychotherapy as a form of treatment combined with the administration of psychotropic drugs is an example of appropriation and transfer par excellence, a case of the pragmatic weaving of select knowledge stocks into West German psychiatry. Treatment with these drugs functioned here virtually as a catalyst. Absent a revision of their somatic presuppositions, West German psychiatrists would have been far less likely to consider psychotherapeutic treatment without this detour via medication.

If we adopt a comparative perspective with regard to articles published on diagnostic classifications and on the clinical picture of schizophrenia, we find that the nature of transfer varied. While the cross-border topics listed above were addressed in connection with this condition, there was no discussion of international classification attempts, at least not in *Der Nervenarzt*. Psychiatric knowledge thus oscillated between local, national, and international (mostly American, but also British and French) discourses, depending on the specific topic and on the discursive context. With respect to both classificatory schemas and schizophrenia, the evidence shows that psychiatrists' practices and self-image were of exceptional importance. The latter included the portrayal of psychiatry as a form of expertise. Comparison with neurology has revealed that this line of argument cannot be explained solely with reference to factual diagnostic difficulties or illnesses that could not be traced back to a single cause. It must be understood as psychiatrists' well-functioning strategy of styling themselves as experts in phenomena that defied attempts at secure "scientific" classification.

Between tradition, Pavlov, and the WHO: multiple diagnostic classifications and the clinical picture of schizophrenia in the GDR

Medical reactions to diagnostic grids

Diagnostic systems and schizophrenia were also widely discussed in the GDR in the 1950s and early 1960s. The debates there featured some similarities and interconnections with the FRG but differed overall in the greater range of perspectives discussed and the higher degree of change.

The starting point for debate was itself different from that in West Germany. In all the West German institutions examined in this book, diagnoses were made at least with reference to the coding of the Würzburg Key. In contrast, from about 1952 onward, the physicians at Greifswald, Rodewisch, and Großschweidnitz started to use a coding system recently introduced by the Ministry of Health.[131] This was not, however, a dedicated attempt to reclassify psychiatric and neurological conditions, but a numbering system for syndromes in all medical disciplines featuring more than 300 items. At Rodewisch and Greifswald, the new coding system began to be used quite soon after its introduction, with both schemas being deployed in parallel between 1952 and 1954. From about 1954 onward, coding systems in alignment with the Würzburg Key then disappeared from the GDR. However, the new system was unsatisfactory from the physicians' point of view, since psychiatric and neurological diseases were listed unsystematically alongside other diseases.[132] Yet a debate on the best diagnostic system for psychiatric and neurological diseases for use in the GDR took off only in the wake of international discussions.

As in the FRG, the debate on diagnostic classifications in the GDR gained traction from 1959 onward. But in contrast to the situation across the border, East German psychiatrists made explicit reference to Stengel's paper for the WHO, *Classification of Mental Disorders*, and from 1960 onward diagnostic systems were discussed beyond the pages of psychiatric journals. The unit for psychiatry within the Ministry of Health's Department of Health Protection Organization wrote to the clinics to find out which diagnostic system they considered useful, enclosing the various schemes and relevant publications.[133] The Würzburg Key, Stengel's proposal for the WHO, Gilyarovsky's Soviet system, the U.S. DSM, and various systems used at the local level were all up for discussion.[134]

Dr. Steinkopff, chief physician of the psychiatric clinic at the Karl-Marx-Stadt/Chemnitz hospital, attached a prefatory letter to his clinic's statement. His apt conclusion was that achieving international convergence was a daunting task for psychiatry since it was impossible to refer even to "national psychiatry." The most one could assert, he underlined, was the existence of "regional psychiatry."[135] Steinkopff came out in favor of the Würzburg Key of 1931. He contended that this classificatory system, which privileged "organic," "endogenous," and "reactive" elements, "of course [bears] the hallmarks of a specific history of science and is therefore not entirely free of presuppositions. The advantages of its practicability, however, seem to outweigh [any disadvantages]."[136] Unlike in West Germany, use of the 1931 scheme required explanation. But the rationale given dovetailed with an argument that attracted support across the border as well, namely, its practical usefulness.

To what extent did the FRG and GDR still form a common epistemic space toward the end of the 1950s? One clue is the fact that the clinic in Karl-Marx-Stadt used a modified version of the Würzburg Key presented in *Der Nervenarzt*, namely, Jung's diagnostic scheme mentioned above, which incorporated neurological conditions.[137] Steinkopff referred to the journal several times in his remarks. In addition to the relevant article by Jung, Steinkopff mentioned a second piece in *Der Nervenarzt*, namely, Scheid's text,[138] which I addressed earlier in the context of diagnostic classification.[139] Scheid too had emphasized the solid practical value of the long-established schema. Like Jung and Scheid in *Der Nervenarzt*, the physician in

Karl-Marx-Stadt underlined the practical necessity of a classification schema that brought together psychiatric and neurological syndromes in one system. He also mentioned that "to meet our own needs, we have made further small insertions."[140] These insertions related, among other things, to "certain transient disorders of schizophrenic character that involve no tangible defect,"[141] which were classified as "episodic psychoses."[142] This shows how a local diagnostic system from West Germany, published in a psychiatric journal to promote its general use, was taken up in a clinic in East Germany and adapted to local interpretations of illness. It is hard to imagine a more impressive demonstration of the relevance of West German psychiatry and its publications to practice in the GDR. It also underscores the high value placed on local knowledge. The first point of reference for many psychiatrists was in fact their clinic or asylum. When they sought concepts relevant to practice, they either drew directly on their own practical experience or relied on that accrued in other institutions. This comes across clearly in all of the responses to the Ministry of Health's inquiry. Patients and their families could thus be faced with differing attributions of illness depending on the receiving facility. The same applies to physicians when their patients had previously been committed to other asylums or clinics. This local specificity entailed more than a pragmatic adaptation to everyday clinic life. In Steinkopff's department, it encompassed a specific focus on and classification of illnesses. Certain schizophrenic syndromes were categorized in new ways as the system proposed by Jung in *Der Nervenarzt* was adapted to the hospital in Karl-Marx-Stadt in light of the perceived lack of long-term after-effects. The prognosis was thus viewed as crucial. This was by no means new,[143] but the asylum in Karl-Marx-Stadt ascribed such importance to it that it was inserted as a separate point into the diagnostic scheme.[144] Much as in the FRG and as emphasized at the Second International Congress of Psychiatry by M. Bleuler, schizophrenia again proved particularly difficult to classify.

Steinkopff thus read the journal *Der Nervenarzt* published in West Germany and implemented its suggestions at his clinic, illustrating once again the substantive exchange between the two German states in the medical field in the 1950s.[145] More astonishing is the fact that the chief physician of the Karl-Marx-Stadt clinic legitimized the use of his classification scheme in a letter to the GDR Ministry of Health by referring to this West German publication. This underlines the strong position of the medical profession in the early GDR,[146] a point reinforced by Sabine Hanrath's finding that psychiatrists in East Germany, in contrast to the FRG, managed to ensure the legal enshrining of their influence in compulsory committals.[147]

Steinkopff briefly discussed the Soviet and American schemes in his reply to the Ministry of Health. He objected to the Soviet system primarily on the basis that it lacked a division of the causes of illness into predisposition and environment and that it was unworkable in practice.[148] The first point, stated in a single sentence, nevertheless struck at the heart of the Soviet understanding of psychiatry: the distinction between predisposition and environment, so important in the German tradition, did not exist in Gilyarovsky's Soviet system. As a result of the new privileging of the cortex,[149] all psychiatric illnesses were declared disorders of the higher nervous system, rendering this division obsolete. Pavlov had assigned the "conditioned reflexes" so central to Soviet medicine to the cerebral cortex. In his Lamarckian worldview, these reflexes enabled organs to adapt unconditionally to the environment[150]; he thus made a direct link between physiological processes and external living conditions.[151] The cerebral cortex was considered fundamental to humans' behavior within their environment, a doctrine whose exclusive validity was proclaimed at the Pavlov conference of 1952. In Soviet medicine, this marked the beginning of the so-called "dictatorship of the cortex."[152] Steinkopff considered the American scheme too fine-grained and therefore impracticable.[153] His criticism of the Soviet classification system was thus more substantial than that of the American one.

The response from the Karl Marx University clinic in Leipzig to the Ministry of Health's inquiry took a different form, contrasting with that provided by the clinic in Karl-Marx-Stadt even in the basic approach taken. Before responding, the clinic consulted several psychiatrists, seven of whom expressed a positive view of the Soviet system, while four favored that of the World Health Organization, and one preferred the American system.[154] Its director, Prof. Müller-Hegemann, then wrote that he had understood the inquiry to mean that everyone should adapt to the WHO classification scheme if possible. He thought this made sense as a means of ensuring greater international uniformity and argued that "only if the WHO classification system should prove completely unsuitable would it be up for debate whether it would be preferable to use one of the other proposed schemes. Only if one of these should then fail to impress could one discuss whether we should return to the old German classification scheme of 1931 or develop a new one."[155] In his clinic, he stated, the conclusion had thus been reached that the WHO scheme was quite workable if it were adapted with respect to certain points. He then stated without transition that the American classification system was quite unusable; it was, he asserted, considered "wrong in its basic layout" because it distinguished fundamentally between organic and psychogenic triggering factors.[156] Psychosocial explanations were rejected in the Soviet approach just as in the FRG. In both cases, they contradicted the basic premise that psychiatric illnesses were somatic in nature,[157] even if the ideas in the USSR and the Federal Republic about exactly what this meant lay far apart. For all their differences, both rejected psychosocial factors in the etiology of illness. In the socialist interpretation, however, these played a decisive role as triggers.

A third point of view was articulated by Hanns Schwarz, director of the Greifswald University Psychiatric Clinic. He considered international uniformity "almost impossible,"[158] arguing that "ideological issues always shine through" in the discipline of psychiatry.[159] Schwarz expressed a critical view of the American system and was most enthusiastic about the Soviet one.[160]

He concluded that his clinic would try to align itself with the WHO system, but he believed that in reality "Germany" needed a classification system of its own.[161]

The diversity of the responses illustrates the broad spectrum of opinion. In no way did the clinic directors feel compelled to embrace Gilyarovsky's Soviet system or even to present it positively in their statements. In some cases, they assumed that the Ministry of Health was urging them to adopt the WHO system.[162] Each of the classificatory models was identified as the favored option at least once in at least one of the replies analyzed here—with the exception of the American schema. While no particular preference for the Soviet system is evident, the American approach was rejected, often quite forcefully. Much as in the FRG, here too we can observe epistemic transfer interwoven with boundary marking. It is questionable whether the psychiatrists would even have engaged with the American model had the Ministry of Health not explicitly asked them to. The preference for the Soviet system articulated by Hanns Schwarz, director of the Greifswald University Psychiatric Clinic, can be explained by his high regard for Pavlov in general—which was rare among psychiatrists in the 1950s, even in the GDR. Schwarz moved for a time between Freudian and Pavlovian positions but mostly embraced the latter from 1952 onward.[163] Generally speaking, the shared German tradition remained an important and mostly positive benchmark.

In addition, all the statements from the clinics or asylums were as one in arguing from their local perspectives. As in West Germany, this underscores the major role of practice in psychiatrists' thinking. Whether schemas were fit for practice was an important criterion in all the responses considered here, with the physicians basing their views on the experience they had gained at the local level. A second key criterion was also tied to local factors. Some of the clinic or asylum directors had differing opinions about which aspects ought to inform a classification scheme, an issue that was also discussed in the journal *Psychiatrie, Neurologie und medizinische Psychologie.* Similar to the contributions in *Der Nervenarzt,* three out of four relevant articles in the journal took the view that a diagnostic system ought to be structured etiologically.[164] In contrast to the FRG and in accordance with the character of the health system in the GDR, however, the importance of prophylaxis was also addressed in connection with classification schemes. Cécile and Oskar Vogt thus described the merits of an etiological classification as follows: "The discovery of triggering factors is of the greatest therapeutic and prophylactic importance, because nowadays the identification of a cause in itself often indicates how it might be combated."[165] This emphasis on prophylaxis also crops up in articles on schizophrenia. Generally, both postwar states were united by a strong focus on this condition. In 1950, Rolf Walther, still working in Uchtspringe at the time and later director of Rodewisch, called for a prophylactic approach to schizophrenia, stating that the goal was to take "remedial measures to improve environmental conditions at work, in families and in society" in order to eliminate "stimuli" (*Reize*).[166] The term "stimuli"[167] already hints at the Soviet perspective.[168] Between 1949 and 1963, essays on schizophrenia were published regularly that drew heavily on Pavlov, though in others the Soviet explanatory models of schizophrenia played no role at all.

Schizophrenia between tradition and Pavlov

In line with Pavlov's views, schizophrenia was interpreted in East Germany in a fundamentally different way than in the FRG. Yet the arguments put forward in the articles appearing in *Psychiatrie, Neurologie und medizinische Psychologie* interfaced to some extent with other well-known explanatory currents, some of which were accepted in the West. There are two reasons for this. First, Pavlov made prominent reference to other researchers, with Ernst Kretschmer being a prime example. Second, explanations that were not genuinely Soviet could still be compatible with Soviet ideas. In his article, for example, Walther took Kretschmer's constitutional theory as his starting point to explain the somatic cause of schizophrenia, relating different constitutions to metabolic disorders.[169] Pavlov had established categories of nervous strength, which, among other things, he matched up with Kretschmer's types: Pavlov's "neurasthenic" type was supposedly equivalent to Kretschmer's schizophrenic.[170] The idea that metabolic disorders might have something to do with the occurrence of schizophrenia was discussed in the FRG; in and of itself, this notion had nothing to do with a Soviet reading of the disease. But Walther went on to argue in a decidedly socialist way:

> As we see it, schizophrenia is rooted in a predisposition as an endogenous element, which is understood as a centrally induced shift of equilibrium in the vegetative system and associated lability of coordination between the brain stem and the cerebral cortex. Whether this endogenous dispositional element manifests depends on exogenous factors, in other words on environmental influences, which we call stimuli. The main sources of stimuli are personal-occupational, familial, and social circumstances.[171]

Walther thus explained schizophrenia as resulting from a malfunction of the area of the cortex highlighted by Pavlov. The "dictatorship of the cortex" took aim at the biologistic interpretation of diseases and undergirded diametrically opposed analyses that privileged external influences rather than the inexorable progress of a disease. Torsten Rüting aptly concludes that this was an attempt to prevent the international paradigm shift toward the autonomous functioning of organic systems.[172] This cortex-focused framework differed fundamentally from the prevailing ideas in the FRG, both in its theoretical premises and in the actions proposed in light of it. The psychoanalytic explanations emanating from the United States, meanwhile, were alien to both the biologistic and Pavlovian positions. Ultimately, both assumed a somatic cause, whereas the U.S. position included purely social-psychological approaches.

Walther was by no means the only author to take this explanatory route in his writings. It should be noted, however, that about half the articles arguing from a "Soviet" perspective were produced by authors from neighboring socialist countries. The same line of argument can be found, for example, in texts by Kiril Cholakov, a native of Bulgaria[173] and in a Hungarian article on "Hallucinosis in Schizophrenia."[174] It may be that the publication of these pieces was an attempt to publicize contributions consonant with the socialist line, since East German psychiatrists were failing to produce them in sufficient numbers.

While the Pavlovian line had been enshrined shortly after Pavlov's death in 1951,[175] until 1963 articles continued to appear that, although they never spoke out against the new doctrine, took no account of it either. These were on topics that could be addressed without necessarily raising questions of principle. For example, Rudolf Lemke of Jena, which happened to be home to a Pavlov Institute, published an article on the incidence of neurological diseases and defects in schizophrenic patients. He concluded that these were highly likely—the data allowed no definitive statements—to occur more often than among psychiatrically healthy people but made no further classificatory moves of any kind.[176] This strategy of avoiding any integration of research results into a wider theoretical framework was far from rare. It did not always involve statistical studies, as in Lemke's article. Another example is an article examining the diagnostic distinction between schizophrenia and obsessional neurosis, which elucidated problems and proposed solutions exclusively with reference to concrete examples.[177]

This approach to schizophrenia, located between the avoidance of ideological statements and explicit adherence to Pavlov's Soviet interpretation, explains why the expertise so often cited in West Germany played no role in discussions or articles in the GDR. The Soviet explanatory framework meant that the issue of expertise, which was associated with the attribution of psychoses to an unknown physical cause, did not arise in the first place. The "dictatorship of the cortex" localized the cause unambiguously in that part of the brain. Since Pavlov could be circumvented but not challenged, at least in *Psychiatrie, Neurologie und medizinische Psychologie*, there was no basis for a discussion of expertise. This, however, tells us nothing about practice, and the medical records at Greifswald and in Saxony show that the problem of differing diagnoses persisted on a significant scale.

Diagnostic practice in the FRG and GDR

Within the committal process, physicians communicated and legitimized their diagnoses in light of those of other physicians, a specific constellation that shaped committal practices. This was unproblematic when the diagnosis made at the inpatient facility and that of the committing physician coincided. But such congruence was far from universal, as already indicated by my analysis of articles in *Der Nervenarzt*. Often, several physicians were involved prior to committal and rarely did they arrive at exactly the same diagnosis. Hence, communicative channels enabling physicians to discuss differing diagnoses were a *sine qua non*.[178] Normally, the asylum or clinic informed the committing physician by letter of the diagnosis made during inpatient treatment. Attempts to legitimize diagnoses can be traced in even greater detail in expert evaluations (*Gutachten*). If diagnoses or assessments of the disease, its course and treatment had already been produced, the evaluation included comments on them.

In the following, I analyze an expert evaluation carried out at Bethel and a doctor's letter from Greifswald. Such missives from Greifswald provide valuable evidence, as they were about two pages long and generally quite detailed. It is apparent from both genres of text that great efforts were made to establish a long-term psychiatric classification for patients. I will also show that, rather than problematizing differing diagnoses, psychiatrists legitimized their diagnosis with reference to their own practices, without relating them to older diagnoses. No differences appear in the practice, communication, and legitimation of diagnosis in the "Third Reich," the GDR, and the FRG, except that doctors' letters and evaluations were typically longer after the war. This is consistent with the finding that diagnostic systems were not debated during wartime; it is hardly surprising given the shortage of physicians during World War II and the focus on danger and security. The relationship between psychiatrists and other physicians was also very similar in the GDR and FRG, but it was much less concerned with maintaining consensus vis-à-vis external actors than in the case of communication among psychiatrists.

Psychiatrists among themselves

The expert evaluation from Bethel and doctor's letter from Greifswald provide insights into the difficulty—often encountered in practical contexts—entailed in arriving at a diagnosis. When the diagnosis had been completed, the clinic or asylum physicians wrote a letter to the referring doctor in which they thanked them for the referral and presented their own diagnosis. The physician's letter considered below, from 1947, set out a diagnosis that clashed with that of the committing colleague. The first three sentences addressed the initial diagnosis:

Thank you very much for referring your patient Mrs. [Anna M.] due to suspected amentia.[179] She was under observation here for four days. This, in connection with the objective and subjective anamnesis, was unable to confirm the tentative diagnosis mentioned above.[180]

Only the new diagnosis made at the Greifswald University Psychiatric Clinic was subsequently discussed, while no reference was made to possible reasons for the difference between the two diagnoses. The cornerstones of the new diagnosis were the statements made by the patient and her relatives along with observation in the clinic. Her file noted that states of weakness, to which the patient had referred, were observed in the inpatient setting on several occasions.[181] In the doctor's letter, the responsible physician gave a detailed account of her medical history, starting with the depressive illness suffered by her mother and ending with her condition upon admission. The anamnesis and observations were summed up diagnostically in the statement that the patient was a "somewhat peculiar, sensitive, romantically inclined personality with a tendency to brood and a constitutionally depressive disposition."[182] Such lengthy descriptive diagnoses, as well as the sole reference to the period of treatment in the clinic in which the letter was composed, were quite common. These phenomena also occurred frequently in the two institutions in Saxony and in their West German counterparts. The following is an East German example of a description given under the heading of "diagnosis": "State of physical and mental exhaustion plus psychopathic personality, 368 K, no mental illness of any kind."[183]

We can gain a detailed insight into how these diagnoses were legitimized and what they signified if we look at the expert report (*Gutachten*) on the revocation of Greta W.'s incapacitation, which included several diagnoses and—since it is an expert evaluation—provided a more detailed rationale.[184] Mrs. W. had been incapacitated in 1961 because of "mental weakness" (*Geistesschwäche*) and arrived at Bethel in 1963 for six months of inpatient observation. This was intended to assess whether her incapacitation was still medically appropriate. Mrs. W. sought to have her incapacitation revoked, which is why the competent court ordered her to be committed for "observation."[185] The evaluating physician, Dr. B., had at her disposal earlier diagnoses and incapacitation evaluations. Since her first inpatient stay in 1950, a total of eight physicians had diagnosed Mrs. W.'s condition in various ways. The several inpatient facilities were first located in the vicinity of Hanover and then in North Rhine-Westphalia after the patient moved there. When she was first committed, the diagnosis given was "abulic [*willenlos*] hypochondriac, querulous psychopath"; about a year later in another asylum, the neurological diagnosis was "myasthenia gravis pseudoparalytica."[186] Another hospital confirmed this diagnosis in 1953. Three years later and the patient had moved to North Rhine-Westphalia, where she attended a hospital and was diagnosed as suffering from a psychiatric disorder, namely, "symptomatic psychosis with a paranoid slant." That same year, another hospital diagnosed "schizophrenia (catatonic stupor)." In 1960, when the first application for incapacitation was submitted, the evaluating clinic attested to her "catatonic condition." In 1962, immediately before Greta W. was transferred to Bethel for evaluation at her own request, the Land hospital in Eickelborn diagnosed "chronic schizophrenia, defective personality."[187]

At the von Bodelschwingh Asylums, Dr. B.'s report concluded with the following diagnostic description: "chronic schizophrenia with relatively frequent acute episodes of a catatonic character."[188]

The eight diagnoses, only two of which were exactly the same, can be divided into three basic groups. The first entailed a psychiatric classification without the status of disease, in other words, reference was made to a syndrome that was not construed as wholly somatic. In the Würzburg Key, such diagnoses came under item 16, "psychopathic personalities." The term "psychopath" (*Psychopathin*) conveyed the cause of the psychiatric abnormality, namely, a blend of constitutional factors and personal attitude toward and approach to life.[189] The three adjectives "abulic," "hypochondriacal," and "querulous" vividly described the specific manifestation involved—and undoubtedly with negative connotations. The second group comprises two instances of the same neurological diagnosis plus "symptomatic psychosis with a paranoid slant." The latter diagnosis was once again drawn from the field of psychiatry; however, unlike "psychopathy," psychosis was considered a full-fledged somatic illness. A symptomatic psychosis was conceptualized as an organic defect, one triggered by an external agency. It is not clear from the file from Bethel why this medical assessment was made almost seven years earlier in a different institution. Again, a description of the patient's condition, namely, "with a paranoid slant," was added to the diagnosis. Crucially, "symptomatic psychosis" was identified the presumed cause. Finally, three diagnoses in the vicinity of "schizophrenia" were given, which differed from the previously diagnosed "symptomatic psychosis" in that the mental abnormalities were not viewed as caused by a direct external influence. While schizophrenia too was conceptualized as somatic, it was regarded as an event within the body, in other words an endogenous disorder. As with the attribution of "psychopathy," the diagnosis of schizophrenia entailed a postulated cause; however, in contrast to "psychopathy," this was assumed to be a somatic, endogenous cause. At the same time, the disorder was described in more detail in various ways, for instance with respect to its course, which was identified as chronic, its specific manifestation, and in terms of the description of the patient's condition as "catatonic stupor" or "defective personality." On one occasion, all that was noted was a "catatonic state." This is not a diagnosis in the strict sense, but a description of a mental state that may form part of various diagnoses. In addition to schizophrenia, conditions such as progressive paralysis or symptomatic psychoses could also lead to a "catatonic state."

Evidently, classifying disease and making a diagnosis proved difficult on a number of levels. The various diagnoses postulated a range of causes. Ultimately, though, even the diagnosis did not provide enough information to determine whether an asylum stay or incapacitation was appropriate or to resolve all treatment-related issues. When schizophrenia was diagnosed without further descriptive additions it remained open which symptoms were involved, how pronounced they were, and how frequently they occurred.

All this, however, was crucial to the proposed revocation of Greta W.'s incapacitation, on which the Bethel physicians were to give their views. In the expert evaluation, Dr. B. referred to the diagnoses and descriptions mentioned above and then reported on her observations. Her arguments drew on the observations made on her ward, not previous diagnoses, although she listed them all. In her evaluation, she described the practical problems entailed in arriving at an assessment of Greta W.'s condition. She noted that the patient had isolated herself from the other patients during the first two weeks, but that this had then ceased without "significant administration of drugs."[190] The physician wrote: "Over the course of 5 months, Mrs. [W.'s] reactions have been virtually free of abnormalities."[191] The doctor noted that her patient showed drive, helped other patients, went shopping alone in Bielefeld, was interested in others' opinions, acknowledged earlier phases of illness, and so on.[192] The Bethel doctors felt that Mrs. W.'s condition had improved so much that they were keen for her to take a leave of absence and believed she could live on her own in the near future. Leaves of absence often served as dress rehearsals for discharge. Mrs. W.'s guardian, however, advised against this course of action.[193] Bethel then wrote him again in an attempt to convince him that a leave of absence and early discharge were medically appropriate and that he should reconsider.[194] The positive impression the doctors had gained can be inferred from the wording: "We would therefore urge you to give your consent [to the leave of absence]. As things stand, there is absolutely no risk involved."[195] The leave was then arranged but did not take place. According to the expert report, a "catatonic stupor" set in "suddenly" immediately before the leave of absence was due to begin. Ms. W. stopped speaking, and refused food, medication, and care.[196] In line with the reasoning of the expert evaluation, these observations led to the aforementioned diagnosis of "chronic schizophrenia with relatively frequent acute episodes of a catatonic character." Greta W. was assessed as "legally fully incompetent" and thus remained incapacitated. This assessment explicitly applied not just to the current phase of the illness, but also to the phases between episodes.[197]

Two important points become clear here. First, the assessment was not only intended to describe the situation at a particular moment but to facilitate the long-term "classification" of the patient. In addition to the diagnosis of schizophrenia, this required a more precise description. The adjective "chronic" clarified that there were no healthy phases and that Greta W. had to be regarded as fundamentally schizophrenic. The five months without symptoms, described in detail in the expert evaluation, only featured in the diagnosis as an absence: they constituted a period to be imagined by the reader between the explicitly mentioned, frequently occurring episodes. The patient was "defined" holistically as a person in light of these episodes. The course of the disease could be described even more precisely through mention of frequently occurring relapses, while the clinical picture could be conveyed in greater detail with reference to episodes of a "catatonic character."

This is not a conspicuously hasty diagnosis. In fact, despite the previous diagnoses and the patient's incapacitation, the physicians at Bethel sought to arrange a leave of absence for her and aired the strong possibility of discharge. What we can discern here, though, is a near-systemic compulsion to classify. The clinical picture of schizophrenia in particular was linked to the idea of certain types of disease course—another classificatory move within the framework of diagnosis—and since it was conceived as endogenous, it was assumed to progress in a more or less predictable way. According to the logic of the psychiatric ordering of diseases, a patient with this condition could not be imagined in the absence of such a course. Inevitably, this entailed not only assigning a disease, but also classifying a person. The often lengthy diagnoses featuring various additions had a paradoxical dual function. They were intended to allow the clearest possible attribution of a syndrome while also including important information about a patient that could simply not be captured in a brief diagnosis. This descriptive diagnostics was consonant with the classical procedure for achieving scientific objectivity. Classification informed by an ideal type was viewed as distorting objective truth. It was assumed that by gearing themself toward such ideal types, the scientist was unconsciously making the object—in this case the patient— conform to the reference system.[198] The lengthy diagnoses thus ensured the "objectively correct" description of a "given case." As the example of Greta W. illustrates, however, in practice this did not lead to the desired objectivity if this implies that the diagnoses were always identical or even similar.

Psychiatry as a science thus used various forms of representation and a range of legitimizing strategies. While the making of a diagnosis was described as expertise, the form of the diagnosis, which took account of a variety of different aspects, was guided by the principle of "objectivity." Hence, in their self-portrayal and in the ways they presented themselves to the outside world, psychiatrists often oscillated between self-stylization as experts in that which defied scientific designation and the idea that they could provide reliable, precise, objective classifications of disease. They themselves, then, constantly traversed the borderline between order and disorder. On the one hand, as noted by Foucault, they were tasked with assigning "madness."[199] On the other hand, as they carried out this classificatory work, they moved back and forth between systematic description and instinctive expertise.

The rationales set out in the doctor's letter and the expert evaluation demonstrate in exemplary fashion just how important the practices of the individual psychiatrist were considered to be. The other physicians' diagnoses were listed, but the assessment in the expert report was based solely on the account of the patient's behavior at Bethel. This dovetails with the importance attached to individual psychiatric practice in the articles addressed above in the psychiatric journals. There was no discussion of why or how different diagnoses came about, or why one's own diagnosis was more convincing than previous ones. It was enough to justify the diagnosis with reference to one's observations and to conversations with the patient and their relatives. The relationship between psychiatrists thus went un-thematized. In the context of expert evaluations, we might presume that highlighting inconsistent diagnoses would place a question mark over the expertise of the profession as a whole. Yet correspondence with other psychiatrists exhibits the same peculiar acceptance of the fact that in practice diagnoses simply differed. The relationship of psychiatrists to other physicians, meanwhile, was quite different.

Psychiatrists and other physicians

So far, we have considered differing diagnoses by different psychiatrists. Committals, however, almost always involved doctors who had no specialist psychiatric training but who played a key part in the process. In the "Third Reich" and West Germany, these were the public health officers (*Amtsärzte*) in the health offices and the general practitioners. In the GDR, physicians in health offices, polyclinics, and rural outpatient clinics or company physicians played a decisive role. Hospital physicians were sometimes significant in this context too. While this state of affairs was not discussed in wartime, at least not in *Der Nervenarzt*, a different situation pertained in the postwar states, in both of which psychiatrists addressed the issue of the involvement in committals of colleagues without psychiatric expertise.

In 1954, an article by Dr. Donalies (1894–1961), head physician of the Eberswalde Sanatorium-Nursing Home, was published in the East German journal *Das Deutsche Gesundheitswesen. Zeitschrift für Medizin* ("The German Healthcare System. Journal for Medicine") entitled "Psychiatrie in der Pflichtassistentenzeit! Eine Anregung" ("Psychiatry during compulsory internship! A proposal").[200] His key contention was that every physician should spend some time in a psychiatric department during their practical training. Donalies justified this by highlighting what he considered to be the disastrous consequences of the lack of specialist knowledge among committing physicians:

> We have our patients coming into the asylum through committals that at times defy description. It will seem crude but at least clear to state that the diagnoses are often on the same level as a general practitioner referring a patellar fracture[201] to a surgeon as suspected appendicitis. [...]
>
> But it is more alarming still if a patient is then wrongly evaluated as a result of all the missing anamnestic indications [...], and finally, these committals also permit highly unfortunate conclusions to be drawn about the psychiatric supervision and control of the population in general.
>
> There is a strong possibility [...] that incipient hebephrenic or paranoid personality changes will result in committal only after a misfortune has occurred, and we recall a case in which a woman came in for her second admission after she had beaten her husband to death. The first time, she

had come to us with no more than a—of course incorrect—diagnostic term of foreign origin, but with no indication at all of the (surely pathological) states of agitation observed in her for some time.

The author then went into more detail about the crucial importance of anamnesis, addressing three further aspects of medical knowledge. First, he contended, psychiatric knowledge was lacking at key points that were crucial to the committal process. Second, in Donalies' view, psychiatric knowledge should be used to control the general population. Third, he attached huge importance to the case history as a means of generating psychiatric knowledge in individual instances. I discuss this in more detail below.

Psychiatrists in the FRG grappled with very similar problems. In 1951, in an article in the *Der Nervenarzt* journal entitled "Vorschläge für den Wiederaufbau der Offenen Fürsorge für Geisteskranke" ("Proposals for the reconstruction of noninstitutional care for the mentally ill"),[202] Hans Merguet, director of the Lengerich Provincial Sanatorium in Westphalia, called for asylum physicians to be placed in health offices:

Only rarely do the health offices have a psychiatrically trained physician on their staff and they are also overburdened with other tasks. Consultations in pertinent cases by an experienced specialist can go a long way toward relieving the pressure they face in this difficult area and enabling them to act quickly, decisively, and appropriately.[203]

Much like the chief physician at Eberswalde, he also addressed the aspect of control:

In principle, it is not only discharged asylum patients and others who are mentally ill in the narrow sense who must be cared for. The social security doctor (*Fürsorgearzt*) ought to be available in all cases in which the health office and local physicians may need his advice with respect to the mentally deviant or abnormal personalities. Such "criminals" and "asocials" or other conflictual people (*Konfliktmenschen*) will not be psychopaths in every case. Likewise, patients slated for committal to an asylum should if possible be presented beforehand. Not infrequently, at that point the asylum psychiatrist can still find ways and means to avoid or postpone admission.[204]

Linked to the aspect of control here is the additional imperative of preventing unnecessary admissions. Hence, the two contributions to the debate mentioned above from the FRG and GDR address the importance of scientific competence to psychiatric control in addition to the lack of specialist medical expertise. Psychiatrists underlined the need for psychiatric knowledge as a means of disciplining the population, and in East Germany, the state held the same view. While the above authors were already lamenting the fact that this need had gone unfulfilled, a different picture pertained when it came to the concern articulated in *Der Nervenarzt* that admissions must be avoided if at all possible. Since the 1920s, psychiatric institutions had been debated primarily in terms of the costs arising for the community as a whole, reflecting the general interest in keeping admissions down. This is why the asylums were keen to shift psychiatric oversight to the preliminary stages of admissions, in the FRG to the health offices and in the GDR to the company doctors, polyclinics, and rural outpatient clinics.

In addition to these aspects, the article in the journal *Das Deutsche Gesundheitswesen* also mentions the importance of the anamnesis to diagnosis and prognosis.[205] This highlights a specific feature of psychiatric knowledge compared to other forms of medical and natural scientific knowledge. Significant portions of this knowledge do not originate in observation, but in interaction with the patient, which is bound up with the fact that once differential diagnosis became established the course of a disease was considered central to diagnosis.[206] Yet in the period at issue here, asylum psychiatrists in particular rarely got to see the sick in the early stages of their condition. Patients often entered clinics or asylums only when, for a variety of reasons, they no longer seemed tolerable to their families or social milieu. This made the assessment undertaken by other physicians, which was criticized in the two articles considered above, all the more important. In contrast to differing diagnoses among members of their own medical guild, psychiatrists cast doubt on the anamnestic and diagnostic abilities of other physicians and made their dissatisfaction public in professional journals. This indicates that the profession's interpretive monopoly was always at issue within the practice of diagnosis.

The relationship between doctor and patient

Journal articles on committal practice highlighted the problem of physicians of a different medical specialism taking the patient's history incorrectly, which hampered the accurate assessment of their condition. Psychiatrists attached much importance to the information provided by laypersons, the patient, and the social environment—and its correct interpretation by physicians. In what follows, then, I probe physicians' approach to the information provided by laypersons and the assessments made by the latter themselves, in other words "lay diagnoses."

The flow of information from family to institution

The information that physicians used for diagnosis came from their patients, their families, and the social environment in two different ways.

First, information and interpretations from laypersons reached asylum psychiatrists via the questionnaires of the welfare associations. (Supra-) municipal authorities and associations were involved in almost all committals to state sanatorium-nursing homes because prior to admission there was a need to clarify who would bear the costs. The health insurance funds usually paid for shorter stays at university psychiatric clinics. In all three systems, the costs of longer asylum stays were at least partly covered by the welfare associations. It was also possible and indeed quite common for welfare associations to pay for a stay in a private asylum such as Bethel.

The welfare associations and municipal authorities thus played a lead role in the admission process. The provincial associations or the administrative district of Upper Bavaria (*Regierungsbezirk Oberbayern*), to which the various welfare associations were subordinate, determined which institution the patient was admitted to and got the welfare associations involved. Since the asylums served specified areas, the choice of asylum was generally based on the patient's place of residence. The relevant authorities were supposed to ensure that a completed questionnaire was submitted to the asylum along with the patient. This provided the institution with information on a number of key points: personal data, how the stay was being paid for, whether the patient was considered a danger to themself or others, and the reason for admission.[207] This information could be relevant to filling out the admission form in the asylum, so it might influence the view of the admitting physician as well. In order to complete the questionnaires, relatives or other members of the social environment, such as neighbors, teachers, and priests, were questioned. The information furnished by the admission forms, which are one of the sources I use in this book, is limited in a dual sense. First, the statements made by members of the patient's social world were geared toward predefined questions. These responses might be provided by a local authority official, in which case, the individual writer was also providing second-hand information.[208] If no relevant person could be found, large parts of the questionnaire often remained blank. What this means is that the information it contained, and thus the data available to the physician, were already filtered by the patient's social milieu, whose members could either try to meet whatever expectations they anticipated or emphasize certain kinds of information while omitting other kinds in light of what they saw as their own interests.

Second, the anamnesis was, as it were, a form of medical appropriation—and thus selection and interpretation—of lay knowledge, which was transformed into expert knowledge. Since the key phases of illness preceded entry into the asylum and could not, therefore, normally be observed by physicians, they had to rely on others' observations. Klaus Konrad, director of the Göttingen University Psychiatric Clinic, stated that "only in light of the coexistence of different symptoms, the sequence of their occurrence, data on individual and family history, and a wealth of additional determinants do we construct the diagnosis."[209] This applies all the more to admission diagnoses, in which the anamnesis effectively replaced medical observation.[210]

The anamnesis was also pre-structured by questions and the medical records obviously contain only what was written down. To give us a sense of how anamneses proceeded and what was supposed to be included, it is helpful to examine textbooks. Here I analyze the guidance on taking a medical history in the popular textbook by Kurt Kolle, which appeared in a second edition in 1943, a third in 1949, and a fifth in 1961. In the GDR, the first Soviet textbook on psychiatry was not published until 1960 and is thus irrelevant to the vast majority of the period under study here.[211] But given the absence of alternatives, we can assume that the accounts provided in the well-known textbooks were still being used in the early East Germany as well. All three editions of the above-mentioned volume included a section on initial contact with the patient, the consultation, and the forming of a medical opinion, and they differed only minimally.[212] Kolle emphasized that there were several crucial levels to consider during the consultation. He began by discussing first impressions, including facial expression, clothing, and posture.[213] He then turned to the consultation itself, distinguishing between the patient's manner of speaking and the content of their speech. The form of what was said included, for example, whether the patient expressed themself "straightforwardly or awkwardly," spoke "haltingly or articulately," and whether they frequently digressed.[214] With regard to the first point, Kolle, writing in the first person singular and thus appearing to share his own experience, noted that the first impression already steered his "diagnostic thinking in certain directions."[215] This is reminiscent of the intuitive expertise emphasized in the articles we looked at in *Der Nervenarzt*. However, he partially revised this initial statement two pages later, writing that "many patients who visit (or are sent to) the neurologist do not initially present anything abnormal even to the trained medical eye. All the essential information is contained in the 'case history [*Vorgeschichte*].'"[216] Here he underlines the tremendous importance of the anamnesis, explaining that a good one must be lengthy and that the best approach is simply to let the patient talk about their life in an unguided manner.[217] Only then, he averred, should the physician steer the consultation, if necessary, by asking questions, and thus address specific topics: childhood, adolescence, parents, economic background, school, occupation, and the patient's relationship with their spouse or with the opposite sex.[218] Then the doctor should turn to their medical condition. Here Kolle addressed an issue of considerable importance to the relationship between physician and patient, one that tells us a good deal about the transformation of lay into expert knowledge: the patient's self-interpretation and the psychiatrist's priorities, which were often at variance.

> I want to know when he first noticed his complaints or the symptoms disturbing him, whether they are constant or come and go, whether he has perhaps felt ill for years or whether there have been many years of health between periods of affliction. Here a problem arises that it is crucial to combat, especially in the case of mental conditions: the patient's

(and his relatives') need to immediately provide an explanatory cause for every occurrence. The sick person knows that his melancholy stems from a quarrel with his mother-in-law and greatly resents the fact that I do not share his opinion.[219]

Psychiatrists were interested in the course of the disease in terms of its form, not in light of the external factors often identified by laypersons as an explanation for it. They thus viewed patients' case history as vital to making an assessment, but they interpreted this information differently than laypersons by looking at the disease in isolation. Psychiatrists' goal was to analyze the disorder and the patient regardless of the rest of their life. They ascribed illness based on its form or course and then linked it back to the patient's life. From psychiatrists' perspective, it was the illness that explained the patient's experiences, while laypersons explained the illness with reference to these experiences. It was through this line of questioning and form of categorization that physicians appropriated lay knowledge. This "pertinacious" medical interpretation turned physicians into experts and opened up the potential for a third mode of self-presentation within the diagnostic process. In addition to the strategy of objectification through meticulous description and self-portrayal as an intuitive expert, this involved self-stylization as an authority in possession of the "correct" scientific knowledge required to classify the illness.

Doctors' and lay diagnoses

Certain questions structured the dialogue that unfolded in the context of the anamnesis, including those concerning the onset (and course) of the disease. This shaped the consultation but did not determine the content of the patient's statements. The anamnesis reveals that laypersons and physicians sought to make diseases comprehensible and manageable by categorizing them. Yet they did this in different ways and to some degree with different goals. Physicians carried out a formal categorization that was intended to classify the individual as comprehensively as possible and to assign them to a category while taking their individual characteristics into account. Especially when preparing expert evaluations, but in other contexts as well, this sorting process was aimed at the future: disease classification and description created a basis for making decisions on asylum stays, incapacitation, and potential treatment.

Lay people too classified diseases, but with far greater reference to the past, seeking explanations that slotted the illness meaningfully into their lives. Patients themselves and their families usually related behavior they saw as abnormal to other events, identifying direct triggers of the most varied kinds. These could be physical illnesses, shifts in the weather, or dramatic political or personal changes, such as the death of a relative.[220] Patients and their relatives almost always embedded illnesses in their life course, unless they expressed no view at all or failed to articulate any kind of coherent interpretation. When it comes to this basic mindset, no gender-, or context-specific differences stand out among lay people. But if we probe what exactly in their everyday lives laypersons linked illnesses to, we can discern certain differences. One key sphere of life in terms of both attributing illness and determining the need for an asylum stay, one in which we can discern both gender- and society-specific characteristics, was "work," which I discuss in the next chapter.

Another topic that both laypersons and physicians discussed in highly gender-specific ways with respect to disease classification was sexuality. This was especially true of the categorizing done by police and physicians, as in the case of forcible committal to prevent transmission of STDs explored in the last chapter.[221] But gender-specific categorizing was hugely important beyond venereal disease, playing a major role in diagnostics in general. Research in the history of psychiatry has problematized gender-specific aspects above all in connection with certain diagnoses. One much-discussed example is the diagnosis of hysteria, which, as Paul Lerner has shown, was also applied to men, especially in the course of World War I.[222] Another disorder that historians have shown to entail major gender-specific differences in social perception and medical diagnosis was alcohol addiction.[223] Beyond individual diagnoses, meanwhile, Ann Goldberg has highlighted gender differences in the nineteenth century in the context of admission to asylums and treatment. The volume *Zwang zur Ordnung* ("The drive for order"), by Marietta Meier et al., states in summary that "gender- and class-specific distortions crop up quite often within the framework of an ostensibly neutral diagnosis and approach to treatment."[224] In line with this, rather than focusing on particular diagnoses as gender-specific, it is worth scrutinizing deeper gender-related connotations of both the medical gaze and lay perspectives.

The committals of Birgit S. to Bethel between 1943 and 1959 provide us with exemplary insights into the differing interpretations made by doctors and lay people as well as the gender-specific evaluation of illness. In 1943, after a suicide attempt, she was admitted for the first of a total of five times. Her husband stated that she had been depressed since her son was reported missing at Stalingrad. "Reactive depression" was the medical diagnosis made at Bethel, placing her under no. 17 of the Würzburg Key, "abnormal reactions."[225] During the next four committals in 1948, 1953 (twice), and 1958, the patient stated in each case that her troubled state of mind had begun immediately after a physical illness. These were flu or a cold, and in 1958 pneumonia. The diagnosis in these cases was "endogenous depression in the post-menopausal period."[226]

While the first diagnosis took up the layperson's reasoning to a certain extent, with the doctors too making a connection between the son's fate and the mother's mental state, this ceased to apply later on. In line with the Würzburg Key and the textbooks cited above, the psychiatrists understood her persistent distress over her son being reported missing at Stalingrad as reactive depression. They thus regarded this behavior not as normal, but as comprehensible.[227] The diagnosis "endogenous depression in the post-menopausal period," meanwhile, neither established a link with any sort of external cause nor with the narrative put forward by the patient and her family. On the contrary, the diagnosis referred twice to developments within the body that were "inescapable" (*schicksalhaft*). The adjective "endogenous" indicated that the depression was understood as an internal somatic event, while "post-menopausal" conveyed the idea that it was directly connected with age-related changes in the female body. In the Würzburg Key, "endogenous depression" came under no. 15, "manic-depressive disorders." As with other diagnoses, in this case the diagnostic system included no additional gender-specific elements. But because psy-chiatrists sought to describe the patient as precisely as possible when they assigned them to a number, they themselves often added terms linking the onset of illness in women to certain physical changes. In the sample of nearly 1,500 medical records, about half of which were for women, diag-nostic additions such as "postnatal" or "post-menopausal" were ubiquitous in all three political systems. In one case in the FRG a woman was ex-amined for unsoundness of mind and to establish whether there was a causal connection between the offenses of which she had been accused, such as lying and stealing money, and the occurrence of her period.[228] As this is the only case of its kind in all the files examined, it reveals the breadth of the possible rather than the typical. In this instance, a link between menstrual cycle and soundness of mind was ultimately ruled out, but not because such a connection was thought unlikely: the dates of the misdemeanors simply failed to match the dates of menstruation.[229] For the expert evaluation, family members were asked about this possible temporal convergence, showing that doctors seriously looked into it.[230] It is evident here that the search for a diagnosis could be specific to women and that at times physicians and laypersons shared the same point of departure. On the other hand, the case of Birgit S. shows that medical diagnoses and lay narratives could differ significantly. It is not possible (least of all for a non-medical professional) to reconstruct from the files how diagnoses were made and whether they were correct, nor is this the goal of the present study. But distinguishing between reactive and endogenous psychoses was traditionally considered difficult.[231] Here, I merely note that the medical diagnosis and laypersons' assessment could differ but did not necessarily do so. Was this discussed and if so, how? To answer this question, I now scrutinize families' communication with physicians.

Correspondence between laypersons and physicians

In the medical records examined here, medical issues played a subordinate role in laypersons' letters—or were not addressed at all. While family members commented on them in the subjective and objective medical history (because physicians always asked about the onset and course of a disease), they did not approach the clinic or asylum themselves with related concerns, questions, or assessments. This stood in contrast with the Nazi regime's focus on health and heredity issues. The state's and the asylums' interest in these matters also finds reflection in the medical records. First, the "medical observation form" featured a box for the physician to tick if they believed the person committed was subject to the provisions of the "Sterilization Law." Second, the page centered on the patient was followed by several pre-structured sections in which information was to be entered about their family, sections that were dropped in the postwar period.

It was in fact the regime's, as well as doctors' and medical institutions', extraordinary focus on illness and heredity that prompted patients to visit the asylums less frequently on medical grounds. In line with this, the topics of illness and diagnosis figured less often in the communication between doctors and lay people. During the war, such matters were regularly negotiated only in the context of clarifying diagnoses, a process that took place in university psychiatric clinics but not sanatorium-nursing homes. At the Greifswald University Psychiatric Clinic, committals for the purpose of clearing up diagnoses mainly involved MS and epilepsy. In the case of MS, patients attended to find out the cause of their condition but not to receive inpatient treatment. Inpatient admission in cases of epilepsy often occurred because a person was hospitalized during or immediately after a seizure, or because they were called in for evaluation as a result of a seizure. Hence, MS sufferers often went to a clinic because they did not know they had MS, while epilepsy sufferers did not present for examination voluntarily. These admissions as a direct consequence of an epileptic seizure were among the rare cases in which the differential classification of a disease constituted a fraught issue between physician and patient during the war period. Those committed were typically desperate to prevent a diagnosis of "genuine epilepsy," which in all cases led to sterilization. This outcome could be avoided if the physician concluded that this was an isolated epileptic seizure triggered by a specific event. Such an assessment led to the less consequential diagnosis of "symptomatic epilepsy." An example of the successful attainment of this diagnosis is Christel D.'s "assessment due to seizures" in 1941.[232] The doctor's summary in the medical record reads:

> She then had a seizure a few days after the miscarriage. She knows she was unconscious but no more than that. She thinks that there was only one seizure but that if there were two they must have taken place on the same day. There have been no further seizures since then.
>
> She has noticed no personality changes of the kind described to her. She has, she states, a clear sense of all her day-to-day business and works as quickly now as she used to.
>
> She smokes about three cigarettes a day.

During the examination and on the ward the patient was entirely inconspicuous. She converses in a lively manner and plays piano. Gives clear, unambiguous answers to questions, is pretty strong intellectually, expresses herself eloquently, and is quite aware of everything. No slowing down, no dullness, no easily provoked irritability.[233]

Christel D. was able to place her seizure in a causal relationship to her miscarriage and, moreover, make a credible case that it had been a one-time occurrence with no after-effects. The connection with the miscarriage was convincing in a context in which psychiatric and neurological patients were always examined for any kind of gynecological or sexual abnormality. Physicians regularly associated unusual behavior, sensations and sensitivities or extreme physical reactions with specifically female events, such as child-birth, miscarriage, pregnancy, menstruation, and menopause.[234] However, the patient also mentioned two other important points, plausibly articulating and demonstrating that she was fully capable of working and thoroughly integrated socially.

During the war, then, lay people rarely came into contact with asylum physicians to clarify medical issues or request help, and when they did this was often an essentially involuntary act. This changed in the postwar period. Wives and husbands, sons and daughters, and fathers and mothers now wrote to asylums not only to expedite or prevent committals, but also with other concerns as well. However, the nature of the communication differed in East and West.

In many of the more than 400 individual case files I reviewed for the early FRG, family members, but also patients themselves, wrote to doctors with requests for help and advice. This usually occurred when a patient had been to the same clinic or asylum several times, in other words, the institution and individual doctors were familiar to them. In the case of Walther M., who had already been committed to the LHA Marburg nine times, his wife contacted the attending physician in 1948. The medical record contains only a carbon copy of the doctor's letter of reply, which addressed the wife's concerns: food allowances and an application for "additional living space." The doctor promised to support her on both fronts by writing to the relevant agencies. He also told her that, in light of her husband's persistent inquiries, he had assured him that he could count on the asylum for help should his condition worsen again.[235]

Far less often than in this typical situation, relatives got in touch with clinics or asylums even before the first committal, in other words with a doctor they did not know in an institution with which they had no previous contact. When this occurred, it often involved a middle-class family and a male family member seeking advice from a physician. In the course of these committals, the medical record almost always addressed the difference in disease classification between psychiatrists and lay people. Stefan A.'s committal is a prime example. This case also exemplifies how the middle classes dealt with sick family members and sheds light on their relationship to psychiatry. In 1947, Stefan A. was a student in his early twenties whose father owned a pharmacy.[236] His committal was initiated when his father wrote to the Munich University Psychiatric Clinic for advice about his son.[237] At the beginning of the letter, the father described his son's behavior and identified a whole series of causes to which it might be attributed:

> Our youngest son [Stefan], a medical student in his third semester, twenty-four years old, evidently suffers from mental disorders of a psychological nature. He was in the armed forces for five years as a radio operator and as such performed arduous service in Russia at Stalingrad, etc., under the group high command and at that time complained in particular about the strenuous and grueling night duty. At the end of the war, he experienced many unsettling situations as a result of flight and capture, then again being handed over to the Russians and another, this time successful, escape, such that it seems reasonable to assume that something may have been left over that disrupted his nervous system. We know of no case of schizophrenia or the like among our relatives. His depression began soon after his return home in 1945, in the July, when he was unable to begin his long-awaited studies for such a long time because it took so long for the lectures in Munich to begin. But then came what we believe to be the decisive factor that triggered his mental depression. He fell in love, which was probably unrequited, and had many occasions for jealousy. He was utterly changed by this, so that he began to behave toward his parents and friends in a completely different way, lost all desire to work, and now spends days on end in a state of lethargy, constantly staring at a book or newspaper without reading it. In short, he often acts toward us in a quite closed-off and obdurate manner.[238]

Stefan's father concluded by requesting that he and his wife be permitted to visit the university psychiatric clinic to obtain advice on how to proceed and how they ought to behave toward their son.[239] The father classified his son's illness in the letter in several ways. He conjectured that various war experiences and war-related stresses might have been causes of his depressive state. He then mentioned two precipitating factors that he and his wife considered decisive, namely, the delay in beginning his studies after the war and an experience of unrequited love. The father also described the ways in which his son's behavior was abnormal: he slept a great deal, took no pleasure in working, and was unapproachable. As his father saw it, this was a depression due to identifiable external circumstances. He sought to buttress this reasoning by stating that there were no mental illnesses, such as schizophrenia, in his family. Unbidden, the father thus sought to ward off any implication of a hereditary disease.

Stefan A. was then admitted to the psychiatric clinic as an inpatient for three days before being transferred to Eglfing-Haar. In the referral letter to the latter asylum, the committing physician at the clinic wrote that his parents were unwilling to acknowledge the severity of the illness and blamed it on external factors, such as lovesickness and jealousy. The physician, meanwhile, assumed the son was suffering from an endogenous psychosis. The physicians at Eglfing-Haar agreed with the view expressed by the university clinic.[240] In this case, then, explicit mention was made of the physicians' and family's different modes of explanation. At Haar, the doctors administered an insulin shock treatment, after which they discharged Stefan A. It is not clear from the medical file how his father reacted to the doctors' conclusion that this was an endogenous disorder rather than a response to a spate of unfortunate events.

All we can state with certainty is that in the long run the parents put their trust in the doctors rather than questioning their assessment: they continued to write letters both to the university clinic and to Eglfing-Haar asking for advice. It is unclear whether the doctors convinced them of the validity of their disease classification or whether they simply needed someone to take the decision off their hands. The latter surely played a role, going by the letters. In December of the same year, the parents again took their son to the university psychiatric clinic. When he was about to be discharged after a few days because he was again "quite calm," his father wrote to Eglfing-Haar.[241] He explained that on this occasion, prior to his admission to the university clinic, they had had even more "difficulties" with their son than before his first committal. In light of this and in view of his discharge from the clinic, the father inquired whether he could perhaps bring Stefan back to Eglfing-Haar, although, as he mentioned, his son was vehemently opposed to this, stating that he had "a horror of Eglfing."[242] Dr. B. answered the same day: "There is simply no other option than to have the patient brought here. He should not be taken home. A lengthy asylum stay is the best option."[243]

With respect to the doctor's intensive communication with the father, we should bear in mind that Stefan A. came to Eglfing-Haar as a private patient. His father displayed trust and a great willingness to accept medical advice, a reflection of the positive relationship between members of the middle class and the institution of psychiatry. The bourgeoisie differed from other population groups in its greater readiness to seek help from psychiatrists, an attitude that extended back to the nineteenth century.[244] It is remarkable that this trust was not fundamentally shaken by the Nazi era. The case described was not an isolated one. One of several other cases was the committal of Elfriede L., whose family doctor and family had jointly initiated her committal to Eglfing-Haar.[245] Much like Stefan A.'s parents, Elfriede L.'s father showed tremendous trust and gratitude toward the attending physician at Eglfing-Haar. This is evident in a letter from father to doctor about six weeks into his daughter's asylum stay:

Dear Dr. L.!

Thank you very much for your letter of January 21, 1949.

In particular, I am deeply grateful for the medical efforts you have made, which have already led to an improvement in my daughter's condition. I am so happy about this that I cannot find the words to express it. I am also sincerely pleased by your assurance that you will do everything to ensure my daughter's recovery. My sister, Mrs. [F.], has already told me time and again about your great efforts to restore my daughter to health. I hope, dear Dr. L., that I will have the opportunity to demonstrate my gratitude to you one day.

Perhaps you will come to our lovely spa town for a little break and would permit me to entertain you. I would also be happy to assist in finding suitable lodgings and making other arrangements.

I will visit the asylum on Sunday, the 30th of this month, from 10–12 o'clock to see my daughter and would be pleased if I could meet you in person.

I cannot comment on the insulin treatment because I do not understand it. This was merely the advice of the departmental physician at the Munich University Psychiatric Clinic. I leave that entirely up to you, dear Dr. L.

Thanking you once again for your dedicated work and for your letter, I remain respectfully yours, […].

The two examples from Eglfing-Haar are also worth mentioning because just four years after the end of the war such a trusting attitude among relatives of middle-class patients might seem surprising.[246] Eglfing-Haar had, in fact, continued to murder the sick on a massive scale even after the termination of the T4 Campaign, by setting up hunger houses for example. Shortly after the war ended in 1945, Bavarian radio reported on this fact, so the establishment's criminal past was hardly a secret.[247]

In the GDR, meanwhile, relatives did more than ask for advice. They made suggestions about treatment far more often than in the West German cases. Asylum staff usually responded to these suggestions, so they found their way into the medical records. A typical example is the correspondence between Rodewisch and Annegret M., whose adult daughter was accommodated there for the fifth time in 1953.[248] In March, her mother wrote that she did not think it was good for her daughter to be "shocked so often" and asked that the staff seek to establish whether she might be fine without shock treatment.[249] In contrast to the two previous examples of committal to Eglfing-Haar, the patient's mother considered herself competent enough to state her opinion on the course of the disease and its treatment. Elfriede's father in the previous example, meanwhile, felt unable to express a view on insulin treatment even when explicitly asked by the physician. Annegret's mother also considered taking her daughter back home and wrote: "As much as I would like to bring my daughter home, I am also anxious about doing so in the near future. Is it reasonable to say that her condition has improved?

Could it be that the summer heat has had an effect on the disease?"[250] The attending physician, Dr. M., responded two weeks later addressing the mother's concerns. She wrote that an attempt had now been made to forgo the electric shocks, but this had proved impossible.[251] The next few letters were focused on a possible leave of absence over Easter. In June, Annegret M. then wrote to the doctor:

> Dear Dr.,
>
> I am writing to you today with a request. Would it be possible for my daughter Mrs. [Marie M.] to be allowed out from time to time? Provided her condition permits it. I think she is in good shape for the most part. Perhaps this might be possible [if she were to go] with a similar patient. It must surely help improve patients' condition if they have something to look forward to. I know this must be a difficult decision for you because my daughter once tried to abscond years ago.
>
> As I see it, however, one cannot always take such a strict approach, and it might be appropriate on occasion to relieve the monotony of asylum life. Especially since my daughter also works there. [...]"[252]

Here the mother again informed the doctor of what she believed might be beneficial for her daughter during her stay at the asylum and what modifications the staff might therefore make. The doctor replied that Marie M. had in fact been leaving the asylum grounds regularly for several weeks together with a fellow patient.[253] She added: "We are of course committed to treating our patients according to their individual characteristics, and we are pleased when the patients' mental condition allows us to grant them greater freedoms."

Relatives' ideas and interventions, of the kind seen in the above correspondence, were not uncommon in the East German institutions studied for the present book. Here we might recall the cases discussed in Chapter 3, including the role of Walpurga R.'s sister in the decision to release her.[254] The findings in the present chapter dovetail with the picture that emerged from analysis of forcible committals in Chapter 3. Significantly fewer patients were formally forcibly committed; instead, committals were decided upon and carried out by relatives and physicians, even in the case of persons of legal age and sometimes against their will. The entire stay was often based on the relatives' wishes and doctors' consent. The duration of the stay was also down to the family. On this point, the GDR and West Germany differed significantly. The initiation of forcible committals in the FRG was comparable to a certain extent with the procedure in East Germany, because in the former, too, the family was often the driving force behind forcible committals and judicial orders were frequently obtained after the event. But the situation after admission was very different in the two states. In the GDR, relatives were in a stronger position vis-à-vis doctors, since they determined the length of stay rather than a police authority, as in the Nazi period, or a court, as in

West Germany. Families' proposals and requests thus reflected the specific power relations in the GDR: on the basis of their greater decision-making power, patients' families penetrated into the realm of medical expertise. Udo Schagen and Sabine Schleiermacher have summarized the structure of the health care system in East Germany as follows: "Though physicians were stripped of their previous organizational and definitional power, which had rested upon their professional prerogatives, a doctorly-medical mindset continued to dominate all matters of health and illness in a surprisingly enduring way."[255] Yet what we have seen is that this is only partially valid when it comes to the practice of committal. It does apply in the sense that psychiatrists were able to fortify their position of power vis-à-vis other institutional actors, be they police or municipalities. But when we consider noninstitutional actors within the practice of committal, it is apparent that medical laypersons in the GDR had a more self-confident attitude and laid claim to interpretive authority in a more assertive way than their West German counterparts.

Circulation of knowledge between East and West: lay demands for "Western" treatment standards

In addition to the advice given to and the demands made of doctors, the medical records often point to another issue that arose between relatives and doctors, one directly related to the division of Germany. Time and again, we find that the patient's relatives sought to procure medicines and medical equipment from the West. An entry in Manfred L.'s medical record following a visit by his son to Großschweidnitz in December 1956 ended with the remark: "His son wishes to attempt to obtain a hearing aid for his father in the West. He also wants to try to procure Raupina and Megaphen."[256] Both drugs were antidepressants, the father's stay at Großschweidnitz being due to depression. In the GDR, psychotropic drugs were far less available in the 1950s than in the FRG.[257] It is unclear here whether the doctor or the relatives came up with the idea of importing the medication. Other files indicate that in some cases it was laypersons that made such suggestions. In addition to the unregulated form of committal, families' potential to secure medical resources, especially psychotropic drugs, blurred the established power relations between physicians and laypersons in East Germany.[258]

The asymmetries of medical care between East and West affected the relationship between laypersons and physicians in other ways as well. It was not just through the procurement of medicines that the two Germanys remained connected. We can also observe a substantial epistemic transfer, with patients repeatedly referring to knowledge, methods, and therapies from West Germany in communication with their physicians.[259] This is particularly striking in letters from patients with MS to the Ministry of Health. I take this disease as an example for three reasons. First, MS always confronted physicians with the problem of incurability and unsuccessful treatment. Second, and directly related to this, people suffering from multiple sclerosis submitted numerous requests. The Ministry had a specific collection of such submissions from MS patients, but among those generally classified under psychiatry numerous cases also involved multiple sclerosis.[260] The stock of letters on psychiatry and multiple sclerosis also adds to our understanding of the issue, discussed earlier, of the differing ways in which neurologists and psychiatrists were stylized as scientific experts. What emerges is that, contrary to the picture painted by neurologists, from patients' point of view it *did* matter where and by whom they were diagnosed and treated for a neurological disease. The letters often embody a thorny issue: patients sought to obtain permission for an inpatient stay in the FRG. This was of course rejected. Instead, the response was to propose committal to a facility in the GDR.

Petitions from patients with MS or their relatives to the Ministry of Health are typified by disappointment at the East German doctors' inability to help them. It was by no means the case that other countries, east or west of the Iron Curtain, had effective treatment methods, let alone successful cures. In their petitions, however, lay people frequently assumed a connection between conditions in the GDR and the lack of help available to them, and they looked for ways to circumvent this perceived problem. Many letters featured requests for treatment in the FRG. In 1961, for example, Margot M. wrote to the minister of health, Dr. Lammert: "I request permission for a course of treatment in West Germany in order to prevent further years of invalidity and return me to the work process."[261] She described the course of her illness and mentioned that she had heard of a woman from Luxembourg who had undergone successful treatment for MS in Paris. This treatment, she stated, was based on the assumption that MS is caused by a virus.[262] She added, "Unfortunately, according to the doctors, this treatment cannot be carried out in this country."[263] But her brother in West Germany had informed her that it was available in Kassel. She concluded her letter with a request that she be allowed to avail herself of this therapeutic option in the FRG. "I ask the FDGB National Executive Committee (FDGB-Bundesvorstand; the FDGB was the Freier Deutscher Gewerkschaftsbund or Free German Trade Union Federation) to help me regain my health and enable me to undergo this treatment."[264] This letter illustrates two points. First, patients acquired a considerable amount of specialized knowledge about possible causes of and treatments for their disorder. Other individuals suffering from MS also requested specific forms of treatment, frequently making inquiries about Dr. Evers' raw food therapy[265] or "hormone refreshment therapies" (*Frischhormontherapien*).[266] The assumption mentioned by Margot M. that MS was caused by a virus was in fact the dominant theory in the Western world.[267] Second, this special knowledge drew on research and institutions outside the GDR. This was knowledge that circulated via personal connections, as in the case of

Margot M., who referred to acquaintances and relatives. Also typical is the remark—likely a strategic one in the "workers' state"—that the treatment would ultimately help restore her ability to work. Margot M.'s request, like all those for treatment abroad, was rejected (and even stays in neighboring socialist countries were out of the question).[268] Instead, replies typically held out the prospect of an inpatient stay in the GDR.[269] But as neurology departments were plagued by a chronic shortage of beds, those affected were often told: "We hope to be able to inform you of a date for your stay in the near future."[270] Unlike Margot M., after a negative answer some East Germans wrote another letter to the Ministry of Health, usually expressing bitter disappointment, but also criticism of the state, as in Irmgart H.'s case:

> I was not in the least surprised about the negative reply. It was bound to come. The government was my last hope. Do you think it is a pleasant thing when you only cost the state money and nowhere receive any help? From one year to the next, you hope that things will get better. Life is so short and when you ask for something from the state, you experience nothing but disappointment. [...] Believe me, Dr., it is terrible to always have to say thank you.[271]

This letter exemplifies the prevailing sense among patients that they could receive help elsewhere. The standard sentence with which Dr. Lammert began all her letters of reply, which sought to forestall this idea, seems to have had no effect on patients: "An appropriate remedy for your illness does not yet exist anywhere in the world, that is, one effective in all cases."[272] In light of the state of research and therapeutic options at the time, the statement that there was no universally efficacious remedy seems staggeringly positive. While the 1950s and 1960s were characterized by scientific optimism, a treatment for MS was no more than a remote theoretical possibility until the late 1970s.[273] Still, researchers across the world perceived the dawn of a new era in medicine. In line with this, in his monograph on multiple sclerosis, Murray notes that in the 1950s citizens of the United States persistently asked their doctors whether there might be potential for treatment after all.[274] In this respect, patients in the GDR behaved in much the same way as those discussed by Murray in the United States. What seems remarkable, though, is that patients in East Germany were so well-informed thanks to links with other laypersons in Western countries and that they believed them far more than the official (and in this case accurate) information they received from their own Ministry of Health, namely, that no successful method of treatment existed. On the one hand, this can be put down to despair in the face of an incurable disease, which was typical of MS patients in the GDR and beyond. The records examined for this book also include a few letters here and there from West German citizens who hoped they might gain access to Soviet methods of treatment via East Germany. One patient in North Rhine-Westphalia wrote:

Dear Sirs,

I have been suffering from multiple sclerosis for a number of years. It has now come to my attention that Russian doctors have already had great success in combating the disease. I would be very grateful if you could suggest to me how I might get in touch with such doctors. I would gladly cover any expenses that might arise. (...)

Respectfully yours,[275]

On the other hand, the many requests for Western treatments also demonstrate the widespread belief in the superiority of Western medicine in the early GDR. This was not due exclusively to the factual superiority of Western medicine, but also to a fundamental distrust of its East German counterpart. The lack of trust, typical of those affected, in "socialist" neurology and the GDR's health care system was so deep-seated that it seemed inconceivable that the information provided by the Ministry, that MS was not effectively treatable, was simply true.

Summary: disease and diagnostics in comparative perspective

During the war and in both successor states, diagnostics was characterized by uncertainty. Patients regularly received several different diagnoses. Physicians tried to overcome the difficult task of assigning a number within whichever diagnostic schema dominated at their institution by recording additional information on the course, prognosis, or cause of the condition.

In contrast to these basic similarities between the three German states, medical aspects were less important in committals during World War II than in the postwar period. It was only in the two successor states that the problems entailed in anamnesis and diagnosis were again addressed within the specialist medical debate. In both East and West, psychiatrists sought to ensure that their professional interpretations prevailed over those of laymen and those of physicians who had undergone no specialized psychiatric training. Meanwhile, the unclear etiology and fuzzy definition of many psychiatric disorders prompted fundamental debates among West German psychiatrists and neurologists on psychiatry's status as a science and on their professional self-image. One concept of science presented objectivity in diagnosis as the clear-cut categorizing of phenomena as illnesses, producing classifications that could, allegedly, be communicated unambiguously to others and that were based on straightforwardly describable and measurable observations. Yet this idea soon came up against the limits of both plausibility and persuasiveness. Despite this, neurologists insisted on a strictly natural scientific concept of objectivity, whereas psychiatric authors propagated the ideal of *expertise* in publications such as *Der Nervenarzt* journal. Due to their alleged special dispositional talent and the tacit knowledge they acquired in practice, psychiatrists as experts were supposedly able to intuitively perceive and identify mental illnesses. No comparable discussion took place in the GDR due to the ideological presuppositions that held sway there. According to the Soviet perspective, based on Pavlov, psychiatric diseases such as schizophrenia could ultimately be traced back to unambiguous origins, namely, malfunctions of the cortex.

Nonetheless, an astonishingly wide-ranging debate on diagnostic classifications was conducted in East Germany from 1959 onward, with psychiatrists often openly embracing Western models in their communication with the Ministry of Health. Even in the journal *Psychiatrie, Neurologie und medizinische Psychologie*, the Pavlovian interpretive paradigm sometimes took a backseat. When it comes to schizophrenia, the evidence confirms Anna Sabine Ernst's finding that in the field of medicine Pavlovian research coexisted with other modes of inquiry.[276]

In the FRG, the debate on diagnostic classifications and schizophrenia was more uniform and more traditional in character. Psychosocial explanations for schizophrenia, much discussed in the United States and Switzerland, were rejected by most West German psychiatrists. Still, the use of psychotherapy was increasingly accepted, at least within the theoretical discussion. This was essentially due to the new treatment options opened up by psychotropic drugs, which enabled German psychiatrists to integrate psychotherapy into their approach without changing their fundamental view of the cause and course of mental illness. The rejection of American research approaches and practices was common to most psychiatrists in both post-Nazi states.

As we have seen, local knowledge was profoundly important in the debates on diagnostic systems in both West and East Germany. Diagnostic schemes were adapted to local conditions. At the same time, many hoped to see a nationally or even internationally uniform system. As apparent in communication about differing diagnoses in specific cases, individual physicians strongly emphasized their practical experience as a means of legitimizing their professional knowledge. They vigorously defended the local—and thus also personnel-based—authority to define disease. Although discussions of this topic were absent during the war period, individual physicians' reference to local tradition and their practical experience shows that the local power base within diagnostics was probably nothing new. Meanwhile, the attitude of clinic and asylum doctors in the GDR as apparent in their discussions with the Ministry of Health—we might think of their open criticism of Soviet ideas—shows impressively that physicians' position of power remained largely intact in both German states.

The way laypersons explained mental illnesses was marked by a high degree of continuity and they inserted them into narratives about their life course and personal circumstances. Beyond this, however, the interaction between lay people and physicians differed in the FRG and GDR. In the latter, laypersons' position of power, strengthened by the vacuum of rules, manifested itself in their more self-confident dealings with asylum physicians. While in West Germany members of the patient's social environment tended to communicate with doctors in the form of questions and requests, relatives in East Germany frequently made suggestions and put forward their own interpretations. Likewise, relatives' initiative in procuring scarce psychotropic drugs from the West—and sometimes other medical products or equipment—points to a blurring of the traditionally hierarchical relationship between physician and layperson with respect to core medical competencies.

Notes

1 Brink, *Grenzen*, 270ff.
2 LHA Marburg, Patient file sign. 16K10740F, Entry, Cover page of medical history, LWV Hesse, 16.
3 Ibid., Certificate, March 15, 1946.
4 Ibid., Entry, April 18, 1946.
5 On the connection between illness on the one hand and societal norms and ideas of order on the other, and on the risk of a truncated view if we try to decipher social concepts of order solely from a medical perspective, see Meier et al., *Zwang zur Ordnung*, 35. Andrew Scull seeks to capture this connection with respect to the United States and the United Kingdom through the conceptual pair "social order/mental disorder": Scull, Andrew, *Social Order-Mental Disorder. Anglo-American Psychiatry in Historical Perspective* (London 1989).
6 For a seminal account and summary of the institutional position of physicians, who classify the "insane" and draw boundaries through their very role as listeners in a specific setting, see Foucault, Michel, *Die Ordnung des Diskurses* (Frankfurt/ M. 2007), 11ff.
7 On the call to refrain from writing history from either the physicians' or patients' point of view, and instead to bring the two together, see Condrau, Flurin, "The Patient's View Meets the Clinical Gaze," *Social History of Medicine* 3, 2007, 536.
8 Christians, *Amtsgewalt*, 17.
9 For more detail on decision making about forced sterilizations as well as their execution, see ibid., 143ff.
10 vBS Bethel, Patient file sign. 9/152, HAB, Patient files Morija I.
11 The limits of the tolerable and the criteria used to determine it are discussed in detail in the following chapter, "Work and Performance." Committals associated with violence, which I discussed in Chapters 2 and 3, are also relevant in this context.
12 Brink, *Grenzen*, 194.
13 On the murder of the sick in its various phases and the varying regional approaches after the termination of the T4 Campaign, see for example Süß, *Volkskörper*, 311ff.
14 Though this is not an endorsement of Szasz's radical claim that institutions create the diseases in the first place. Szasz, Thomas, *The Myth of Mental Illness. Foundations of a Theory of Personal Conduct* (New York 1961).
15 LHA Marburg, Patient file sign. K12962F, Entry, December 1951, LWV Hesse, 16.
16 Schizophrenia was defined in various ways. The absence of a coherent personality was considered to be one of its main features in different conceptions of the disease. See Fabisch, Hans et al., "Schizophrenie. Zur Geschichte der Schizophrenie Diagnostik," *Psychopraxis. Zeitschrift für Psychiatrie und Neurologie* 1, 2000, 26–32. I did not decide to focus on schizophrenia because I assume that this syndrome and the changes it underwent are exemplary of all psychiatric diagnoses. On the contrary, the next two chapters will show that continuities and ruptures in clinical pictures and in their practical application

clearly depended on the syndrome involved and its significance not only within psychiatry but also in political discourse. The diagnosis of schizophrenia is examined here because it was common, particularly widely discussed, and fell within the core area of the discipline of psychiatry.

17 See Murray, *Multiple Sclerosis*; Bernet, *Schizophrenie*.

18 Hess and Majerus, "Writing," 142.

19 At Greifswald, physicians began working with this schema in 1948. There are no indications as to why this switch occurred in that particular year.

20 Ehlerding, Mark, *Sind Klassifikationen sinnvoll? Zur Anwendbarkeit des Person-In-Environment System in der Klinischen Sozialarbeit* (Munich 2002), 12.

21 Kolle, Kurt, *Psychiatrie. Ein Lehrbuch für Studierende und Ärzte* (Berlin 1943), 376 f.

22 Thus, Kraepelin already distinguished between MDI and dementia praecox/schizophrenia with reference to the poorer prognosis for dementia praecox. See Arenz, Dirk, *Eine kleine Geschichte der Schizophrenie* (Bonn 2008), 14.

23 Oswald Bumke took over Kraepelin's chair in Munich in 1924. Many of the committals to Eglfing-Haar analyzed in this book were referrals from the Munich University Psychiatric Clinic that he directed. A short biography of Bumke can be found in Klee, Ernst, *Das Personenlexikon zum "Dritten Reich." Wer war was vor und nach 1945* (Frankfurt/M. 2005), 84 f.

24 Bumke, Oswald, *Lehrbuch der Geisteskrankheiten* (Munich 1936), 2.

25 Ibid., 2 f.

26 Ibid., 3.

27 Ibid.

28 Kurt Kolle was head of the Munich University Psychiatric Clinic from 1952, having previously been a professor in Frankfurt am Main. See Klee, *Personenlexikon*, 329.

29 Kolle, *Lehrbuch*, 372.

30 Ibid., 382.

31 Ibid., 380.

32 See Chapter 1 and Engstrom, *Psychiatry*, 24.

33 This reference to the "humanities" meant that there were no measurements to draw on.

34 Kolle, *Lehrbuch*, 380.

35 Ibid.

36 Lorraine Daston and Peter Galison bring out the close relationship between notions of the scientific self, scientific practice, and particular styles of generating scientific knowledge. See Daston and Galison, *Objectivity*, 32.

37 Ehlerding, *Klassifikationen*, 12.

38 Stengel, Erwin, "Classification of Mental Disorders," *Bulletin of the World Health Organization* 21, 1959, 601–663.

39 Such a connection could be demonstrated, for example, by analysis of psychiatric networks in the 1950s and 1960s, which is far beyond the scope of this book.

40 Richard Jung was, among other things, the first president of the German Society for Clinical Neurophysiology (Deutsche Gesellschaft für Klinische Neurophysiologie). See Grüsser, Otto-Joachim, "Richard Jung (1911–1986)," *Neuropsychologia* 4, 1987, 739–741.

41 Jung, Richard, "Ein neurologisch-psychiatrisches Diagnosenschema," *Der Nervenarzt* 12 (1948), 552–559.

42 Ibid., 552.

43 Ibid.

44 Scheid, Werner, "Diagnose, Aufbau der Diagnose und Differentialdiagnose in der Neurologie," *Der Nervenarzt* 3 (1959), 97–110.

45 Ibid., 97 (original emphasis).
46 Jung, Richard, "Ein neurologisch-psychiatrisches Diagnosenschema," *Der Nervenarzt* 12 (1948), 552–559, 552.
47 The terms morphological and topographical are an attempt to assign disorders to specific areas within the body. In contrast, an etiological system is geared toward the cause of diseases, while a symptomatological approach foregrounds the external signs of illness.
48 Jung, "Ein neurologisch-psychiatrisches Diagnosenschema," 552.
49 Scheid, "Diagnose, Aufbau der Diagnose und Differentialdiagnose," 97.
50 Tabes dorsalis is a long-term consequence of syphilis, which entails damage to the spinal cord. It is the cause of the progressive paralysis mentioned earlier in connection with venereal disease.
51 Ibid., 99.
52 Jung, "Ein neurologisch-psychiatrisches Diagnosenschema," 552.
53 Daston and Galison, *Objectivity*, 27.
54 As early as the final third of the nineteenth century, the inability to classify and understand illnesses in such a way as to facilitate a cure sparked off discussions about what psychiatrists were in fact capable of doing and what the point of asylums was. See for example Walter, "Fürsorgepflicht," 83.
55 Conrad, K., "Das Problem der 'nosologischen Einheit' in der Psychiatrie," *Der Nervenarzt* 11 (1959), 488–494.
56 Ibid., 490 f.
57 Ibid., 490.
58 Ibid.
59 Ibid.
60 Ibid., 491ff. The other two articles are Bash, K.W., "Koordination psychiatrischer Ordnungsschemata," *Der Nervenarzt* 8 (1963), 352–359; Mechler, Achim, "Degeneration und Endogenität," *Der Nervenarzt* 5 (1963), 219–226.
61 Kraemer, Richard, "Zur Diagnose der Schizophrenie," *Der Nervenarzt* 5 (1960), 203–207.
62 Ibid., 204.
63 Ibid.
64 Ibid.
65 On Jaspers' influence and the definition of schizophrenia as the illness that defies understanding, see Arenz, *Geschichte der Schizophrenie*, 88.
66 Kraemer, "Zur Diagnose der Schizophrenie," 204.
67 A short biography of Kurt Schneider can be found in Schott, Heinz and Tölle, Rainer, *Geschichte der Psychiatrie. Krankheitslehren, Irrwege, Behandlungsformen* (Munich 2006), 150ff.
68 Schott and Tölle, *Geschichte der Psychiatrie*, 147.
69 Jaspers, a psychiatrist and philosopher, introduced the distinction to which Kraemer refers here, that between "static" and "genetic" understanding (*Verstehen*). "Static understanding" is purely descriptive, whereas "genetic understanding" presupposes empathy. The idea that it is impossible to achieve the genetic understanding of certain psychiatric illnesses also comes from Jaspers. Delusion, for Jaspers, is a somatic, ultimately inexplicable phenomenon. See Kupke, Christian, "Was ist so unverständlich am Wahn? Philosophisch-kritische Darstellung des Jaspers'schen Unverständlichkeitstheorems," *Journal für Philosophie & Psychiatrie* vol. 1, 2008, 1–12.
70 As already mentioned, the disease later known as schizophrenia first went by the name of "dementia praecox." The naming reflects its "splitting off" from "Alzheimer's disease" as a disorder of old age.

71 Nikolaus Petrilowitsch (1924–1970) was a Jaspers-oriented psychiatrist who became a professor in Mainz in 1964.
72 Henricus Cornelius Rümke (1893–1967) was a Dutch psychiatrist.
73 Kraemer, "Zur Diagnose der Schizophrenie," 205.
74 This classification as intuitively alien was not limited to schizophrenia. Much like the "praecox feeling," reference was, for example, also made to a similar feeling vis-à-vis epileptics. Kraemer too makes mention of this. See ibid.
75 On Kurt Schneider and the longevity of this concept in the second half of the twentieth century, see Moldzio, Andrea, *Schizophrenie—eine philosophische Erkrankung?* (Würzburg 2004), 161.
76 Polanyi, Michael, *Personal Knowledge. Towards a Post-Critical Philosophy* (Chicago 1958).
77 Collins, Harry M., "Tacit Knowledge, Trust and the Q of Sapphire," *Social Studies of Science* vol. 3 (2001), 72.
78 Kraemer, "Zur Diagnose der Schizophrenie," 205.
79 Ibid., 204.
80 Daston, Lorraine, "On Scientific Observation," *Isis* vol. 1 (2008), 98. A practical example of this would be taking a patient's temperature with calibrated measuring instruments. See Hess, Volker, "Die moralische Ökonomie der Normalisierung. Das Beispiel Fiebermessen," in Werner Sohn and Herbert Mehrtens (eds.), *Normalität und Abweichung. Studien zur Theorie und Geschichte der Normalisierungsgesellschaft* (Opladen 1999), 222–243.
81 Daston and Galison, *Objectivity*, 27–28.
82 Ibid., 311.
83 Engstrom, *Psychiatry*, 88.
84 "Psycho-physical experiments were designed to measure psychological reaction times to external stimuli, as well as various mental functions and capacities such as memory, decision making, attention span, etc." Quoted in ibid., 131.
85 Ibid., 12.
86 Ibid., 48ff.
87 Hess and Majerus, "Writing," 142.
88 In most articles in *Der Nervenarzt* this was not done in the same detail as in Kraemer's account of the "praecox feeling." However, expertise was often given positive emphasis.
89 Trigeminal neuralgia refers to an extremely unpleasant facial pain, the cause of which is still unknown.
90 See for example Scheid, "Diagnose, Aufbau der Diagnose und Differentialdiagnose in der Neurologie," 97.
91 Kraemer, "Zur Diagnose der Schizophrenie," 205.
92 Kaufmann, *Aufklärung*, 101ff.
93 On the impossibility of empathizing with endogenous psychoses, see also, for example, Bumke, Oswald, *Lehrbuch der Geisteskrankheiten* (Munich 1936), 3.
94 On Griesinger and his importance to psychiatry, see Engstrom, *Psychiatry*, 51 and 60 f.
95 Roelcke, "Etablierung," 119; Ayaß, *Asoziale*, 13.
96 Neuner, *Politik*, 71ff.
97 The fact that expertise cannot be attributed exclusively to established experts is highlighted by Emma C. Spary for the early modern period, in which expertise played a more widespread role, with reference to the field of food. Spary, Emma C., "Kennerschaft versus chemische Expertise," in Kaspar von Greyerz et al. (eds.), *Wissenschaftsgeschichte und Geschichte des Wissens im Dialog—Connecting Science and knowledge* (Göttingen 2013), 37.

98 Spary also emphasizes that experts were sometimes interested in having certain "knowledge stocks" in common with their "target group," without this implying that these experts did not chiefly have their own interests in mind. Ibid., 41.

99 On the difference between "communitization" (*Vergemeinschaftung*) and "sociation" (*Vergesellschaftlichung*), see Weber, *Wirtschaft*, 21ff.

100 Bajohr, Frank and Michael Wildt, "Einleitung," in Frank Bajohr and Michael Wildt (eds.), *Volksgemeinschaft. Neue Forschungen zur Gesellschaft des Nationalsozialismus* (Frankfurt/M. 2009), 11.

101 Herbert, Ulrich, "Liberalisierung als Lernprozeß. Die Bundesrepublik in der deutschen Geschichte—eine Skizze," in Ulrich Herbert (ed.), *Wandlungsprozesse in Westdeutschland. Belastung, Integration, Liberalisierung 1945–1980* (Göttingen 2002), 23.

102 Szöllösi-Janze, "Wissensgesellschaft," 284.

103 In this chapter, see the section "Diagnostic practice in the FRG and GDR."

104 See Kleist, Karl, "Die paranoiden Schizophrenien," *Der Nervenarzt* 11 (1947), 481–493.

105 Among other things, cerebrospinal fluid helps maintain the metabolism of the central nervous system.

106 See for example Duensing, Friedrich, "Die Absorption der Liquorultrafiltrate Schizophrener im ultravioletten Licht," *Der Nervenarzt* 6 (1947), 277.

107 See for example Runge, Hans, "Zur Prognose der Schizophrenie. (Nachuntersuchung schockbehandelter Psychosen)," *Der Nervenarzt* 4 (1942), 151–157.

108 Hess and Majerus, "Writing," 142.

109 A typical example was the account in Walter von Baeyer's (1904–1987) article of 1950, in which he emphasized numerous differences between "Europe" (by which he meant Western Europe) and "America," but in reality mentioned examples only from German psychiatry. But as we will see in the following, major differences existed, for example between German, Swiss, and British psychiatry. Baeyer, Walter von, "Gegenwärtige Psychiatrie in den Vereinigten Staaten," *Der Nervenarzt* 1 (1950), 2–9.

110 Schildt, Axel, *Zwischen Abendland und Amerika. Studien zur westdeutschen Ideenlandschaft der 50er Jahre* (Munich 1999).

111 Sullivan had considerable influence on U.S. psychiatry and psychology. However, his major work on interpersonal theory, published in the U.S. in 1953, was not translated into German until 1980. For a detailed account of Sullivan and his reception, see Conci, Marco, *Sullivan neu entdecken. Leben und Werk Harry Stack Sullivans und seine Bedeutung für Psychiatrie, Psychotherapie und Psychoanalyse* (Gießen 2005).

112 Gilman, Sander L., "Constructing Schizophrenia as a Category of Mental Illness," in Edwin R. Wallace and John Gach (eds.), *History of Psychiatry and Medical Psychology. With an Epilogue on Psychiatry and the Mind-Body Relation* (New York 2008), 469.

113 Ibid.

114 Well-known psychiatrists, such as Kurt Schneider and Kurt Kolle, whose textbooks are used as sources in this study, were still fighting vehemently in the 1960s against the recognition of psychotherapy in the statutes of the health insurance companies. Roelcke, Volker, "Psychotherapy between Medicine, Psychoanalysis, and Politics. Concepts, Practices, and Institutions in Germany, c. 1945–1992," *Medical History*, vol. 4, 2004, 486 f.

115 This is for example the main result of the research presented in the following article: Loch, W., "Zur Behandlung fortgeschrittener Schizophrenien mit Megaphen und Reserpin," *Der Nervenarzt* 10 (1956), 463–467, 466.

116 On Eugen Bleuler's influence on the conception of schizophrenia, see Bernet, *Schizophrenie*.

117 Bleuler, M., "Die Problematik der Schizophrenien als Arbeitsprogramm des II. Internationalen Kongreßes für Psychiatrie," *Der Nervenarzt* 12 (1957), 529–533, 529.

118 Ibid.

119 This corresponds to the state of the textbooks of the Nazi era. See for example Bumke, *Lehrbuch*, 533.

120 Internationally, Kurt Schneider was unable to gain widespread acceptance for his ideas in the postwar period, but his work played a significant role in the updating of the American Diagnostic and Statistical Manual of Mental Disorders (DSM) from 1980 onward. Schott and Tölle, *Geschichte der Psychiatrie*, 155.

121 See Schneider, Kurt, "Kritik der klinisch-typologischen Psychopathenbetrachtung," *Der Nervenarzt* 6 (1948), 6–9, 7.

122 This made psychotherapy theoretically tenable. However, this tells us nothing about how it was applied in the 1950s. On the establishment of psychotherapy, see Roelcke, "Psychotherapy."

123 Rosenkötter, Lutz, "Zur Psychodynamik der Schizophrenie. Amerikanische Auffassungen zur Entstehung der Schizophrenie," *Der Nervenarzt* 10 (1961), 467–470, 467.

124 Ibid.

125 According to Kury, the lack of reception of Selye's stress research can be attributed to three factors. After World War II, the field of medicine in Germany chiefly prioritized disease control; instead of stress, "managerial disease" (*Managerkrankheit*) rose to prominence; and endocrinology, on which Selye's research was based, was in a weakened state in postwar Germany due to emigration during the Nazi period. See Kury, *Der Überforderte Mensch*, 109.

126 Rosenkötter, "Zur Psychodynamik der Schizophrenie," 468.

127 Stierlin, Helm, "Familie und Schizophrenie," *Der Nervenarzt* 11 (1963), 495–500.

128 See for example Meerwein, F., "Klinisches und psychotherapeutisches Anliegen im Spiegel der diagnostischen Frage," *Der Nervenarzt* 5 (1960), 207 f.

129 Bernet, *Schizophrenie*, 12.

130 The thematization of psychoanalytic and psychotherapeutic concepts in *Der Nervenarzt* reflects the journal's original orientation. When it was founded in 1928, it was expressly intended to publish articles on these topics together with neurological and psychiatric ones. Roelcke, "Psychotherapy," 475. On psycho-therapy, its recognition and use in the Weimar Republic and the "Third Reich," see Cocks, Geoffrey, *Psychotherapy in the Third Reich. The Göring Institute* (New York 1985); Zeller, Uwe, *Psychotherapie in der Weimarer Zeit. Die Gründung der Allgemeinen Ärztlichen Gesellschaft für Psychotherapie* (AÄGP) (Tübingen 2001).

131 This was the *Verzeichnis der Krankheiten und Todesursachen für Zwecke der Medizinalstatistik* (Catalog of Diseases and Causes of Death for Purposes of Medical Statistics). See PsychN Greifswald, Letter to MfG, August 16, 1960, BAB, DQ 1/22109, fol. 1.

132 Ibid.

133 Neurological-Psychiatric Clinic, Karl Marx University Leipzig, Letter to MfG, November 21, 1960, BAB, DQ 1/22109, fol. 1.

134 The responses analyzed in what follows were either from the three facilities studied in this book or from the clinics and hospitals in Saxony that referred patients to Großschweidnitz. Großschweidnitz itself did not respond to the inquiry.

135 Dresdner Strasse Hospital, Letter to MfG, August 31, 1960, BAB, DQ 1/22109, fol. 2.

136 Ibid., fol. 3.

137 Ibid., fol. 3 f.

138 The publications in *Der Nervenarzt* are the two articles already mentioned, which I cite again here for the sake of clarity: Jung, Richard, "Ein neurologisch-psychiatrisches Diagnoseschema," *Der Nervenarzt* 12 (1948), 552–559; Scheid, Werner, "Diagnose, Aufbau der Diagnose und Differentialdiagnose in der Neurologie," *Der Nervenarzt* 3 (1959), 97–110.

139 Dresdner Strasse Hospital, Letter to MfG, August 31, 1960, BAB, DQ 1/22109, fol. 3.

140 Ibid., fol. 3 f.

141 Ibid., fol. 4.

142 Ibid.

143 On the contrary, Kraepelin already distinguished between MDI and dementia praecox/schizophrenia with reference to the worse prognosis for dementia praecox. See Arenz, *Geschichte der Schizophrenie*, 14.

144 Dresdner Strasse Hospital, Letter to MfG, August 31, 1960, BAB, DQ 1/22109, fol. 3.

145 See Ernst, *Sozialismus*, 333.

146 Ibid.

147 Hanrath, *Euthanasie und Psychiatriereform*, 366.

148 Dresdner Strasse Hospital, Letter to MfG, August 31, 1960, BAB, DQ 1/22109, fol. 4.

149 Rüting, Torsten, *Pavlov und der Neue Mensch. Diskurse und Disziplinierung in Sowjetrussland* (Munich 2002), 279.

150 Ibid., 123.

151 Ibid., 114.

152 Ibid., 279.

153 Dresdner Strasse Hospital, Letter to MfG, August 31, 1960, BAB, DQ 1/22109, fol. 4.

154 Neurological-Psychiatric Clinic, Karl Marx University Leipzig, Letter to MfG, November 21, 1960, BAB, DQ 1/22109, fol. 1.

155 Ibid., fol. 2

156 Ibid.

157 Both the idea that psychiatric disorders had to do with malfunctions of the cortex and the view, dominant in the FRG, that they were endogenous, were as one in postulating a physical cause.

158 PsychN Greifswald, Letter to MfG, August 16, 1960, BAB, DQ 1/22109, fol. 2.

159 Ibid.

160 Ibid., fol. 2 and 3.

161 Ibid., fol. 3.

162 The Ministry of Health's request itself is not included in the BAB, DQ 1/22109 holding, so this cannot be verified.

163 Schmiedebach, Heinz-Peter, "Psychoanalyse, Psychotherapie und die Lehre von Pawlow im Werk von Hanns Schwarz," in Wolfgang Fischer and Heinz-Peter Schmiedebach (eds.), *Die Greifswalder Universitäts- und Nervenklinik unter dem Direktorat von Hanns Schwarz 1946 bis 1965* (Greifswald 1999), 32.

164 Vogt, Cécile and Vogt, Oskar, "Vorbemerkungen zu einer ätiologischen Klassifikation der Schizophrenie und anderer 'funktioneller' Psychosen," *Psychiatrie, Neurologie und medizinische Psychologie. Zeitschrift für Forschung und Praxis* 1 (1953), 4–7; Joschko, H., "Vorschlag einer ätiologisch begründeten Klassifikation neuropsychiatrischer Leiden in Verbindung mit einer Einteilung neurologischer und psychopathologischer Syndrome zum Zwecke der Dokumentation," *Psychiatrie, Neurologie und medizinische*

Psychologie. Zeitschrift für Forschung und Praxis 9 (1963), 341–346, 345; Müller-Hegemann, D., "Zur Klassifikation neurologisch-psychiatrischer Krankheiten. Vorschlag eines Diagnoseschemas," *Psychiatrie, Neurologie und medizinische Psychologie. Zeitschrift für Forschung und Praxis* 9 (1963), 350–356, 350.

165 Vogt und Vogt, "Vorbemerkungen," 7. K. Leonhard expressed similar views: Leonhard, K., "Diagnoseverzeichnis psychiatrischer und neurologischer Krankheiten," *Psychiatrie, Neurologie und medizinische Psychologie. Zeitschrift für Forschung und Praxis* 9 (1963), 346–350, 346.

166 Walther, Rolf, "Überlegungen zur Pathogenese der Schizophrenie," *Psychiatrie, Neurologie und Medizinische Psychologie. Zeitschrift für Forschung und Praxis* 8 (1950), 225–231, 230.

167 In Pavlov's construction of the conditioned reflex, specific reactions are triggered by external stimuli. On environmental stimuli in Pavlov's theory, see Rüting, *Pavlov*, 114.

168 When I refer to the Soviet position in what follows, the reader should bear in mind that it did not correspond one-to-one to Pavlov's views. Pavlov's legacy was in fact administered by Konstantin Bykov from 1949 onward, who interpreted it in accordance with the tenets of Stalinism: ibid., 273.

169 Walther, "Überlegungen zur Pathogenese der Schizophrenie."

170 Rüting, *Pavlov*, 150.

171 Walther, "Überlegungen zur Pathogenese der Schizophrenie," 226 f.

172 Rüting, *Pavlov*, 285.

173 Kiril Cholakov, "Zur pathophysiologischen Analyse einiger Frühsymptome der Schizophrenie," *Psychiatrie, Neurologie und Medizinische Psychologie. Zeitschrift für Forschung und Praxis* 4 (1955), 97–101, 99.

174 Gyula Nyírő and Jenő Drietomszky, "Halluzinose und Schizophrenie," *Psychiatrie, Neurologie und Medizinische Psychologie. Zeitschrift für Forschung und Praxis* 3 (1959), 66–75.

175 On the introduction of Pavlov in the GDR, see Ernst, *Sozialismus*, 311ff.

176 Lemke, Rudolf, "Neurologische Befunde bei Schizophrenen," *Psychiatrie, Neurologie und Medizinische Psychologie. Zeitschrift für Forschung und Praxis* 8 (1955), 226–229.

177 Steiner, U., "Beitrag zur Differentialdiagnose zwischen Zwangsneurose und Schizophrenie," *Psychiatrie, Neurologie und Medizinische Psychologie. Zeitschrift für Forschung und Praxis* 1 (1956), 1–11.

178 Since committals and discharges or further transfers often occurred "after notification by telephone"/"after a telephone conversation with … ," we may assume that explanations of divergent diagnoses were also given verbally.

179 Amentia was a synonym for feeble-mindedness.

180 PsychN Greifswald, Patient file prov. sign. 1947/351, Letter, July 9, 1947, UA Greifswald, PsychN, 1.

181 Ibid., 2.

182 Ibid., 1.

183 KA Großschweidnitz, Patient file sign. 754, Entry, June 5, 1956, HSta Dresden, 10822. The code 368 K refers to the diagnostic key of 1952.

184 vBS Bethel, Patient file sign. 84/995, Evaluation (*Gutachten*) by Dr. Sch. and Dr. B., HAB, Patient files Mahainam II.

185 Ibid.

186 Myasthenia gravis pseudoparalytica is a weakness of the muscles that is now known to result from problems in the transmission between nerve and muscle.

187 vBS Bethel, Patient file sign. 84/995, Evaluation by Dr. Sch. and Dr. B., HAB, Patient files Mahainam II.

188 Ibid.
189 On notions of degeneration and constitution already widespread in the German Empire, see Engstrom, Eric J., "'On the Question of Degeneration' by Emil Kraepelin (1908)," *History of Psychiatry*, vol. 3, 2007, 392.
190 vBS Bethel, Patient file sign. 84/995, Evaluation by Dr. Sch. and Dr. B., Sub-item "Progress of Observation," HAB, Patient files Mahainam II.
191 Ibid.
192 Ibid.
193 Ibid., Letter from guardian, September 17, 1962.
194 Ibid., Letter to guardian, October 8, 1962.
195 Ibid.
196 Ibid., Evaluation by Dr. Sch. and Dr. B., Sub-item "Progress of Observation."
197 Ibid., Sub-item "Final Evaluation."
198 Daston and Galison, *Objectivity*.
199 Foucault, *Psychologie*, 132; see also Meier et al., *Psychiatrie*, 41.
200 Donalies, G., "Psychiatrie in der Pflichtassistentenzeit! Eine Anregung," *Das Deutsche Gesundheitswesen* 51 (1954), offprint.
201 A broken kneecap.
202 Merguet, Hans, "Vorschläge für den Wiederaufbau der Offenen Fürsorge für Geisteskranke," *Der Nervenarzt* 4 (1951), 150–153.
203 Ibid., 151.
204 Ibid., 152.
205 Donalies, "Psychiatrie in der Pflichtassistentenzeit!"
206 See Arenz, *Geschichte der Schizophrenie*, 14.
207 These forms have not always been preserved. They were usually placed in the administrative files, but some archives preserved only medical records and not administrative ones (Eglfing-Haar for example).
208 On the informative value of medical records as a source, see also the introduction and conclusion of this book.
209 Conrad, "Das Problem der 'nosologischen Einheit,'" 490.
210 For a summary account of the way in which, according to Foucault, direct observation supplanted the medical history as the starting point for the medical determination of illness in the mid-nineteenth century, see for example Raffnsøe et al., *Foucault*, 145.
211 Giljarowski, W. A., *Lehrbuch der Psychiatrie* (Berlin 1960). It is quite possible that admission interviews changed in the course of the 1960s in part due to the translation of psychiatric texts from the Soviet Union. As early as 1960, we find for example that at the Greifswald University Psychiatric Clinic these consultations upon admission were adapted to the "socialist" conception of psychiatry. The heading "social anamnesis" appears for the first time and repeatedly in the files from 1960, whereas previously—as in all the other institutions examined here—the medical history began with the so-called "self-anamnesis" (*Eigenanamnese*) and the "objective anamnesis." The term "social anamnesis" in itself emphasizes the importance of external factors to the genesis of mental abnormalities in line with Soviet psychiatry. In terms of content, however, these are narratives put forward by the patient or their relatives, as previously found under the other two headings. To what extent this new rubric was related to changes in medical assessments or treatments in the clinic is impossible to say, since the present book's main focus is on the committal process. In Großschweidnitz this regrouping did not occur until 1963 at the earliest. The rapid change in Greifswald makes sense given that its director Hanns Schwarz, unlike most other psychiatrists in the GDR, had a genuine interest in Pavlov and Soviet psychiatry.

212 The chapter entitled "Vom Untersuchen seelisch Kranker" ("Examining the mentally ill"), which remained unchanged in all versions of the book, formed its final section in the third and fifth editions, while appearing somewhat earlier in the second. The 1962 textbook additionally includes a brief section on psychological testing procedures. Kolle, *Lehrbuch*, 370–377; Kolle, *Lehrbuch* (1949, three print runs), 394–404; Kolle, *Lehrbuch* (1961, five print runs), 348–353.

213 Kolle, *Lehrbuch*, 334. In the following, the page references refer to the 1943 edition. Unless explicitly stated, these references can usually be found verbatim in the other editions.

214 Ibid., 335.

215 Ibid., 334.

216 Ibid., 336.

217 Ibid., 335 and 337.

218 Ibid., 337.

219 Ibid., 338.

220 The death of a father, for example: KA Rodewisch, Patient file sign. 7424, Anamnesis, SächSta Chemnitz, 32810, 1.

221 This is context-specific only in that psychiatric establishments were no longer involved in combatting STDs in the postwar period. The focus on women as carriers pertained both before and after this era. Lindner, "Traditionen," 222; Lindner, *Gesundheitspolitik*, 298.

222 Lerner, *Men*.

223 Hauschildt, *Trinkerfürsorge*, 24.

224 Meier et al., *Psychiatrie*, 44.

225 vBS Bethel, Patient file sign. 3766, Entry, July 3, 1943, HAB, Patient files Gilead III.

226 Ibid., Entry, August 18, 1958.

227 Bumke, *Lehrbuch*, 2.

228 LHA Marburg, Patient file sign. K9944F, Evaluation, December 6, 1941, LWV Hesse, 16.

229 Ibid., Evaluation, December 6, 1941, 29.

230 Ibid., Evaluation, December 6, 1941, 1ff.

231 Fabisch et al., "Schizophrenie," 29.

232 PsychN Greifswald, Patient file prov. sign. 1941/770, Entry, January 6, 1941, UA Greifswald, PsychN.

233 Ibid., Entry, January 22, 1941.

234 It is undisputed in the research that psychiatric diagnoses have gender-specific aspects. For a summary, see for example Meier et al., *Psychiatrie*, 44.

235 LHA Marburg, Patient file sign. K10563M, Letter to wife, December 15, 1948, LWV Hesse, 16.

236 HPA Eglfing-Haar, Patient file sign. EH 4383, Admission form, January 25, 1947, AB Upper Bavaria, EH.

237 Ibid., Letter from father to the Munich University Psychiatric Clinic, January 18, 1947.

238 Ibid.

239 Ibid.

240 Ibid., Entry in the medical history, January 16, 1947.

241 Ibid., Letter from father to HPA Eglfing-Haar (undated, receipt stamp: December 9, 1947).

242 Ibid.

243 Ibid., Letter from Dr. B. to father, December 9, 1947.

244 Goldberg, "Conventions of Madness," 178; for a summary, see also Chapter 1 in this book.

245 HPA Eglfing-Haar, Patient file sign. EH9682, Entry, December 9, 1948, AB Upper Bavaria, EH.
246 Numerous comparable cases can be found in the medical holdings of Bethel and the LHA Marburg.
247 Stockdreher, "Heil- und Pflegeanstalt."
248 KA Rodewisch, Patient file sign. 4895, Letters from the mother, March 2–September 10, 1953, SächSta Chemnitz, 32810.
249 Ibid., Letter from mother, March 2, 1953.
250 Ibid.
251 Ibid., Letter from Dr. M. to the mother, March 16, 1953.
252 Ibid., Letter from the mother, June 19, 1953.
253 Ibid., Letter from Dr. M. to the mother, June 24, 1953.
254 KA Großschweidnitz, Patient file sign. 2741, HSta Dresden, 10822.
255 Schagen and Schleiermacher, "Gesundheitswesen," 423.
256 KA Großschweidnitz, Patient file sign. 686, Entry, December 27, 1956, HSta Dresden, 10822.
257 See *Klöppel,* "Brigade Propaphenin."
258 On the significance of the availability of resources from the West to real-world power relations in the GDR, see Fulbrook, *Leben,* 63 f.
259 West German citizens less often placed their hopes in "Soviet" treatment methods.
260 See BAB, DQ 1/3902; BAB, DQ 1/21228; BAB, DQ 1/21230.
261 Letter to minister, August 15, 1961, BAB, DQ 1/21230.
262 Ibid.
263 Ibid.
264 Ibid.
265 Many patients embraced the assumption that significantly reduced fat consumption would lower the relapse rate. See Murray, *Multiple Sclerosis,* 87.
266 BAB DQ 1/3902, Requests Psychiatry 1952–1954, an example being Request, July 28, 1954.
267 Murray, *Multiple Sclerosis,* 252.
268 I reviewed all requests concerning multiple sclerosis. I was not, however, able to inspect every general request relating to psychiatry, which included some relating to MS in the following periods, which I did examine: 1952–1954 and 1959–1963: BAB, DQ 1/3902; 21228; 21230.
269 An example being: Letter from Dr. Lammert, April 3, 1962, BA Lichterfelde, DQ 1/3902.
270 Ibid.
271 Letter, December 22, 1961, to Dr. Lammert, BAB, DQ 1/3902.
272 As in: Letter, January 6, 1962, BAB, DQ 1/3902.
273 Murray, *Multiple Sclerosis,* 224ff.
274 Ibid., 224.
275 Letter, June 12, 1961 to Health Minister of the GDR, BAB, DQ 1/3902.
276 Anna Sabine Ernst assesses the Pavlov campaign as unsuccessful. According to her, Pavlov research in the 1950s was conducted alongside but not integrated with other research and had no impact. See Ernst, *Sozialismus,* 335ff.

5 Work and performance

Ability and inability to work in committal rationales

As we have seen throughout this book, if we wish to grasp the complexity of a committal, we need to think about more than the criteria of illness or danger to self and others. Diagnosis and insight into illness were not usually decisive to the committal behavior of patients nor did their relatives consider them the most important aspect. The key factor was how to cope with those everyday realities that made a person's illness or behavior seem intolerable within their social milieu, and the core benchmark in this regard was whether they were capable of performing everyday work routines. In 1946, Martina R.'s mother-in-law concluded that her relative was no longer competent in this respect and she presented this as grounds for committal:

> Over the last few weeks her condition has worsened. She believed she had to starve herself and, without discussing it with the family, got herself a job waiting tables, yet when it came to wanting to work, she didn't think about the most obvious thing, such as washing her own child's diapers, and so on, all of which my eldest daughter took care of.[1]

In addition to her oldest daughter, her mother-in-law contrasted Martina R.'s behavior with that of her sister, who was also married to one of her sons. She

> has acquitted herself marvelously. My son died on his estate in Mecklenburg due to mistreatment by the Russians. His wife (the patient's sister) now runs the estate all on her own and keeps herself and her children going without assistance, although she never studied anything of that sort, but is trained as a craftswoman.[2]

She complained that her daughter-in-law was failing to smoothly carry out her household and child-rearing duties amid the trying circumstances of the postwar period. A "healthy" person was expected to be able and willing to work under all conditions, with disruptions to the work process in the broadest sense playing a key role in prompting people to conclude that someone they knew required institutionalization. This could relate to both

DOI: 10.4324/9781032716237-6

the individual's perceived responsibilities and the work of those in their social environment. The latter came into play, for example, if a sick family member had to be looked after. Work, ability to work, and willingness to work, unlike danger and illness, were not official reasons for psychiatric committals but were frequently mentioned in the context of committals.[3] Yet the assessment of work ability and performance as indicators of illness, like the attributions of illness in the previous chapter, depended in large part on the speaker's perspective. These concepts were fundamentally open to interpretation and had to be linked with concrete criteria. Inevitably, within this framework, the patient was interpreted in terms of others' needs and wants. Here, quite different aspects, varying according to perspective, could function as comparators. Laypersons often drew on their own experience, while physicians' expert evaluations indicated degrees of ability to work in percentage terms, as measured against a nominal value. Diagnoses were products of their time, incorporating expectations of "normal" behavior deemed beneficial to society.[4] Some diagnoses even articulated an evaluation of work and performance semantically, as in the notions of the "asocial psychopath" and "pension neurosis."

In this chapter, I begin by analyzing statements made in favor of or against asylum stays by different actors. I then shift focus away from the need for institutionalization to definitions of illness: the attribution of a psychiatric disorder and the subsequent identification of a need for a stay in an asylum were two separate and not necessarily related processes. In the context of the attribution of illness, I shed light on two different relationships between work and health: inability to work as a sign of illness and "overwork" (*Überarbeitung*) as a cause of psychological afflictions. To this end, I first analyze discourses about work and health among patients and their relatives before turning to the physicians' perspective. I examine the medical gaze both in the scholarly discourse on work and performance and in committal practice, with admissions to assess a person's capacity for work being particularly relevant to the latter.

Sources and what they can tell us

I base my analysis here on psychiatric journals, textbooks, patient files, and, in a few cases, statistical data from medical records. These sources allow me to reconstruct different actors' perspectives on work-related issues, including patients' ideas. Here, in addition to first-person documents, I draw on medical histories and diagnostic exploration as it appears in the records. This raises the question of whether patients' thematization of work in their medical histories might be due solely to physicians having a special interest in this topic. In fact, this is not what a close inspection of the sources and their context of origin suggests. The manifold ways in which work was addressed in medical laypersons' first-person documents indicate that statements on this topic were at the very least not exclusively due to external prompts.[5]

In addition, a close look at diagnostic exploration reveals that while physicians regularly elicited facts about work, they did not ask about the relationship between work and illness from the patient's point of view.[6] This is consonant with the guidance provided in psychiatric textbooks. Such publications were much the same in this regard in the Nazi period and the early FRG, while the GDR gained its own textbook, translated from Russian, only in 1960.[7] According to the instructions on anamnesis provided in such texts, the patient ought to be asked about their school performance and occupational history.[8] The physician was encouraged to let the patient talk in an undirected manner and to take down their words as accurately as possible, ideally verbatim.[9] Practice seems largely to have conformed to the textbooks. This, at least, is suggested by case histories from the LHA Marburg, Rodewisch, and Großschweidnitz, in which doctors' questions were typically inserted into the medical record in parentheses and in abbreviated form.[10] They routinely asked questions about work, but such inquiries were an attempt to illuminate the structure of the patient's life course and were of a general nature. The following sequence of questions was typical:

> (Did well in school?) "I have to say, I never really paid much attention." (Ever repeat a year?) "No, but I easily might have done." (Learnt a trade?) "No, I've only been at the company." (What kind of company?) "Brush factory and then at Knorr, those are the two factories I have worked at." (How long working there?), [etc].[11]

Hence, there is evidence to suggest that when it came to self-attributions of illness or health, the evaluation of a person's work was not a topic raised chiefly by physicians. Going by the medical records, it is not obvious that physicians explicitly asked patients how they evaluated their work in connection with their state of health. Still, work was a theme in medical records beyond the facts that doctors asked about. References to work and performance can, therefore, be read predominantly as a lay perspective, while the interpretation of work and performance tells us something about the psychiatric knowledge of the time that was applied in practice.

At the threshold: work and institutionalization, 1941–1963

Inclusion and exclusion: work in families' committal rationales during the war

Especially for the World War II period, the category of work facilitates the exploration of psychiatric history and the history of society as they relate to one another. Work and the ability to work were of crucial importance during the war in several respects. Both research on the Holocaust and on the murder of the sick have shown that the ability to work was an important, though by no means conclusive, criterion for selecting those to be murdered in asylums and concentration camps.[12] At the same time, the extraordinary emphasis on the individual's usefulness constituted a key component of "internal racism." In connection with the category of work, this manifested itself, for example, in the campaigns against so-called "asocials" and the "work-shy" in the immediate run-up to World War II.[13] A Nazi-specific change also took place at the legal level, with labor law being removed from the sphere of civil law and incorporated into criminal law. "Failure to fulfill a service obligation [*Dienstverpflichtung*] or leaving an assigned post [became] punishable offenses."[14] Previously, responsibility for dealing with misconduct on the job had rested with the company.[15] In addition, the world of work was characterized by an extreme performance-centered ideology, with company-based health care making the largest contribution to its practical implementation.[16]

Less is known, however, about whether and if so how, work, the ability to work, and performance shaped everyday life in families during the war.[17] To investigate this, I now scrutinize the role of work in rationales for committal.

Although argumentative references to work were not unique to Nazi Germany, they had war-specific features in the period from 1941 to the end of the war for two reasons. First, war and work were often linked quite directly, and second, committal during the years in question must be interpreted against the background of widespread knowledge about the murder of the sick.[18]

The distinction between the ability and inability to work marked a threshold of belonging and not belonging that affected almost every area of life. This distinction is, therefore, of crucial importance to understanding inclusion and exclusion in everyday practice. The patient's labor, as well as that of family members, played multiple and important roles in the negotiation of both committal and length of stay. Police and health offices often placed great emphasis on people's ability to work and their usefulness in the course of committals, as we saw in Chapter 3, "Danger and Security." But relatives too argued—sometimes successfully, sometimes unsuccessfully—that the patient was needed at home to work, that they could not stay at home because they were unfit for work, or that their committal was preventing them from contributing to the work of the "community." Work and performance were thus central to argumentative strategies of inclusion and exclusion. I will illustrate this with reference to arguments made by relatives that were typical of the evocation of work and performance in committal procedures during World War II. I begin by describing committals that shed light on the use of "inability to work" as a committal rationale, before going on to analyze an example in which a husband wished to prevent his wife's institutionalization by claiming that her presence was vital to his ability to work.

Marie H.[19] was committed to the Leipzig University Psychiatric Clinic in 1942 before being transferred to the Untergöltzsch Sanatorium-Nursing Home. In 1942, she was 28 years old, married, and had two children. Her husband was serving at the front. She was taken to the university clinic in

Leipzig by her sister, who stated that the patient was talking "a lot of twaddle"[20] and was convinced that her husband was cheating on her. Marie H. herself said that "she felt hypnotized."[21] After seven days she was discharged, and her file remarks: "Her husband, who had returned from the field, took his wife home at his own request and at his own risk. He was informed that [his wife was suffering from] an incipient mental illness."[22] Two months later, the husband took his wife back to the Leipzig clinic. Among other things, it was noted that:

> He had taken the patient out on his own responsibility on September 9, 1942, after a few days' stay in the clinic. However, things had gone badly at home. She had neglected the household and failed to take care of the children. Everything had been left undone, and the patient herself had been completely intransigent and indifferent, showing no concern for anything. They had had intercourse, but the patient had been cold during it, in sharp contrast to the past. Now he had to return to the front, so he thought it best to bring the patient back to the clinic. It was impossible for her to cope at home alone. The two children were with the grandparents.[23]

The patient stated on the same day:

> But it had gone very well at home. She doesn't even know what her husband's problem is; she had taken good care of everything. She no longer feels that she is sick at all. She would like to go back home to help her mother do the washing. [...] She has no idea why she is being locked up here when she could do so much work at home ... .[24]

After this man had initially taken his wife home from the clinic at his own risk, he now brought her back. Her failure to perform her household duties played a major role for him, as typical of many husbands' committal rationales. In the course of the committal of another woman to Bethel in 1942, it was noted: "Husband asks that we 'strive to educate his wife to become a socially responsible Christian housewife' and hopes 'that this goal can be achieved in the asylum, if [her condition] is not wholly hereditary, and only there' (!)."[25] It was also quite common for a husband to link his wife's ability to work and what he considered "abnormal sexual behavior." Hence, it was not only the police and health offices that made connections between gender, sexuality, ability to work, and willingness to work.

The wife in the first example argued—unsuccessfully—that she had "taken good care of everything" at home and that her labor was needed there. Both parties sought to use the argument from work capacity to their own ends. Both referred to specific spheres of work. The husband expressed frustration about the fact that his wife had failed to take care of the children, while she talked about doing the laundry. We can see here that, for the patient and her husband, the unofficial threshold between the ability and inability to work was directly anchored in everyday life. They took this threshold as a given and referred to it in their arguments as a matter of course. This is particularly significant in that the (in)ability to work was not an official criterion for committal and thus provides deep insights into behavioral norms within society. As a rationale put forward by the patient and her relatives, the ability to work was a concretization—closely bound up with everyday life—of the need for institutionalization that enjoyed wide recognition within society. In terms of its persuasiveness, the reference to performance in the household was in turn linked with intra-family and societal power relations. Ultimately, the husband and the doctors decided his wife's fate. While we have no clear evidence that there was greater cooperation between male family members than between female relatives and physicians, we can discern gender differences in the issues central to such cooperation. It was quite common for husbands to classify their wives' housework and sexual behavior as unacceptable and for physicians to go along with this. Women, on the other hand, initiated committals in collaboration with physicians almost exclusively with reference to physical violence. One example is the case in Chapter 3 in which the army doctor discharged a soldier home and his wife then initiated committal on the basis of his violent behavior.

The ability and willingness to work were key characteristics of acceptability within family and society, not only, but especially under wartime circumstances. Marie H.'s husband, whom we encountered a moment ago, cited his return to the front as the reason why his wife's household management had finally become unacceptable. His rationale, which he considered both sayable and powerful, arose from linking his wife's "unwillingness to work" to wartime conditions.

The ability to work and performance of Minna W.,[26] who was admitted to the Eglfing-Haar Sanatorium-Nursing Home in March 1944 as dangerous to the public, were crucial to her committal in a completely different way. Her evaluation by the public health officer, which was meant to explain why the patient was a danger to the public, reveals that she had been reported to the health office several times by her neighbors since 1941. She was certified as suffering from delusions, which manifested themselves in the conviction that her neighbors were planning to kill her. The patient's husband, another soldier at the front at the time of her committal, sent a letter to the asylum. He stated that he had been at the front since 1939 to "protect homeland and family."[27] He explained his wife's behavior in this context: "It is not hard to understand why my wife went to pieces in these difficult times. It was her worry over me."[28] Then he requested her release:

> As I am suffering very badly due to my wife's downturn and this has caused my performance to decline noticeably, I have been granted twelve days' special leave to care for her. I ask you, dear directors, to give my

children back their mother by releasing her from the asylum, thus restoring my former strength and allowing me to perform my duties in the way so crucial to achieving final victory for all of us.[29]

This letter reveals room for argumentative maneuver in the context of psychiatric committals even during the Nazi era, as families tried to prevent or shorten their relatives' committals. In contrast to the two previous examples, the primary concern here was not the patient's ability to work, but her husband's. While the first source brought out the distinction between ability and inability to work as a concretization of the more abstract tolerable/non-tolerable boundary, this source points to a different function of psychiatric institutions. The invoking of non-patients' ability to work alerts us to an understanding of these establishments that was closely linked to the functioning of society. The idea here was that removing "disruptive elements" must not lead to a loss of efficiency. Here, once again, it becomes clear how deeply rooted the practice of committal was in everyday (wartime) life. The husband understood the asylum as a solution to disruption and inappropriate behavior. His concerns were focused on the fact that his wife's committal would cause more disturbances than it would eliminate. Since her husband was a soldier, an issue that was often highlighted in other contexts is thrown into particular relief: the work of the committed person's family and thus its contribution to the "National Community" (*Volksgemeinschaft*) and to achieving "final victory." The patient's husband described his activity as a soldier using terms from the world of work, referring for example to his declining performance.[30] At the same time, he emphasized the importance of his activities to the community by stressing his desire to achieve "final victory for all of us." The acceptance of the work impairment argument is also evident in the fact that the husband was given special leave to care for his wife. In committal rationales, work often formed part of a larger argumentational complex that foregrounded several different spheres of life. Reference was made to wives' housework and above all to child rearing, as well as to war-related work. The patient files from the war period also contain examples of committal in which women tried to prevent their husbands from being admitted to an asylum by highlighting their work for the family.[31]

Overall, the category of work casts much light on behavioral expectations in everyday life and helps us grasp the social practice of inclusion and exclusion during World War II. In committal practice, rationales that foregrounded work and the ability to work gained special persuasive power precisely because of their connection to wartime tasks and circumstances. From the vantage point of committal practice, what we find is that from 1941 to the end of the war, that conflict influenced the scope for negotiating the tolerable in two ways. First, non-institutional actors now had no room for maneuver at all in certain constellations, as in the case of women declared "asocial" who were forcibly committed due to venereal disease.

Second, the paradigm of the national comrade (*Volksgenosse*) who was able and willing to work opened up room for maneuver. Arguments focused on the notion of "willingness to work and performance" were used not only in exclusionary practices, but also to inclusionary ends. Relatives could point out that committal might have a negative impact on another person's ability to work and thus impair the functioning of the "National Community." The scope for argumentation was thus multi-directional. The multifaceted significance and context-specific role of the category of work in committal rationales during World War II shows that work played a key role not only in the asylum, in Nazi propaganda, and in extermination processes, but also in everyday notions of belonging and tolerability.[32]

Restoring capacity for work, safeguarding work processes: familial reasoning about committals in West Germany

In the FRG, too, patients and their families frequently couched their arguments in terms of work and performance in the course of committals. Relatives' rationales were structurally similar to those put forward during the war, though less drastic. Three points are particularly pertinent to the analysis of continuities and discontinuities between wartime Germany and its western successor state. First, in the latter people no longer evoked connections between individual committals and the good of society as a whole, as occurred, for example, in references to wartime military service. Second, the focus was firmly on the family. Finally, a parallel to the Nazi period can be seen in arguments centered on wives' neglect of household duties.

In continuity with the past, relatives in the FRG cited both the patient's inability to work and the effects of their illness on their own capacity to work. But in contrast to committals between 1941 and 1945, which must be read against the background of the murder of the sick, family members no longer used the argument from work to reverse committals as quickly as possible. Typical was the committal rationale put forward by Miranda L.'s family, mentioned in Chapter 2, namely, their claim that they could no longer carry out their daily work because someone always had to take care of the patient. Since all of them were engaged in farming from dawn to dusk, they were unable to supervise her at home when she became agitated.[33]

There would appear to be two main reasons why arguments centered on work and performance shifted away from foregrounding the "National Community" to emphasizing the immediate social environment in West Germany. For some patients or their relatives, it may be that references to the *Volkskörper* or "national body" in wartime were an instrumental appropriation of propaganda. In addition, the sources indicate that people in the Nazi era expected the "National Community" to have real effects in their own everyday lives and, especially toward the end of the war, were disappointed when these failed to materialize. Patients stated, for example, that they would have liked to have seen more "comradely" behavior during aerial bombardment.[34] The sources do not allow us to determine how notions of individual and society interacted in committals after the war but prior to the founding of the FRG. Due to the rudimentary patient records and the special psychiatric clientele of the years immediately after the war, medical histories cannot be meaningfully examined to reveal patients' and relatives' expectations of "community" or society.[35] However, for many, the "society in a state of collapse" (*Zusammenbruchgesellschaft*) was undoubtedly characterized by the loss of relatives, hunger, flight, homelessness, and dependence on the black market.[36] All of this suggests that, until the foundation of the two German states, people increasingly felt thrown back on themselves and, at best, on their families. While the new paradigm of the socialist community was propagated quite rapidly in the GDR, the early FRG lacked an equivalent, vigorously promoted, unifying social self-image. It is true that West Germans were invited to integrate themselves as individuals into larger wholes, by embracing one of the Christian communities for instance. Yet such options did not encompass every citizen of the new state—Catholics and Protestants were, for example, addressed separately—nor were they articulated with the same validity claim as in the case of the *Volksgemeinschaft* or, in the neighboring state, the "new man in the socialist world."[37] It was in fact the family that functioned as the most important unit in early West Germany. Defining oneself within the small family unit took on tremendous importance. Studies of advertising and consumer behavior, for example, have shown just how much the individual acquisition of gender roles matched the division of tasks in family life.[38] The family, a crucial benchmark in multiple spheres of life, thus makes its presence felt in many medical histories and ego-documents.

In the 1950s and early 1960s, patients in the FRG often highlighted the fact that their families were participating in an advancing economy and that they were hard-working and had successful careers. Hence, while family members often underlined patients' work performance, time and again patients vicariously underscored their relatives' diligence and success. A 25-year-old blacksmith, committed in 1961 for "alcoholism" (*Trunksucht*), for instance, stated that none of his three siblings drank and that they "had all worked their way up."[39] He then provided precise details of his siblings' occupations, which he described as "respectable": they were in the air force, machinists, and commercial clerks.[40]

Within the West German family, expectations and assessments of individual family members' ability to work resembled those of the wartime period. Men's and women's work capacity continued to be addressed but in different argumentational contexts. Relatives of female patients, and above all husbands, focused on household management. As during World War II, they cited household neglect as a pragmatic reason for committals. References to the war, which cropped up frequently in committals before the end of that conflict, were supplanted by other arguments. A typical rationale for the committal of women was that they were neglecting their domestic tasks and their husband "had had to take care of the household over the last few weeks."[41] From relatives' point of view, one key purpose of committal was to restore the capacity for housekeeping.

In the context of the committal of men, too, relatives in the FRG brought up ability and willingness to work. But in such cases, arguments about work did not serve as the main justification for institutionalization. Max T., for example, was admitted to the LHA Marburg nine times between 1952 and the end of 1956. His mother, with whom he lived, was involved in initiating all of his committals. These were a response to domestic violence and increasingly to the fact that this man, who was already thirty years old in 1956, had no job; they also made a connection between his unemployment and his violence.[42] When he was admitted in 1956, his mother related that he had until recently "helped out as a laborer and earned his money in a construction firm" before he "got out of hand," began drinking, hit his mother, and smashed a window pane.[43] During wartime and in the FRG, the topic of women's domestic work was more important and came up more often than male gainful employment. This is probably due in part to the fact that housework fell within the family sphere. In addition, the significance attached to female- and male-dominated spheres of work points to power relations within families and highlights arguments that were considered compelling. Women—often with little or no choice—tended to put up with more than men did.

In the FRG, patients themselves continued to argue with reference to their capacity for work. In contrast to the wartime situation, however, they not only alluded to what they considered their intact ability to work to argue *against* committal. Now both men and women used work and performance as arguments *for* admission, hoping that a stay in a clinic or asylum would restore their working capacity. For example, Frank M. stated of treatment at Bethel: "I would so much like to be free of this ailment and help my family with the work (which there is no lack of."[44]

A double-edged sword: work in East German committal rationales

In the early GDR, the ability and willingness to work remained key criteria for or against committal in the arguments of relatives and the social environment, to an even greater extent than in the FRG. In this context, ideally speaking, there were three variants. First, the ability to work was seen as an indication of mental health and of tolerability within society and the family, in other words, it was addressed as an inclusive factor. Similar to the Nazi period to some degree, but in contrast to West Germany, the ability to work played a role in family members' and patients' attempts to obtain discharge and avoid lengthy asylum stays. Second, conversely, a lack of ability or willingness to work was cited as a reason for excluding people from the world of work and from society. Here, too, similarities with the Nazi era rather than with the FRG are apparent. Third, there was an argumentational logic specific to the GDR, which entailed deriving patients' rights from their work performance.

An example of the discourse on work and performance as signs of mental health are the letters received by 25-year-old Frank A. from his parents after his committal to Rodewisch Hospital in 1953. Frank A. was diagnosed with schizophrenia and had been subjected to electroshock treatment at the asylum without improvement. He was admitted due to sensory illusions (*Sinnestäuschungen*) and delusional ideas (*Wahnideen*), under the influence of which he had, among other things, broken windows. The police had apprehended and forcibly committed him. The patient himself stated that he wished to learn violin in Italy.[45] In the first instance, the initiation of this committal had nothing to do with work or performance. However, the notion of an orderly working life played an important role in his parents' reaction to the committal. They lived separately. Both wrote to their son, each explaining what needed to happen if he was to be discharged and if he was to "be reasonable (*vernünftig*) and a normal person."[46] In both letters, work is presented as a key to this.

His mother wrote: "[...] Look for work here, let go of this idea of yours, be kind and good my child I love you. [...] There is only one thing for it come to me and work so that you can make some money and have a life. [...]"[47]

His father wrote:

Dear [Frank],

You went away without even saying goodbye to me and you can see where you ended up.

I consider it my duty to inform you that you have it in you to be reasonable and a normal person. It is true that your nerves are quite frayed, but with a little good will you can arrange your situation there such that you can be released again shortly as healthy. [...]

And this illusion, which your mother has ingrained in you, that you will then get a pension, is nonsense. There is no reason to believe that anyone will receive a pension due to mental illness. Now it is up to you what you prefer. Your freedom, surely?

Warmest regards,
Your father.[48]

Both parents talked about work. Implicit in their words is the assumption that their son did not wish to get a "sensible" (*vernünftig*) job and that it was now imperative to convince him that this was the only valid course of action. The father mentioned that his son believed he could use his illness as grounds for a pension. He himself considered this absurd but in any case, did not believe his son was suffering from a serious illness, but that he would become "normal" again with some effort of will. This alleged shirking of work was also addressed by his mother. At the beginning of her letter, she stated that Frank had to work if only because she could not provide for him financially. In the further course of the letter, however, she also mentioned gainful employment as an expression of normal and appropriate behavior: "Look for work here, let go of this idea of yours, be kind and good my child." Here, we can detect something of the folk wisdom that people who work tend not to get silly ideas.

Much as during wartime, the ability and willingness to work were interpreted as a sign of the capacity to lead a normal life. In the same vein, patients too continued to cite work to explain why they could not remain in the asylum. Expressions of the desire for discharge similar to the following appear regularly in files from the GDR: "[W]ould like to be released as soon as possible to get on with his work."[49] Much as in the Nazi era, patients keen to leave an asylum sought to appropriate the state's intense focus on work to their own ends.

At the same time, in continuity with the Nazi period, work and performance remained an important criterion of exclusion in East German society. It was not only patients' relatives who understood work in this way. But in contrast to the "Third Reich" and the FRG, in the GDR the firm was more often involved in committals and discharges. Companies presented the will to work as a virtual precondition for social acceptance and social aid. A prime example is the negotiation of Martin W.'s stay at a clinic. In 1949, the 25-year-old was to be released from the Greifswald University Psychiatric Clinic following a suicide attempt. However, the process of discharge dragged on because it proved difficult to find a dwelling and job for him. Finally, he was released despite lacking work. At the suggestion of the Stralsund Municipal Hospital (Städtisches Krankenhaus Stralsund), a doctor from the Greifswald clinic wrote to the People's Solidarity welfare organization (Volkssolidarität) in Stralsund:

> The ward physician of the Städtisches Krankenhaus Am Sund, Stralsund, asked us to contact you prior to the patient's discharge. They wished to try to improve the patient's housing situation and possibly find him a position at the Volkswerft [shipyard]. We would therefore like to inquire as to whether you can do anything of this kind for our patient and hope to receive your reply shortly.[50]

The answer was as follows:

> Regarding the above letter, we regret to inform you that we can no longer provide support for the above-mentioned patient. Despite several promises to cease attempting suicide, [Martin W.,] has done so again and we therefore find ourselves unable to continue to provide yet more assistance to such weak-willed individuals.[51]

Here, the patient was excluded from the world of work with the argument that "such weak-willed individuals" did not deserve a job. In the eyes of the People's Solidarity, Martin W.'s suicide attempts had shown that he was of no value to society. The reply sounds almost like the meting out of punishment for deliberate, malicious misconduct toward the Volkssolidarität, which had provided him with a job on a previous occasion. The wording also perpetuates conceptions firmly entrenched in the Nazi era (and earlier): "weak-willed" (*willenlos*) was an adjective typically applied to "psychopaths."

The workplace as a symbol of belonging crops up at later times as well, as does exclusion from work, and both are evident in a 1962 letter from a company vocational school (*Betriebsberufsschule*) in the district of Neubrandenburg advocating the committal of 15-year-old apprentice Paul C.

> The only reason we took [Paul] into our training center in the first place was because we hoped that the collective of teachers and apprentices would be able to educate and improve him. Unfortunately, our expectations have gone unfulfilled because [Paul] exceeds the bounds of the normal. He behaves completely differently from other youngsters, completely abnormally. We thus find ourselves compelled to terminate [Paul's] apprenticeship, since the risk of accidents due to his behavior is particularly high and no one can take responsibility for this young man.
>
> [Paul's] behavior is not malicious, nor does he consciously wish to irritate his teachers and instructors; he is simply incapable of critically assessing his actions and conduct. [...]
>
> With respect to work too, [Paul] does not work like all the other apprentices but tries to disturb the other apprentices while they are working or keep them from working. [...]
>
> He always arrives late at the start of the work or school day. [...]
>
> In school his performance is not bad at all, he is even strong in math class, but [Paul] is not able to concentrate [...].
>
> At work too, [Paul] has no tenacity and can never be left unsupervised. [...] [Paul's] work performance is far lower than that of all the other apprentices. [...]
>
> Since [Paul] cannot be changed or improved by normal educational methods, we would like to support his mother's request that he be placed in a psychiatric home.[52]

Here, a whole slew of work- and performance-related reasons are cited as to why 15-year-old Paul not only lost his apprenticeship but was also committed in a joint effort by his mother, his training company, and the Neubrandenburg District Policlinic: his inadequate work performance, his inability to fit in, and the risk of accidents. The company also cited as a powerful argument the fact that Paul was behaving "abnormally" and differently from others and refused to be corrected by the collective (*Arbeitskollektiv*). "Normal" is interpreted in this letter as the capacity for adjustment to norms, work ability, and performance. Here we can see the flipside of the GDR's ideology of equality.

Both examples confirm Lindenberger's thesis that the official fight against "asocials" in East Germany enjoyed broad support within society.[53] Here, a wartime discourse of exclusion was perpetuated while also being further undergirded by the GDR's ideology of equality. Conversely, it was precisely this connection between work and equality that spawned a new argumentational schema to the benefit of patients. In line with the doctrine of equality and work-centered propaganda, at times relatives demanded improvements for sick family members working in asylums, deriving pa- tients' rights from their labor in some letters from the 1950s. One mother, in lengthy correspondence with Rodewisch, tried to obtain better treatment for her daughter in this vein.[54] She repeatedly pointed out in her letters that her daughter was not only being treated but also worked at the asylum and therefore deserved better treatment. This woman cited her daughter's labor, for example, when she complained that—according to her child's own account—she had been overpowered by four people during an outburst of rage and was kicked in the belly:

> People will now refer back to this and say that Fr. [P.] is ill and you can't believe a word she says. As a mother, I know my daughter and it is unfortunately very regrettable that she is usually in good shape but suffers from occasional seizures. I know from reliable sources that my daughter is very hard-working and obliging. This is surely also evident in the very fact that she gets up early every day, does the laundry for boiling, and helps out with other work as well. I have nothing whatsoever against this, because such sick people need diversion, which contributes to their recovery. But on the other hand, she should also be provided with distraction by granting her, in light of her condition, a little more freedom to go out.[55]

The argumentational strategy deployed by the patient's mother is typical of the appropriation of work-centered rhetoric. To back up her argument that her daughter ought not to be suffering physical attacks, she drew on the fact that she was, after all, deploying her labor in the asylum. The mother did not emphasize abuses in the asylum in general but derived the right to "good" treatment from her daughter's willingness to work and work performance. Whether used in a consciously instrumental way, intuitively, or out of per- sonal conviction, this mother drew on the state's doctrine of work and equality in pursuit of the pragmatic goal of attaining better treatment for her daughter. The appropriation of socialist rhetoric impacted areas of life in which ruler and ruled did not encounter one another directly. In the case we have just examined, this entailed an epistolary exchange exclusively between nursing staff and Mrs. P's mother. In a small way, this corroborates the finding of GDR research that the communist dictatorship was based—though not solely—on "social acceptance" as well as on its "political and cultural binding force."[56] The mother's line of argument shows that there were forms of acceptance and appropriation beyond direct power relations that undid the dichotomy between rejection and support of SED rule. Whether the mother rejected or supported the system or was completely indifferent to it is irrelevant to the finding that, however motivated, she used tropes typical of the "official" socialist line to achieve personal goals within the immediate family sphere.

When it comes to continuities and ruptures, to summarize, rationales changed in both German states, but in different ways. In the GDR, work and performance remained more important than in the FRG. In the latter, these two factors only played a role in the arguments made by patients and their relatives. In West Germany, work did not represent a link between the individual and society in committal discussions; the focus was on the relationship between the patient, the family, and the social environment. In East Germany, meanwhile, work continued to constitute a link between the state and the individual on the discursive level. Because the socialist state had departed from some of the inhumane aspects of the Nazi era, this link did not have the same relevance to patients' fate as during the murder of the sick. But the argumentative connection was evoked even more frequently, as it was privileged by firms involved in committals and—in contrast to the Nazi period—sometimes used to patients' advantage.

The healthy self during World War II, in the GDR, and in the FRG

We have already seen that patients themselves argued with reference to work when it came to the need for an asylum stay. However, work and performance were even more important in the self-attribution of illness—at least in wartime and in the early FRG. In the GDR, meanwhile, the construction of a healthy or sick self was far less often imbricated with ideas about work and performance.

In individuals' self-description of their state of illness, work could play an important role in two ways. First, inability to work or impaired performance were considered signs of illness. Second, "overwork"[57] was viewed as a cause of illness.

"Overwork" in wartime and in the early FRG

Among those who felt affected by it, "overwork" was a frequently suspected cause of illness in wartime and in the FRG. Mention of this phenomenon during the war ran along gender-specific lines: only women described themselves as "overworked" during this period.

The self-attribution of an excessive workload is virtually absent from the medical records of men during the war.[58] But rather than assuming that "overwork" did not affect men in the 1941–1945 period, especially in view of the high demands on labor during that conflict, it seems more likely that male overwork exceeded the limits of the sayable. This is consonant with the observation that a consistently negative view of mentally ill soldiers had taken hold by the time of World War II.[59] The symptoms of psychologically damaged soldiers were now put down essentially to innate inferiority. At the same time, company-based health care had been introduced on the "home front," with the goal of expediting peak performance among workers and keeping absence due to illness to an absolute minimum. In the wartime context, "overwork" thus lay beyond the realm of the communicable when it came to males. Further evidence for this conclusion can be seen in the fact that "overwork" was mentioned among men in both the eastern and western zones immediately after the war. "Overwork" featured in medical histories in both the GDR and the FRG and, in contrast to the Nazi era, it was addressed by both genders.

Women, meanwhile, frequently cited "overwork" as a cause of illness both during the war and after it. Many files from the period between 1941 and 1963 include statements by women themselves and those around them that they were suffering from "overwork." When Berta K. was committed in 1957, for example, her husband attributed his wife's anxiety and sleep disturbances to the fact that she had "taken on too much work at the factory."[60] It was particularly common for husbands to ascribe "overwork" to their wives. Another example is Felix L.'s assessment of the reasons for his wife's admission in 1957: "He had been far from agreeable to her working at the dressmaker's during the past year and took the view that she had overdone it there."[61] "Overwork" as a cause of mental illness seems to have been so self-evident to female patients themselves that prior to diagnosis they often attributed exhaustion to "overwork" even in cases of organic illness.[62] Maria T., for example, who died of a brain tumor shortly after admission in 1948, attributed her "severe headaches" to her occupational activities:

> Starts with feeling of weakness, severe headache, 'her nerves were shredded' [*mit den Nerven fertig*]. She worked in the municipal cash department and thought she had overdone things, the figure-work had become too much for her. Patient is alone here—evacuated from Silesia— she got herself certified as unfit for work; took to her bed at home and exhibited apathy with intermittent stupor, little food intake when urged, at night she was found lying under a cow in the cowshed of the farmer whose house she lives in. No delusional ideas, speech disorders, or cramps.[63]

During the war, too, female patients and those around them articulated the idea that they were suffering from an excessive workload, though this was diametrically opposed to the concept of the person extolled under Nazism. Two typical examples are the medical histories of Sophie L. and Maria T. Sophie L., who was committed to Bethel, was, according to her own assessment and that of her husband, so overworked in her job at a uniform factory that she felt completely run down and had pains all over her body.[64]

When Maria T. was admitted, her stepmother mentioned overexertion as the reason for her illness:

> Otherwise very capable, [... .]. Married for six years, no children or miscarriages. Good marriage. Husband is perhaps a little soft and yielding. At present he is on active duty. Patient worries about him a great deal. She is highly overstrained by her job. Suffers from sleep disturbances, anxiety, and indecisiveness. Outpatient medical treatment had been unsuccessful.[65]

The regime's call for women to take on more burdens during the war[66] came up against certain limits in reality, which they themselves sometimes articulated. The demand for women to work stood in stark contrast to the housewife model privileged and practiced since industrialization, especially in bourgeois households but even to some extent in working-class families.[67] "Overwork," then, could be ascribed to women yet new ideas about work were to some degree eliminating gender-specific attributions of health. This confirms Sybille Steinbacher's finding on gender stereotypes in the World War II era. She notes that while "stereotypes became more flexible," their basic structure remained intact.[68] Even if women's relationship to work increasingly matched that of men, the spatial separation between gender-specific spheres of work retained its significance in the rationales aired by patients and their relatives—even when it had been largely eliminated in everyday working life. We see an indication of this in the very fact that women could be regarded as suffering from "overwork" during the war and also in the fact that husbands often regarded their wives' complaints about their employment as legitimate, while taking a far dimmer view of any expression of discontent with or neglect of their household duties.

The third important aspect of the construction of work as a cause of illness among both men and women is that the discourse on excessive workloads was about more than extreme physical demands. We find evidence of this in the reasoning of Maria T.'s stepmother, who explained her stepdaughter's condition as a result of her worry over her husband at the front and exhaustion due to work. In other medical histories, too, "overwork" was presented as more than just a consequence of physical exhaustion. Expectations about work in a broader sense also played a role in some narratives. During the war, women complained, among other things, that they did not experience "community" at work. One 24-year-old signal-communication woman auxiliary (*Nachrichtenhelferin*) stated that in addition to the strenuous work, she had been very unhappy in military intelligence and anti-aircraft defense for other reasons, namely, because "no one cared about each other."[69] Propaganda-fueled expectations of a lived experience of *Volksgemeinschaft* or National Community, for which individuals should be willing to work to the point of exhaustion, were disappointed. But the disappointment Maria T. felt about the fact that "no one cared about each other" also shows that she had seriously expected to experience a genuine "community."[70] This is a point of considerable relevance to research on the *Volksgemeinschaft*. It is also worth noting in connection with the fact that expectations about and attitudes toward work—as we will see later in this chapter—possessed a special significance for attending physicians too. Furthermore, the recognition of work and the way reality deviated from people's expectations were later to become crucial to the conception of stress and, to an even greater extent, that of burnout.[71]

Work capacity as a sign of health during World War II and in the FRG

Even more widespread than the thematization of "overwork," in both the Nazi era and in West Germany, was the tendency to link work capacity and health. This could involve housework, work in the factory, and work in the office. It was a connection made in virtually every medical history—a cross-class pattern that shows up regardless of gender. In what follows, I illustrate the argumentative production of this linkage by looking at an example from the war period and another in the FRG. I then explore the connection between work ability/performance and the notion of a healthy self in West Germany in greater depth by probing psychiatric committals subsequent to suicide attempts, before presenting an interpretation of my findings.

Both in wartime and in the FRG, patients who considered themselves ill almost always stated that their illness had become apparent to them partly because it was impairing the performance of their work duties. People with various illnesses linked a variety of symptoms to their diminished work performance, such as an inability to concentrate, listlessness, hearing voices, and anxiety. In 1943, for example, patient Lisa B. persistently pressed for admission to Bethel though her family doctor did not consider this a necessity. Her reason for wishing to stay at Bethel is given as follows in her case history: "She has consistently maintained that she could not cope with her work due to restlessness (*innere Unruhe*) or inner vibrations (*innerliches Vibrieren*). But she stated that she had always been able to manage her household up to the very last moment. Her mother-in-law [she said] had therefore stated that she could not be in too bad a condition. She herself felt constantly depressed and was worried about her condition."[72] She was diagnosed with mild depression at Bethel. This example brings out the importance of work capacity to attributions of illness by patients and members of their social milieu. At the same time, it shines a light on two levels that do not necessarily coincide: the individual's sense that their work ability was limited and external perceptions of their capacities. Both women used working ability as a yardstick of health, but the patient and her mother-in-law came to different conclusions, pointing once again to the negotiated element in efforts to establish the presence of mental disorders. It was not only physicians and laypersons that sometimes had quite different ideas about what illness could be linked with and in what ways: as in this case, laypersons' assessments too could diverge considerably.[73]

With respect to the FRG, one of many possible examples is the line of argument put forward during the admission of married coachbuilder Hannes F. to the LHA Marburg in 1962. Hannes F. was committed by the police after destroying furniture and smashing windows in his home in a fit of rage.[74] He and his wife related this incident, which they described as a "nervous breakdown," to his work in two ways. First, when asked if and when he had noticed changes in himself, Hannes F. responded that he had felt dizzy at work several days before the committal and had been unable to concentrate.[75] Second, he and his wife identified the cause of his "nervous breakdown" as his finding out that laws were being broken at his company; he had been terribly afraid that he himself might be falsely linked with these infringements. He underlined that he condemned these "crooked" (*unehrlich*) machinations at his company with every fiber of his being. In this connection, his wife praised his exceptionally "upright and decent character."[76] Both wife and husband feared that the latter's reputation as an "honest worker" was at risk. This explicit connection between work activity, recognition, and psychological well-being crops up repeatedly in the medical records from Bethel and Marburg but is less ubiquitous than the linkage of "feeling unwell" (*Unwohlfühlen*) and work performance, which appears in almost every medical record. Lack of work motivation or lack of enjoyment of work were also frequently taken as signs that something was amiss. In self-descriptions, this was often conveyed in the statement that the individual was merely carrying out their work "mechanically."[77]

In the FRG, unemployment was also cited on several occasions as the cause of suicides or suicide attempts.[78] In 1959, for example, 51-year-old Jens T. was committed to the LHA Marburg after attempting to end his life. Subsequent to an operation four years earlier, he had been unable to find a full-time job and was doing temporary work. "When he had no roof over his head for weeks on end, it [suicide] went through his mind and he finally reached for the pills. He cannot deny it, only now does he realize how dearly he paid for this. He was simply too old and no one was willing to take him on."[79] Here, the patient not only mentioned his current situation as a homeless person but also built his entire explanation around the topic of his unemployment. He underlined his fear of being unable to find any work at all in the future as a key motive for his suicide attempt.

This rationale does not appear in the files from the Nazi period and the GDR reviewed for this book. In the latter case, this is hardly surprising, since involuntary unemployment did not exist there.[80] With respect to the Nazi period, it should be noted that all the files examined were from during the war. In light of this, I suspect that this finding tells us nothing about patients' self-assessment in connection with their performance and the recognition of their work. It seems more likely to be down to changing standards during the war, when occupational success tended to be less of a priority.[81] Right from the start of the Nazi era but prior to the war, meanwhile, Christian Goeschel notes a particularly high number of suicides that were described as caused by unemployment.[82]

The sample studied here, it should be noted, does not allow for systematic statements about motives for suicides in the "Third Reich," the GDR, or the FRG. While committals due to suicide attempts do appear frequently in the cases selected for this book, the files I examined were not chosen in order to illuminate this issue.[83] The only point that stands out is that it was exclusively in the case of suicide attempts in West Germany that prominent mention was made of work and performance. Unlike the "Third Reich" and the GDR, there is no study of suicides in the FRG in which this finding might be embedded. At the very least, though, these suicide cases tend to corroborate the idea that work, performance, and the recognition of both shaped notions of the self in West Germany. The findings in this chapter confirm the assumption, widely shared among researchers, that the performance ethos extended from the Nazi era into the FRG.[84] The medical records suggest that this was not a class-specific, elite phenomenon in that country, as the debate triggered by Wehler on a "de-browned achievement-focused society" might suggest.[85] The documents show that in the late 1950s, factory workers too regarded performance as essential to a healthy self.[86]

As evident in the first example above, it was not only employed men that made the connection between health and work capacity: I deliberately presented a case in which two women defined health and illness with reference to "ability to work." Nicole Schweig's history-of-medicine study on men's health behavior interprets the association between ability to work and health during the first half of the twentieth century as a specifically male phenomenon.[87] The sample taken for this book, meanwhile, contains many cases in which women make the same connection. Against the background of the "Taylorization of the housewife" since World War I, this finding seems more logical than surprising. Via the "home economics" originating in the United States and adopted in Germany, performance and time-saving in the household rose to the status of desirable goals.[88] While not all the objectives of the new "home economics" were achieved, what matters with regard to the relation between work and the healthy self is that the housewife's role was conceptualized in novel ways and that housewives embraced this new attitude with positivity and pride.[89] Borscheid's findings on the "Taylorized" housewife are doubly significant in the context of this chapter. First, it is consonant with the image of the housewife sketched by Borscheid that she evaluated her health by alluding to her housekeeping performance. In the "Third Reich," this was probably reinforced by the "race-based promotion of housework and motherhood," which led to recognition and an enhanced social status even in the public sphere.[90] Second, under Nazism, the model that had been established as desirable in the realm of the household may have facilitated the acquisition and internalization of similar expectations and the same kind of rationalization of labor when it came to paid work for women. With respect to the Nazi era and especially wartime, we might also bring in an observation made by Sybille Steinbacher: while the impact of the cult of motherhood on the realities of women's lives was long overestimated, for many women gainful employment was in fact a dominant feature of their everyday existence. This prompts her to conclude that the "division into male and female spheres [...] increasingly [diminished] as the totalization of war advanced."[91] A different picture pertained when it came to third parties' perceptions within committal practice. Husbands, for example, accepted and supported the notion of "overwork" in connection with their wives' gainful employment but not in the context of housework. I found no differences, however, in patients' self-attribution of "overwork." One key finding of my analysis of medical records in this context, then, is that this privileging of work and performance was neither class- nor gender-dependent.

Ability to work and "overwork" in the GDR

In East Germany, the situation was completely different. On the one hand, work played a huge role at the organizational level, in contrast to the wartime period and the FRG. On the other hand, committal rationales involving work hardly ever appeared in connection with gainful employment from the early 1950s onward. Here, I discuss the new significance of work at the organizational level before scrutinizing changing patterns of argumentation.

In contrast to the wartime period and the situation in West Germany, committals by the company doctor and admissions directly from the workplace accompanied by work colleagues were frequent in the GDR. The committal of 60-year-old Janosch Sch. to Untergöltzsch in 1950 is a prime example. The first entry in his medical record reads:

> Committed by Dr. L.-C. as per the attached medical certificate. Is accompanied by a work colleague and arriving direct from the company. Somewhat detached, quiet, and withdrawn upon admission. Is said to have suddenly changed while working. Was walking repeatedly in circles, raising concerns that he might get caught in the engine of the rotating machine.[92]

Descriptions of sudden change at the workplace and the dangers associated with this were typical in the GDR and beyond. However, the way the situation was handled, as described above, was specific to East Germany and is an indication of the comprehensive change in lifeworlds arising from the dependence of all other areas of life on the company. Janosch Sch. was not only committed by the company doctor but also arrived for admission directly from his workplace with a coworker accompanying him. None of these three elements was commonly found in the FRG. During the war, meanwhile, the sample shows that committals by company physicians did occur, but only sporadically. In East Germany, they took place more often at the Greifswald University Psychiatric Clinic, at Rodewisch, and at Großschweidnitz.[93]

In particular, the fact that the patient mentioned above did not return home prior to committal—despite the absence of any acute emergency, such as a suicide attempt or violence against those around him—and he was not accompanied to the asylum by a relative[94] brings out the key importance of the social environment of the workplace to existential decisions in situations of personal crisis. Moreover, in such committal constellations, work colleagues provided the initial information for the so-called "objective anamnesis." In this instance, then, the first information the physician received in the asylum came from the company physician and a work colleague. This altered the point of departure for both asylum physician and patient compared to a scenario in which the information sources were a family member and the family doctor, with the latter committing the patient. The initial details provided were of crucial import to the patient's fate, since the asylum doctors made decisions that shaped their stay there quite quickly after admission—often before family members had been consulted in the case of committals from the workplace. These early decisions included assignment to a ward, that is, deciding whether to place the patient in a "calm" (*ruhig*) or "restless" (*unruhig*) ward, whether they were classified as "fit for work," and whether they were permitted to leave the asylum grounds, to run small errands for example.

Although coworkers and the company played a comparatively large role in committals, an excessive workload, the capacity for work, and the social constellation at the workplace were not emphasized by the individuals committed. In Janosch Sch.'s case, it appears to have been a mere coincidence that he exhibited outlandish behavior at the workplace. Nor did the doctor's questions induce the patient to relate his afflictions to his job. The causes in this case thus remain obscure. In other cases, people who were committed gave reasons for their condition, but these were not usually related to their work. One example of a committal from the workplace without reference to work is that of 34-year-old Frank G., who is quoted in his medical history as follows:

Yesterday at lunchtime his wife had come home at 1 p.m. with a letter stating that she had been sentenced to a year in prison. She had received this punishment for terminating a pregnancy. They have four small children at home. He had to start his shift at 1.45 p.m. so he was unable to talk to her further. During the shift, he stated, he had the most distressing thoughts, especially about his wife, who might never come back, and also about the children. He then fainted. It was only in Obergöltzsch that he regained consciousness.[95]

Here, as in many other committals from the workplace, the cause of the mental breakdown was to be found in the family sphere. The fact that the patient came from the workplace merely shows—in line with the research—the great importance of workplaces to every area of life.[96]

From the early 1950s onward, "overwork" and attributions of illness due to limited ability to work were only very rarely linked with gainful employment in the GDR. Illness was increasingly attributed to other phenomena that also cropped up on a regular basis during wartime and in the young FRG in addition to the sphere of work—such as sleep disorders and loss of appetite. East German housewives, meanwhile, continued to state regularly that they had noticed their illness primarily through a decline in their performance and hoped to get well so that they could work effectively. The argumentative link between "failure" in the household and psychological breakdowns, up to and including suicide attempts, remained quite common. Housewife Regina M., for example, was admitted to the Greifswald University Psychiatric Clinic in 1954 and, according to the case history, stated that she had been unable to manage her household and take care of her child for some time due to depression:[97] "I could not cope with my work, so I tried to slit my wrists."[98]

In contrast to the Nazi period, however, mentions of work beyond the realm of housework were far rarer in the GDR and, when they did occur, indicated connections with specific occupations and situations. Not uncommon was the self-attribution of "overwork" in direct connection with the opportunities for advancement offered by the new order in the Soviet occupation zone and early East Germany. While the patient records feature no mention of "overwork" in enterprises, they do make reference to "new farmers" (*Neubauer*) and political climbers in the late 1940s. The fact that these groups talked about negative consequences of their work shows that "overwork" was not absent from the other patient files for reasons of non-sayability alone. It should be noted that the sample contains comparatively few files of "new farmers" and political activists, and my selection of files did not take account of occupational distribution. Allusions to "overwork" are not, therefore, representative of these two groups. All we can say for certain is that "overwork" was not mentioned in workers' files but occurred in those of "new farmers" and political activists; this allows for no definitive conclusions about the extent of this phenomenon.

One example of an individual suffering symptoms of overwork in the context of political activity is Ferdinand H., who was admitted to Greifswald in 1955 in a "state of total exhaustion due to political work." In addition to his job as a sales representative, Mr. H. worked as a lecturer at the district party school (*Kreisparteischule*). Both he and the doctors considered this highly time-consuming sideline, along with the political training courses he had also completed, to be the cause of his disorders.[99]

The overwork suffered by "new farmers" and political activists fits the picture painted by previous research. In the case of the former, studies have revealed that many were quick to abandon their land due to a lack of materials and livestock, as well as a dearth of agricultural knowledge.[100] Research on the cadres has shown that they were under constant pressure to undergo time-consuming training.[101] Against this background, it is hardly surprising that these two groups complained of psychological stress arising from their work. This does not mean that the political climbers complained about the work *per se*. Ferdinand H., for example, had no wish to work less but was eager to be rapidly restored to health so he could return to his numerous activities.[102] The concept of the socialist self elaborated by Jochen Hellbeck for the Soviet Union on the basis of autobiographical testimonies sheds light on the political climbers' attitude.[103] Hellbeck argues that the Soviet self, in continuity with self-concepts spawned in the nineteenth century, aimed to subordinate the life of the individual to a higher goal. The Soviet self thus retained the missionary aspirations of the nineteenth century but now the higher goal was the establishment of a communist social order.[104]

"Overwork," however, was not mentioned solely in connection with opportunities for advancement, but also in the context of social decline, for example, among people whose careers had been derailed for political reasons. In these cases, "overwork" was an aspect of general dissatisfaction with the realities of work and occupational advancement in the GDR. Upon admission to the Großschweidnitz Sanatorium-Nursing Home in 1956, 49-year-old Herbert B.[105] was quoted as follows:

> His nervous breakdown, he stated, is no doubt caused by overwork, as he has a family of three to look after. One son is studying at the Technical University in Berlin. Patient is ambitious and suffers from the fact that as a former member of the Nazi Party he had been dismissed from the civil service and all opportunities for career development were closed to him. He had been poised to become a *Reichsbahninspektor* [a senior railway official].[106]

In 1956, Herbert B. worked as a commercial clerk. Unfortunately, no further details about his work can be found in his file. Significantly, this was not just a matter of physical "overload" (*Überlastung*) but of concern for family finances and a lack of opportunities for personal development. The connection between work and health remained significant for both the socialist self and the disappointed middle-class self.

Interpretation: differing perceptions in East and West

Developments in the postwar period differed markedly in the East and West. Without considering findings on the GDR, we might be tempted to conclude that work's importance to notions of a healthy self was a basic feature of the modern industrialized and increasingly rationalized working world. In this regard, we should note that notions of work significantly influenced people's sense of self even before the Nazi era, namely, in the nineteenth century.[107] In any case, this perspective fails to explain the findings of the present book. The linkages between work, performance, and health described here do not entail the internalization of a work- or performance-centered mentality over generations. In the *Annales* tradition, mentalities are understood as "collective patterns of thought and forms of consciousness"[108] that are prior to individual consciousness, and they are assumed to change only gradually. They are typically presented as *explanans* rather than *explanandum*.[109] Since mentalities change slowly,[110] the fact that work-focused rationales disappeared in the GDR suggests that we are not dealing with a performance-centered mentality formed during the Nazi period or even earlier. In what follows, I attempt to analyze continuities and changes in the performance ethos and suggest how we might explain them. The contrasting findings for the GDR indicate that external circumstances exerted a major influence on the idea of the healthy self as a hard-working and performance-oriented self; the immediate circumstances of working life are in fact crucial to explaining the differences between East Germany and the FRG. My thesis is that notions of the healthy self involve the internalization and rationalization—not necessarily subject to conscious reflection—of circumstances. Ideas about work and performance were part of individual worlds of meaning,[111] which retained their relevance only if regularly updated.

The pressure to work and perform during the war was intense. Within the "Aryan" population, a strong performance by men and women in the household, warfare, or gainful employment enabled them to assert their "belonging," whereas a lack of ability to work or willingness to perform provided strong grounds for exclusion from the "National Community." The ability to work also played a key role in patients' self-perception as healthy. This remained the case in West Germany, but the core benchmark changed. West German committal rationales lend support to Michael Wildt's objection to Wehler's idea of a "de-browed performance ethos," namely, that Wehler failed to acknowledge the difference between a racial-biological and individual performance orientation.[112] Committal rationales during wartime and in the FRG differ on precisely this point. Whereas in wartime individual performance was often tied to the "National Community" as a whole, in West Germany only the patient themself and their immediate environment were mentioned in rationales for committal. The "people" or "nation" (*Volk*) and the "community" soon fell away as points of reference, at least in West German medical records.[113] This difference in the prevailing benchmark suggests that immediate social and political circumstances were quick to impact on notions of the self. The postwar conditions of a "society in a state of collapse" (*Zusammenbruchgesellschaft*) prompted the individual to concentrate on their immediate social environment: of necessity, they were thrown back on themself and their family. In fact, the medical records indicate that wartime circumstances had already contributed to this process. The discrepancy between the anticipated experience of the "National Community" and the way the individual was forced to rely on themself during the war was addressed in medical histories, such as that of signal-communication woman auxiliary Maria T., who complained that her colleagues did not care about each other. Further evidence of this is the radical boundary-marking evident in arguments for committal, as described in Chapter 3, "Danger and Security," along with the research findings on denunciation and people's behavior in the bunkers.[114]

An even clearer indication of the relevance of everyday life and work is the fact that, despite propaganda on a massive scale encouraging people to identify with the socialist work-oriented society, patient files in the GDR are virtually devoid of references to work. The finding that workers in East Germany had largely ceased to connect ability to work and health, at least in the medical records analyzed here, supports the thesis that the role played by work in the individual's world of meaning was closely related to concrete realities. These limited the potential role of gainful employment in the construction of the self. In the GDR, working life changed very quickly,[115] with work processes being altered through the introduction of the planned economy and guaranteed work. Workers easily kept the targets that had been introduced to increase productivity artificially low. Moreover, as a result of the planned economy, there were more interruptions to the working process and "under the soft budgetary constraints typical of actually existing socialist enterprises," labor was hoarded even "where there was no constant need for it."[116] Earning more money, furthermore, did not immediately improve living standards, given the limited supply of goods. At the same time, for political reasons, many people were now unable to pursue the careers they aspired to. In the GDR, the carrying out of work as such thus became less important to ideas about the self.

The finding that patients in specific occupational or work situations— especially in the context of social and political advancement or decline— continued to thematize "overwork" can also be explained most convincingly in light of the valorization of immediate circumstances and worlds of meaning. In this regard, three different conceptions of the self can be identified in the early GDR: the "hard-working" (*arbeitsam*) Soviet-influenced self of political climbers, the "hard-working" self of the downwardly mobile, and the self of real existing socialism, which was by far the most common model, for which work activities now played virtually no role. In the FRG, meanwhile, the hard-working self, which Peter-Paul Bänzinger has identified in the 1950s across all social classes, clearly predominated when it came to attributions of a healthy self.[117]

Paradoxically, then, despite the propagandistic valorization of work in East Germany, performance in gainful employment was no longer an apt criterion of health for many people. The political-economic system had entirely unintended side effects on many citizens' conception of the healthy self. This finding confirms the observation made by a number of researchers that the "centrality of labor relations"[118] in the GDR did not mean that work *per se* was especially important to the worker.[119] The decreasing relevance of work to the construction of one's health, as evident in the patient files from Greifswald, Rodewisch, and Großschweidnitz, further fleshes out this finding.

It shows that the differing evaluation of gainful employment in East Germany exercised an impact on fundamental ideas about one's identity and also highlights just how much constructions of identity may depend on tangible political and economic conditions—and how quickly they can change under certain circumstances.

The medical perspective on work and performance between 1941 and 1963

In all three German states, we can read the interpretation of work and performance in psychiatric concepts of illness as indications of the field of tension that existed between the individual and society. This relationship is thrown into particular relief in pension evaluations, as they addressed whether the patient was sick enough to be awarded welfare benefits. Of crucial importance to the concepts of work and performance was their class- and gender-specific selectivity within scientific discourse and on the level of practical application.

Given that patients used the term "overwork" to describe complaints that were not always solely about physical overload but that could sometimes be placed under the rubric of "stress," a term that only emerged later, we might wonder how these complaints were classified and evaluated by physicians. Though it is hardly surprising that self-attributions of stress existed even before that term was coined,[120] how physicians and laypersons dealt with this discrepancy tells us a great deal. The medical interpretation of the "overwork" that patients complained of turns out to be a crucial topic from the psychiatric perspective: differing and to some degree contradictory psychiatric assessments and interpretations of society had clashed since the days of the German Empire. Physical symptoms of fatigue that restricted work were already the subject of studies in labor science carried out in the early twentieth century.[121] Drawing on thermodynamics and notions of the body as analogous to a machine, here physical exhaustion was conceptualized as a natural process. It was assumed that exhaustion protected the body from overwhelming degrees of strain.[122] Physical exhaustion was thus detached from a moralizing discourse and became part of a natural scientific and technological discourse.[123] In line with the prevailing psychiatric doctrine, however, no psychological effects of work on health were recognized. Still, the working person was the subject of psychiatric discussions. Under the German Empire and until the beginning of the Weimar Republic, this working individual was addressed in three psychiatric discourses: on so-called "asocials" and "psychopaths," on traumatic neurosis, and on neurasthenia.

Under the diagnosis of "traumatic neurosis," in the German Empire some nervous disorders were still recognized as occupational diseases, with sufferers potentially receiving financial support. But this was not a matter of psychological effects, since traumatic neurosis was considered a somatic disease.[124] The recognition of nervous disorders construed as somatic, moreover, affected only male-dominated occupational groups such as railroad workers. Female postal workers, conversely, fought in vain to have their nervous complaints recognized as somatic occupational diseases.[125]

Work-related mental disorders among middle-class women, meanwhile, were diagnosed as "neurasthenia," with scientific studies presenting this condition as a consequence of female "overwork" (although most neur-asthenic patients were not engaged in paid employment). The reason for this "overwork" was seen as women's gender-based unsuitability for gainful employment. Here too, then, physicians postulated a physical cause.[126]

In the public discourse on "asocials" and "psychopaths" in the German Empire and the Weimar Republic, the "lower class" was imagined as a danger to the well-being of the entire "people" or "nation" (*Volk*). This "lower class" was regarded as degenerate almost in its entirety[127] and in psychiatric discourse, too, "asociality" and "psychopathy" were attributed to certain groups of people within this social stratum, such as prostitutes and "vagabonds."[128]

"Psychopathy" as a diagnosis in the Nazi era

Psychiatric discourse

By the time of World War II, the class- and gender-specific thematization of work had changed markedly. In the early twentieth century, at Kraepelin's instigation, the neurasthenia discourse was reinterpreted in biologistic terms. Sociogenetic explanations rapidly lost importance and "neurasthenia" was now interpreted as a consequence of degeneration.[129] In this reading, "neurasthenia" and "psychopathy" could be traced to the same cause. By the 1920s, however, "neurasthenia" was being diagnosed far less often and had waned as a subject of public debate.[130]

With the disappearance of the diagnosis of traumatic neurosis after World War I, limitations in men's ability to work not only ceased to be accepted, but were also branded as a refusal to work and as "pension neurosis." In this context, in contrast to Oppenheimer's conception, neu-rosis did not imply somatic change in the brain. As Oppenheimer's diag-nosis fell out of favor, the consequences of war and psychiatric work-related illnesses were largely addressed under the rubric of "psychopathy." The prevailing doctrine, then, no longer acknowledged the psychological effects of a heavy workload as symptoms of illness. Instead, the diagnosis of "psychopathy" classified those claiming to suffer from these complaints as pathological and reprehensible—"overwork" was often equated with unwillingness to work.[131] Where a variety of explanatory approaches had coexisted, the "psychopathy discourse" now reigned supreme.

Yet even in the Nazi era, the term "psychopathy" lacked a clear definition. The only thing everyone agreed on, as Donalies summed it up in 1942 in *Der Nervenarzt,* was that "the field of psychopathies is unlikely ever to see agreement on concepts and terminology."[132] Major points of contention were the exact classification of "psychopathies" and the question of which subsets of "psychopathies" were hereditary and to what extent, as well as how to demarcate them from other clinical pictures.[133] Since the time of the German Empire, the psychopathy discourse had addressed a variety of "social problems" that remained decisive during the Nazi era, without undergoing any specific development in terms of content. The "wrong" attitude toward work was one of the leading topics considered under the rubric of "psychopathy," along—and in connection—with addiction, prostitution, and non-sedentarism (as in the case of the Roma). Ever since Kraepelin described "psychopaths as community aliens" (*Gemeinschaftsfremde*), authors with differing basic assumptions about "psychopathy" had considered a person's relationship to work important. In particular, textbooks—which focused less on academic controversy and more on descriptions of applied relevance—outlined the work behavior ascribed to specific "psychopathic types." For example, in the fourth edition of his highly successful textbook first published in 1936, Oswald Bumke (1877–1950) described the "unstable [*haltlos*] psychopath" as failing to pass muster "wherever serious reflection, purposeful work, or simply the regular performance of duties are required."[134] He then gave specific examples of failure in discrete fields of activity, such as agriculture and office work in a government agency.[135] This description was not Nazi-specific or new. Crucially, though, it was now the only accepted reading of mental complaints in connection with work.[136]

Physicians' diagnostic practice

Whereas patients described their illnesses as work-related states of exhaustion, during World War II doctors overwhelmingly diagnosed these conditions as "psychopathy" across all social classes in accordance with the prevailing medical ideology. It should be borne in mind that this diagnosis was particularly often applied to members of lower social classes, as they made up the majority of the clientele in state asylums. In accordance with the now extremely negative classification of "overwork" within the dominant scientific dogma, medical assessments differed significantly from the self-assessment of those treated. To take one example, the doctor in charge described Sophie L.'s complaints, which she and her husband attributed to severe "overwork" in a uniform factory, as follows in the epicrisis:

> Primarily neurotically fixated on the idea of being a seriously ill woman. Certainly overstates existing complaints considerably. The role of the

wretched, feeble woman has become a way of life for her over the years, one her husband has strongly encouraged her to embrace. No indication of endogenous depressive disorders.[137]

Given the plethora of definitions of psychopathy and the ill-defined borderline mental states that were not considered psychoses, it is not always obvious how best to interpret a given diagnosis or medical description or to determine which tradition it should be placed within.

Overall, it was the concept of "psychopathy" that held sway within diagnostics, though sometimes the doctor identified merely a "state of nervous exhaustion" (*nervöser Erschöpfungszustand*) or described the patient as "neurotic," as in Sophie L.'s case. However, this did not involve a fundamentally different interpretation or evaluation of the illness. In practice, both attributions were often directly related to the diagnosis of "psychopathy." The ascription of a "state of nervous exhaustion" was usually seen as caused by a "psychopathic personality," though not always. The following neurological report from the Ziegenhain Prison and Penitentiary (Gefängnis und Zuchthaus Ziegenhain) concerning the transfer of an inmate to the LHA Marburg is a typical medical description:

> According to the papers presented to me, patient was discharged from the Wehrmacht in '44 as unfit for military service due to severe mental deviance (*Abartigkeit*). A certificate from the doctor who treated him in '40 states that patient suffered from nervous exhaustion and depression (*Gemütsdepression*).
>
> In-depth exploration has revealed that this is a psychopathy of the severest kind featuring obsessive thoughts (*Zwangsvorstellungen*) and suicidal impulses. It cannot be determined with certainty in an outpatient setting whether the clinical picture corresponds to an endogenous psychosis of the schizophrenic type.
>
> In any case, there is a constant risk of suicide; patient therefore belongs in an insane asylum (*Nervenheilanstalt*) and is certainly not fit for prison at present.[138]

This example illustrates once again the fine line between "psychopathy" and psychosis in diagnostic practice.

The other, far less typical end of the spectrum is illustrated by the medical assessment of the condition, described earlier, of signal-communication woman auxiliary Maria T., who felt overwhelmed by her work. The attending physician at Bethel, Dr. G., informed her committing colleague that:

> Observation here revealed no evidence of psychosis. The patient was merely in a state of nervous exhaustion. [...]
>
> It might be advisable to place the patient in a job that would not require her to work night shifts and in which she could perhaps spend

more time doing office work, which seems to suit her better than exclusive reporting duties.[139]

In this case, the physician, Dr. G., did not relate the nervous exhaustion to "psychopathy" and assigned no blame.[140] Instead she attempted to improve the patient's situation. Her assessment did not deviate seriously from the prevailing doctrine on a semantic level, since she used the compound term "state of nervous exhaustion," which, as mentioned, was also a popular label within psychopathy discourse. Yet her assessment and recommendation were unusual. This was a significant departure from standard practice but not completely outlandish. Despite the hegemonic discourse, then, there was still room for maneuver in diagnostic practice and the assessment of patients. Evidently, though, this was rarely deployed to the benefit of those affected.

Managerial disease, "psychopathy," and "exhaustion" (Erschöpftsein): medical interpretations of "overwork" in the FRG

Theoretical concepts

In contrast to the Nazi period, in early West Germany the topic of work and "overwork" again took a more multifaceted form. It was addressed through three different concepts. The psychopathy discourse (1) remained crucial but continued to develop. In connection with this evolution, an alternative interpretation of psychological stress due to work as "exhaustion" (2) gained traction in the 1950s. The notion of "overwork" as a managerial disease (3), meanwhile, was a new phenomenon.

The establishment and function of managerial disease in the postwar period has recently been analyzed in detail by Patrick Kury,[141] who emphasizes that this was a specifically German (and Austrian) diagnosis that did not build on U.S. psychiatric research on stress during World War II.[142] In any case, managerial disease was discussed more by nutritionists and performance physicians (*Leistungsmediziner*) than by neurologists and psychiatrists.[143] There was disagreement over which symptoms formed part of the disease. Still, both physicians and the public agreed on who was affected, namely, the postwar German elite, in other words men in leadership positions. Kury notes the development of a kind of "idée fixe" according to which there was a particularly high mortality rate among the top performers of the postwar period, despite a lack of empirical evidence for this.[144] This prompts him to interpret the debate on managerial disease as a discourse of exoneration for the elite, one that shielded them from accusations of underachievement—much like Roelke's interpretation of the neurasthenia discourse in the German Empire.[145] "The interpretation of managerial disease by contemporaries as a disorder afflicting the elites does not stand up to empirical scrutiny, especially in light of the case studies I have presented here. Nevertheless, and despite some critical voices, in the postwar period managerial disease was construed as a problem affecting elites, probably, at least in part, as a way of cementing existing social hierarchies."[146]

While managerial disease presented an excessive workload virtually as proof of outstanding performance among the elite of the young FRG, the established and prevailing, albeit less vocal, psychiatric discourse on the topic of "overwork" and performance differed in two respects: it was in no way concerned with the elite and it constructed "overwork" and/or a declining performance as due to a mixture of character weakness and hereditary predisposition. This was a slightly modified version of the psychopathy discourse. In the postwar period, Kurt Schneider's previously popular, ten-part "psychopath classification" grew increasingly dominant. In widely read textbooks, the classic chapter on the "clinical pictures of psychopathic personalities" was now "based on Kurt Schneider."[147] What remained unchanged, however, was the way that work and performance were closely connected with certain forms of "psychopathy." This is hardly surprising in that Schneider's typology was not new but had existed in a very similar form since 1923. In particular, the "unstable" and "weak-willed psychopaths" continued to be judged in an extremely negative way with respect to their willingness and ability to work and perform. Similar to the textbooks of the Nazi period, in Ewald's 1959 textbook the "type of the weak-willed"—immediately after the introductory remark that they lack drive—is described in terms of their relationship to work:

> Under favorable conditions, they are sometimes reasonably useful employees in subordinate positions without independence, who get through their daily quota at a very subdued pace, tend to turn up late because they cannot muster the effort to be punctual, just as they give every other difficulty a wide berth. They generally take the *path of least resistance*, will never *overexert* themselves, often appear *truly lazy*, spending their time achieving precisely nothing. [If located] on the middle social level, they are stuffily conventional and petty-bourgeois, sluggish, and devoid of drive. In unfavorable circumstances, they are highly susceptible to influence and can easily be exploited in pursuit of minor acts of malfeasance. Should they be economically secure, they are happy to let others work for them and turn into drones who hang around in sanatoriums during summer vacations, sit around in coffee houses with a blasé air, smoke cigarettes, participate in aesthetic circles if they have a craving for validation, but usually in an entirely passive role, at most play a little tennis, enjoy dressing up nicely and having their hair done, while in the evening they amuse themselves superficially in bars. Women not infrequently descend into a life of prostitution.[148]

Here, the individual was pigeonholed within society in light of work and performance. On this view, depending on the social and economic status of the "psychopath," they harmed society in various ways, for example, by being unreliable employees and contributing little to productivity, or by devoting themself to idle pursuits, if they could afford it. In this typical definition of the "weak-willed psychopath," the lack of a performance orientation was condemned regardless of class.

The postwar period saw two other innovations, and they too were linked with Kurt Schneider. The previously dominant concepts of psychopathy, including the leading conception expounded by Kraepelin, assessed the "psychopath" as deviant within a Lamarckian worldview. Kraepelin condemned "psychopaths" from a moral standpoint, construing them as "degenerates" who posed a threat to the entire *Volkskörper* or "national body."[149] Schneider too described the "psychopath" as deviant but unlike Kraepelin, he based his assessment on a normative conception of the average rather than a value-based norm.[150] In addition, Schneider urged psychiatrists to avoid the term "psychopathy" in their communication with other agencies of the welfare system. This must be seen in the context of recurrent criticism of the compiling of "psychopath typologies."[151] Most importantly, Schneider believed that the term "psychopathy" would soon disappear, contending that while it was still being used in psychiatric practice, it was already "ailing."[152] Hence, as he argued, it was best to use the term "psychopath" only in an in-house psychiatric context: "It is thus advisable, for example in reports to physicians, youth welfare offices, and in expert evaluations of all kinds, to avoid referring to 'psychopaths.' One should describe as vividly and graphically as possible and without 'technical terms' what kind of person one is dealing with."[153]

Despite these changes, it was the continuities with previously prevailing conceptions of psychopathy that predominated. Heredity was still seen as an important cause with respect to certain "psychopathic types"—including the "unstable" and the "weak-willed" psychopaths—while physicians continued to assume individual culpability, especially in the context of work. These views were directly related to the distinction between form and content in psychiatry. The old subdivision still held sway: mental deviations such as the "psychopathies," which were counted among the neuroses as opposed to the psychoses, were determined by their content. This meant that the illness lacked both course and form; instead, the "deviation" was viewed as dependent on the patient's evaluation of the situation.[154] This individual evaluation of situations as a decisive criterion also allowed for personal guilt. Due to the permanent lack of clarity over the extent to which this attitude was inherited or not, the demand that the patient themself strive to improve their condition was always hanging in the air. Particularly in expert evaluations of the entitlement to welfare benefits, the establishment of individual guilt had substantial consequences. This is evident in the article "Die ärztliche Begutachtung von Neurosen für die unterstützende Arbeitslosenhilfe" ("The medical assessment of neuroses for unemployment benefits") by Dr. Paul Hülsmann, who worked at the Essen Labor Office, which was published in *Der Nervenarzt* in 1953.[155] The author addressed the problem that "neurotic people" who applied for pensions often became unemployed during the process. Hülsmann came to the conclusion that "neurotic failure in the work process [is] personality-bound."[156] He freely conceded that there were cases in which the sick person was de facto unavailable on the labor market, despite having been assessed as "fit for work," if their complaints were of a "psychopathic" or "neurotic" nature. In these cases, using a classic argument, he underlined that "practical experience shows—as it did after World War I in the case of the war neurotics—that denial of unemployment benefits can lead to the abandonment of neurotic maladjustments resulting from desire-based representations (*Begehrensvorstellungen*)."[157] The "psychopath" was thus "cured" by stripping them of the underpinnings of their "misconceptions." So-called "pension neurotics," then, continued to be problematized and combated through the tried-and-tested approach. Key elements of the psychopathy discourse remained in place, especially with respect to the evaluation of work and performance, although innovations in the conceptualization of psychopathy and neurosis certainly occurred in other respects.

In the early 1960s, a tiny number of scholars presented declining performance or limitations on the ability to work due to an excessive workload as legitimate, at least in certain cases, rather than as the fault of the individual or primarily the result of "hereditary degeneration" (*erblich entartet*). The director of the Heidelberg University Psychiatric Clinic, Walter Ritter von Baeyer (1904–1987), expressed views of this kind in an article published in *Der Nervenarzt* in 1961.[158] By no means did he dismiss the common constructs of the "parasitic psychopath" (*schmarotzender Psychopath*) or the "pension neurotic," but he pointed out that not every problem described by patients as a "state of exhaustion or overwork" was covered by them. He made his arguments with reference to cases from his practical psychiatric work, effectively challenging the established interpretation that a "misplaced desire" (*Fehlbegehren*), laziness, and the like were the leading cause of self-attributions of "overwork" or inability to work. He underscored that it was also possible for this condition to be triggered by a lack of purpose or recognition, emphasizing that at times the patient might be genuinely "incapable of volition" (*Nichtwollenkönnen*). As examples, he cited refugees who felt that on the whole their new life was meaningless and whose work now lacked any sense of purpose as a result. He gave a similar assessment of the condition of a worker who had worked particularly hard to build a house for himself, but whose elderly in-laws then moved in against his wishes. He regarded as comparable the situation of "many middle-ranking white-collar workers and civil servants who, although they are quite happy to do their work *per se*, cannot enjoy it in an unqualified sense due to their dependence on difficult superiors or rivalry among colleagues."[159] Baeyer charted a middle course here, conceding that, across social classes, patients who suffered from "exhaustion" (*Erschöpftsein*) were not necessarily "psychopaths." However, he distanced himself from functional interpretations of overexertion—that is, a focus on form—that failed to recognize its content.[160] To conceptualize overexertion or "exhaustion" in terms of form would have entailed a substantial valorization of exogenous factors, which would, in turn, have meant problematizing the world of work rather than the individual working in it.[161] Nor did he believe that "exhaustion" or "overwork" constituted the stress syndrome described by Hans Selye that had made such a splash in Anglo-American psychiatry. In the course of World War II, Selye had defined stress as an endocrinological disorder, and his conception had rapidly become established in the United States.[162] Baeyer did not endorse the North American research but pointed out that the phenomenon of "exhaustion" that he was describing was consistent with the neurasthenia familiar from the days of the German Empire. However, he considered it to be ubiquitous—not only in the middle classes, but also in all social strata.[163]

In the early FRG, even the most cautious assessment of an excessive workload without the immediate apportionment of blame had no chance of gaining wide acceptance. This is evident in the fact that a response to Baeyer's article appeared in *Der Nervenarzt* before the year was out, in which Johannes Heinrich Schultz (1884–1970) criticized Baeyer's use of the term "exhaustion" (*Erschöpftsein*). He argued that the use of such terms could culminate in physicians conceding that patients needed more rest and recuperation rather than to change their attitude. To avoid this, he suggested the term "state of failure" (*Versagenszustand*), which he thought far more appropriate.[164] It should be borne in mind that Schultz was a psychiatrist and psychotherapist who had become known chiefly for inventing autogenic training, that is, a method of "working" on the individual. He was among the politically conformist psychotherapists under Nazism.[165] When it came to work, psychiatrists and psychotherapists, who otherwise often held very different points of view, found common ground, since both professions identified the working person rather than their circumstances as the cause of problems.[166]

Overwork, "psychopathy," and legitimate exhaustion in diagnostic practice

Both physicians' descriptions of patients and diagnostic practice correlated with the three research perspectives discussed in *Der Nervenarzt*. The use of terms and the evaluation of complaints, meanwhile, varied greatly from doctor to doctor, even within the same asylum. In what follows, I demonstrate this by looking at the example of committals for pension assessment, which are particularly enlightening for two reasons: they can be clearly assigned to a specific doctor and the assessment had clear consequences for the patient in each case. All these expert evaluations were carried out at Bethel, which I selected because, according to my sample, 20 percent of committals to this institution between 1950 and 1963 were for pension assessment. The sample thus includes several expert evaluations from each doctor whose duties included providing them.

The procedure was always the same. An insurance office—in the case of Bethel, this was often the Detmold Insurance Office (Oberversicherungsamt Detmold)—arranged for a patient's "pension affairs" to be examined at Bethel. The von Bodelschwingh Asylums then contacted the patient, requesting that they appear on a specific date for three days of inpatient observation. The examining physician was also provided with statements from other physicians and the patient's medical record if they had been in an asylum before. This was also the case if previous inpatient treatments had taken place at another institution: the file was then sent to the asylum providing the expert evaluation.[167]

An example of the continuity within medical practice of core elements in the psychopathy-oriented discourse on ability to work is a pension evaluation by Dr. K. from 1952. It is significant in two respects: with regard to the patient's account of her complaints and in terms of the doctor's assessment. The patient stated that she was no longer able to work, as she "always went straight to bed completely exhausted, worn-out, and weak" every day immediately after work.[168] Verena M., a former seamstress, explained her exhaustion as follows:

The demands of a modern business are simply too great. She could no longer keep up with the pace of the work, and in the end she had to sew buttons on by hand, on a piecework basis, and she managed to do less than the young girls. That rankled with her, especially since she earned less.[169]

Signal-communication woman auxiliary Maria T. had put forward similar arguments in 1943, not only complaining about the physical workload, but also explaining that things were particularly unsatisfactory due to the dearth of cooperation and the fact that no one cared about each other.[170] Despite all the differences, in Maria T.'s case, too, self-perception in the context of the working environment, not just the execution of tasks, played a key role. The statements of former seamstress Verena M., meanwhile, make it clear that in her case it was not just the direct physiological consequences of work that were at issue, but also its indirect physical consequences, such as exhaustion; in addition, she felt that her work was valued less than others'. This frequently occurring explanation—the feeling of constant exhaustion and the impression that one's work was not appreciated by those around one—is noteworthy because both elements, which were already being discussed in the 1940s and 1950s, are acknowledged in the concept of stress, which began gaining ground in the 1970s.[171]

After ruling out neurological causes, Dr. K. wrote in his evaluation:

The present psychological findings too contain nothing to indicate the presence of a psycho-cognitive [*seelisch-geistig*] illness, either in the sense of organic-cognitive [*organisch-geistig*] changes or in the sense of an endogenous psychosis of a depressive or schizophrenic nature. Rather, on the basis of our investigations, we believe that Miss [M.] is a personality from a family with weak nerves, who has always been somewhat deviant [*abartig*] and, moreover, intellectually limited, even if not feeble-minded, and has undoubtedly undergone a fateful decline in performance associated with reaching the involutional age (*Rückbildungsalter*). [...] Even today, due to her primitive basic structure and her simple-mindedness, Mrs. [M.] exhibits evident demonstrative and psychogenic traits, while in addition her thinking is clearly dominated by desire-based representations centered on acquiring a pension [*Rentenbegehrungsvorstellungen*]. It is, however, credible that this woman, who in all likelihood has always been a low performer and easily exhausted, having reached involutional age, does in fact no longer feel fully able to cope with the demands of a modern company that chiefly provides piecework. However, it is due to her personal response that she is now reacting to this by concluding that she is completely unable to work.[172]

In the last sentence of the expert evaluation, Dr. K. summarized that: "... if she now considers herself to be an invalid due to her deviant character [*Wesensabartigkeit*] and her desire-based representations centered on acquiring a pension (*Rentenbegehrvorstellungen*), then these are deviant personal reactions that, in the present case, cannot be considered to have any pathological value. From a neurological point of view, based on the aforementioned findings, the examined individual is not an invalid."[173] However one might assess the medical validity of Dr. K.'s evaluation of these complaints, terminologically and analytically he built seamlessly on the Nazi period.[174] He cited family strains, declared the patient's mode of reaction the main problem, and described her condition with reference, among other things, to her "deviant" (*abartig*) status and her "desire-based representations centered on acquiring a pension." As apparent in this expert evaluation—and as confirmed by other expert reports by Dr. K.—he did not use the term "psychopathy," but described the patient by drawing on typical elements of the psychopathy discourse. In other expert evaluations from 1950 and 1960, he described male patients using terms such as "abnormal oddball" (*abnormer Sonderling*), "deviant"[175] (*abartig*), and "unstable personality."[176] Dr. K. thus conformed to the prevailing doctrine, as did most of the physicians at the asylums analyzed here. Some doctors continued to use the term "psychopathy," but their evaluations were otherwise very similar to the example given here both in terminology and explanatory approach.[177]

It is striking that the ascription of character deficiencies that supposedly led to "deviant behavior" was not class-specific: the "deviant, abnormal oddball," for example, was a vocational school teacher.[178]

Yet some expert evaluations composed at Bethel not only avoided the term "psychopathy" but also refrained from taking the associated explanatory approach. Dr. R. provides us with a case in point. For example, he identified a "state of nervous exhaustion," that "does not presently, however, result in occupational disability or incapacity to work. In order to prevent this, we would like to recommend several weeks of treatment. Upon its completion, a final conclusion should be reached about the issue of occupational disability or incapacity to work."[179] Dr. R. thus referred to a state of exhaustion as envisaged by Baeyer, advocating exactly what Baeyer's critic Schultz had feared in his response in *Der Nervenarzt*: a curative procedure lasting several weeks. Instead of helping the patient "realize" that "desire-based representations" (*Begehrvorstellungen*) would lead nowhere by refusing state aid, he advised treatment for a "state of nervous exhaustion" to which most physicians assigned no pathological significance. This was not a completely new approach at the level of practice: we might recall the diagnosis of a "state of nervous exhaustion" and Dr. G.'s associated assessment and recommendation during the war.[180] As explained in Chapter 4 on "Disease and Diagnostics," typically, diagnoses, clinical pictures, and ways of dealing with patients first appeared in contexts of practice and later entered scientific discourse with reference to this practice.[181]

"Overworked" diagnostics: a new scientific discourse with consequences for psychiatric practice in the Soviet occupation zone and GDR

Work in the committal: questions about salary and occupation in medical histories

Admissions to Rodewisch and Großschweidnitz contrasted with those during the Nazi period and in West Germany due to a different approach to the initial interviewing of the patient. This was in line with the findings of psychiatric research carried out in the Eastern Bloc on the role of work and the work environment. Both a poor attitude toward work as well as the conditions and reputation of the enterprise were seen as causes of mental illness. The importance attached to concrete working conditions is exemplified by an article on the medical evaluation of work neuroses by Werner Hollmann, chief physician at the Potsdam Municipal Hospitals (Städtische Krankenanstalten Potsdam).[182] On the causes of work neuroses, Hollmann stated:

> But when it comes to the disorders arising from the enterprise itself, other key factors are its reputation, the local ranking of enterprises and the general evaluation of their product; here, relations with the foreman and supervisor [*Meister*] and with the other employees of the enterprise emerge as significant, as well as the atmosphere in the team [*Arbeitskollektiv*], which in turn depends on a humane attitude on the part of the management. Also important are social institutions, instances of recognition, role models, differences in remuneration, prospects in life, the aesthetics of the workplace, and so on ... .[183]

The physicians at Rodewisch, Großschweidnitz, and Greifswald did not inquire into all the aspects mentioned by Hollmann, but they covered the field of "work" by asking three standard questions during the initial diagnostic exploration: about the amount of the last salary, whether the patient got by on it, and how they liked the work. The answers were carefully noted down. Usually, this took the form found in Janosch Sch.'s medical history: the doctor asked how the patient liked their current work at an appropriate point during the interview, and either at the beginning or end of the exploration they asked about wages and getting by, in this case as the final question: "(Last wage?)[184] '90 pfennigs an hour, 60–70 M every ten days.' He had gotten by on this."[185] A few lines earlier, the patient spoke about himself in the work context: "He no longer got along very well with his workmates. (?)[186] The work situation had turned out just like it does everywhere."[187] Despite this greater attention to work and work circumstances, however, patients were not asked directly whether they saw any connection between their illness and their work.

"Overwork" in medical diagnostics: from "psychopathy" to organ neurosis

The questions asked about income, job, and job satisfaction were consonant with changes in psychiatric research in the GDR. In what follows, I focus on the question of how and why, and in which fields, the scientific conception of work under socialism differed from that of the Nazi period and the FRG. In this context, I also analyze whether this had an impact on medical practice in psychiatric committals.

Under Nazism, both "unwillingness" (*Unwille*) and "inability" (*Unfähigkeit*) to work were subsumed under the diagnosis of "psychopathy" or—making the blend of social exclusion and medicalization even clearer— patients were classified as "asocial psychopaths." In the GDR, the diagnosis of "psychopathy" quickly lost its meaning in this context. Perusal of the journal *Psychiatrie, Neurologie und medizinische Psychologie* reveals just two articles with "psychopathy" in the title between 1949, the year of first publication, and 1963, one in 1951 and another in 1953. The 1951 article on "Psychopathische Persönlichkeiten, ihre Kriminalität und ihre Stellung vor dem Gesetz" ("Psychopathic personalities, their criminality, and their legal status")[188] presented a statistical study of the so-called "pathological material" (*Krankenmaterial*) held by the Jena University Psychiatric and Neurological Clinic. Here, the focus was on the proportion of "psychopaths" among convicted criminals between 1920 and 1950. The article thus took up the other major strand of psychopathy discourse that existed alongside its focus on work and performance, namely, the pathologization of criminals. While alcohol abuse, age, and gender played prominent roles in the analysis, work was of no interest. The 1953 article, entitled "Zur Frage der Psychopathie" ("On the question of psychopathy"),[189] whose author worked at the University of Leipzig, sought to re-locate "psychopathy" within Pavlov's system of higher nervous activity. Following detailed discussion of various approaches in West Germany and the Pavlovian perspective, he concluded: "In Soviet psychology, the direction of research is clearly determined by the dialectical method and materialist theory. In bourgeois psychology, things are essentially chaotic."[190] After expressing commitment to a socialist methodology presented as goal-oriented and useful, the last sentences of the article summarized once again the substantive innovations occurring in the study and treatment of "psychopathy."

The theoretical orientation toward the average as the 'normal' is also outdated in light of practice. This is a bourgeois (*spießbürgerlich*) point of view that cannot hold up against the law of development in nature and society.[191] Another issue is also undergoing change with respect to psychopathy. Among other definitions of the term, a low level of adaptability (*Anpassungsbreite*) was considered a key criterion of psychopathy. Today, in Soviet science and beyond,[192] the role of the psychopath's active behavior and the potential to shape it through work, and indeed collective work, is also being recognized.[193]

A major innovation in the Soviet concept of psychopathy, as well as in socialist psychiatry as a whole, was the emphasis on exogenous factors and the possibility of societal education.[194] In neither article does refusal to work or the like play a role. The second article addressed work only as an aspect of treatment within the socialist collective.

But this does not mean that work and performance were no longer discussed in the journal *Psychiatrie, Neurologie und medizinische Psychologie*: they were, but they were classified in quite different ways. If we again use the titles appearing between 1949 and 1963 as an indicator, what emerges is that work as a topic appeared on a regular basis.[195] Now, however, it was no longer the "inferiority" of "asocials" and "psychopaths" that was thematized, but rather the influence of working conditions on people; work attitudes; and exhaustion in the course of work. In a 1951 article, Werner Hollmann (1900–1987),[196] who published regularly on the subject, set out every conceivable connection between work and illness, his focus on both somatic and mental disorders.[197] With respect to mental illnesses, he cited an explanatory model found in Soviet psychiatry that had emerged from the further development of Pavlovian research and that other authors subsequently drew on repeatedly in numerous articles. His starting point was so-called "organ"[198] and "work" neuroses: "Organ neuroses encompass diseases that have no morphological basis, in which physiological functions are operating abnormally, and whose symptoms are not an expression of organic changes but of psycho-cognitive (*seelisch-geistig*) disturbances."[199]

The connection asserted between physical dysfunctions and the psyche was not in itself specific to the GDR. It was also made in the FRG within the framework of the psychiatric interpretation of mental abnormalities in war returnees but with the opposite meaning. The psychological symptoms of this group were called "dystrophy" and put down to organic damage caused by malnutrition.[200] In West Germany, increasing attention was then paid to social factors from the mid-1950s onward. But it was mainly internists who considered this dimension rather than psychiatrists.[201] Hollmann endowed social factors with tremendous relevance. He had already been interested in the connection between life courses and illness in the 1930s.[202] In his article of 1951, he fused this older interest with the new requirement of socialist research that greater emphasis be placed on external factors and that they be assumed to exercise an influence on the organs in line with the Soviet Pavlov school.[203]

Hollmann identified social conflicts that impacted on the vegetative nervous system as the origin of "organ neuroses."[204] According to the author, while organ neuroses did not necessarily arise in connection with gainful employment, this was frequently the case. The cause of these neuroses, he contended, was excessive ambition, which sometimes occurred not just at work but also in the family. As an example of patients suffering from gastric neurosis (*Magenneurose*), Hollmann cited "particularly ambitious young people who, for example, want to make their mark as skilled workers or foremen vis-à-vis their comrades and, in this way, seek to stand out from the mass of unskilled workers."[205] The author saw the ambition that supposedly triggered the disorder as caused by the ambitious person's status as a closet introvert. They supposedly hoped, by means of their ambition, to attain an elevated position that, consonant with their introverted tendency, would detach them from the collective.[206]

"Work neuroses" were not viewed as organic neuroses, but as a form of neurasthenia. Rapid fatigability during the work process was established as their main symptom. Thus, physicians used the term "work neurosis" for the state that patients called "overwork" when talking to physicians.[207] The condition of "overwork" was thought to be due fundamentally to the patient's incorrect relationship to work or to the transferring to work of dissatisfaction in other areas of life, such as family or sexuality.[208] In addition, a distinction was made between drive fatigue (*Antriebsermüdung*) and overtiredness (*Übermüdung*). Drive fatigue supposedly occurred in workers who needed a particularly large number of "stimuli" to motivate them. They were therefore seen as lacking in drive. If they tried to overcome this lack, they might quickly overexert themselves. Overtiredness, meanwhile, was seen as caused by excessive motivation on the part of the worker. Finally, Hoffmann noted that work neuroses were more common among women, while organ neuroses were more typical among men.[209]

In contrast to the discourses on "psychopathy" and the neurasthenia discourse of the imperial era, class affiliation, logically enough, played no role in the socialist conception and, unlike the idea of the "degenerate psychopath," heritability was not relevant either. As noted by Patrick Kury, managerial disease did not fall on fertile ground in the GDR.[210] Still, the journal *Psychiatrie, Neurologie und medizinische Psychologie* did publish an informative article on this disorder. It began by showing that Western living conditions contributed to the disease and, contrary to its name, it existed in all classes.[211] In conformity with Cold War logic, the author identified Western social conditions as the cause of the illness.[212] But she then stated that the symptoms of so-called managerial disease did in fact occur in the GDR among those in management positions.[213] This she attributed to two factors: the many new appointments that had to be made after 1945, and second, an incorrect attitude to work.[214] In the context of the latter, she conceived of the condition as a form of excessive motivation resulting in a lack of time to relax, in line with the concept of work neurosis developed in Werner Hollmann's article. Among other things, she suggested autogenic training as a solution.[215] As mentioned earlier, autogenic training was an invention of Johannes Heinrich Schultz, who had made a career as a psychotherapist at the "Göring Institute." His method continued to spread on both sides of the Iron Curtain.[216] Directly bound up with this, one feature common to the psychiatric conception of "overwork" in the GDR and the FRG was the importance ascribed to the patient's attitude.

Three points in particular stand out in the recasting of work-related afflictions East Germany.

First, neurasthenia, which was viewed as the cause of inappropriate overtiredness at work, was already *the* bourgeois affliction among mental illnesses in the German Empire.[217] This diagnosis captured the states of insecurity and nervousness at large in the bourgeois world, which patients and physicians then jointly converted into a legitimizing psychiatric discourse. After World War II, the diagnosis of neurasthenia was already predicted to disappear, having steadily declined after its mass dissemination at the turn of the century. In the psychiatry of the GDR, however, neurasthenia underwent a renaissance, at least in the scientific debate—coupled with a reevaluation of its content. The notion of people suffering from the rapid and threatening concomitants of high industrialization was out. Now, in the socialist reading, neurasthenia bracketed together people who were not motivated enough for gainful employment or who pursued overly ambitious individual goals and sought to stand out from their fellows. The socialist concept of neurasthenia thus carried forward certain aspects of the old concept of "psychopathy." I have already highlighted the way in which Kraepelin's biologistic reinterpretation brought the concept of neurasthenia closer to that of psychopathy. Although there was no further uptake of this biologistic reading, the connection between the individual's attitude to work on the one hand and society on the other was a core trope of the psychopathy discourse, which always foregrounded the consequences for society, never the patient's condition.

The second key development is the assignment of organ neuroses to men and neurasthenic drive exhaustion to women. The psychiatric view of women in employment built on and resembled that of the Nazi period. The assumption that women suffered more often from work neuroses in the special form of "drive fatigue" highlights once again psychiatrists' belief that housewives lacked the motivation to pursue gainful employment.

In the case of men, meanwhile, "overwork" lay beyond the realm of the sayable during the Nazi era: any kind of exhaustion syndrome was regarded as a sign of biological inferiority and/or as a refusal to make full use of one's labor power in support of the "National Community." This changed when the psychopathy discourse was supplanted by the fatigue discourse within psychiatric research. Work and performance certainly continued to be held up as imperatives in the life of the individual, as vital to building the socialist state, and they were propagated accordingly. Yet even the propaganda acknowledged that workers first had to acquire the new socialist attitude toward work.[218]

The socialist conception of work, moreover, differed significantly from that of the Nazi regime in two respects. First, the reasons for "insufficient" work performance and individual exhaustion were construed differently. The patient's attitude, which was seen as alterable, played a key role, as did external circumstances. Thus, the steps that could be taken were different as well. Second, men who were not "fully productive" (*voll leistungsfähig*) were no longer stigmatized in psychiatric discourse to the same extent as during the Nazi period. While their disorder was not condoned and it was debated as a social problem, the possibility of recovery was acknowledged, and the importance of social conditions was highlighted. Articles on work in psychiatric journals also backed the idea that the citizens of the GDR must be granted a learning period so that they could develop the correct, namely, socialist, relationship to work.[219]

Third, these articles were greatly influenced by Soviet research, both in terminology and content. Not only is overtiredness interpreted in a Pavlovian way, but the language is riddled with Pavlovian terms, such as "stimuli" and "inhibitions."[220]

In contrast to the development of research views on schizophrenia analyzed in Chapter 4, "Disease and Diagnostics," research on work and health broke more clearly with the Nazi era and with older research traditions. While some researchers in the Weimar Republic explained neuroses in the work context as a result of exogenous factors,[221] the articles on work in the journal *Psychiatrie, Neurologie und medizinische Psychologie* did not reference them. As evident in the text "Zur Frage der Psychopathie"[222] ("On the question of psychopathy"), Western research was highly present in certain articles, always functioning as a negative foil though one that was often discussed in detail. More space was available for research from neighboring socialist countries. Regular contributions from other Eastern Bloc states were published, especially on the topic of work, with examples including "Die Doppelbelastung der Frau im Arbeitsprozeß" ("Women's dual burden in the work process") by E. Klimková-Deutschová[223] of Prague and "Das Erlebnis der Arbeit" ("The Experience of Work") by Stephan Török of the Simaság Institute for the Employment of the Sick (Institut für Krankenbeschäftigung

Simaság), Hungary.[224] In this regard, the selection of articles resembled that on other topics, such as schizophrenia. What is remarkable is that no even slightly divergent opinions appeared in the articles written by German authors. The Pavlovian tradition and the Eastern Bloc as a scientific space were of crucial importance, at least to research on the socio-politically vital issue of work. In contrast to the construction of the health care system in the GDR, psychiatric research on this issue did not draw on the traditions of the German Empire or Weimar Republic. There was no strict separation between psychiatry in the two young German states—as apparent in articles that sometimes referred to Western research views for pages on end, and the fact that physicians from both states could regularly attend conferences together until the building of the Wall. Still, decidedly "socialist" research positions were espoused, at least on the subject of work. While the reception and regular positive mention of Pavlov's ideas make sense given the regime's censorship, the complete break with older research is surprising, especially when set against the marked continuities on the subject of schizophrenia. My evaluation of journal articles on the latter subject showed that, despite censorship, it was possible to maintain aspects of the old doctrinal system and that different strands of explanation, not all of which were oriented to the dogma privileged under socialism to the same degree, could coexist.

A slew of reasons can be put forward for the striking rupture in psychiatric research on "work." Below, I first identify the causes of the break with the previous doctrine and then reasons for the failure to take up alternative research views found in the Weimar Republic.

Unlike research on schizophrenia, studies centered on work tended to be the focus of political and public attention: they related to a core area of socialist ideology. We may assume that this upped the pressure to fit in. This is corroborated by the fact that while the concept of "psychopathy" as a whole was not altered or replaced, it no longer covered "work and health," while "sexuality and health" continued to be subsumed under "psychopathy."

With regard to the topic of work, however, the new political environment opened up opportunities for psychiatry and neurology. During the Nazi era, work, performance, and health mainly came under "psychopathy," which, as a "syndrome"[225] (*Krankheitsbild*), formed an interface between psychiatry and social hygiene, placing it at the margins of the medical domain. While this provided an opportunity to extend the psychiatric field to social issues, it also meant that psychiatry had to tolerate the presence of other expert groups within the same discursive space. The consistent reinterpretation of the fraught interstices of work and health in accordance with the socialist notion of the "dictatorship of the cortex" contributed significantly to processes of somatization and thus to clearer pathologization. Mental abnormalities related to work and performance were now shifted from the boundary between psychiatry and society to the threshold of psychiatry and neurology, placing them wholly within the medical domain.[226] The link to society was still there, of course, and was emphasized incessantly. But now it was clear that other fields, such as occupational and social welfare, had to assist the medical experts. Had research on schizophrenia been Pavlovized in a similar way, meanwhile, there would have been no equivalent increase in power for the psychiatric and neurological professions. That syndrome had already been "somatized." With respect to schizophrenia, East German psychiatrists and neurologists needed to mark their boundaries with the established view chiefly vis-à-vis American perspectives, in which this view was being challenged profoundly. This interpretation is not meant to suggest that no scientist in the early GDR believed in the Soviet-style theories they espoused. There were certainly some convinced Pavlovians among psychiatrists, with Hanns Schwarz, director of the Greifswald University Psychiatric Clinic, being a prime example.[227] Still, given the high degree of continuity of personnel between physicians in the Nazi era and the GDR, it makes sense to try to identify the reasons for changing interpretations of work, reasons that go beyond an ideological shift.[228]

Two key factors explain the lack of continuity not only with Western positions and those of the Nazi period but also the Weimar era. First, few of the psychologists who had offered an impactful alternative to the prevailing doctrine in the Weimar period remained in the GDR: many had emigrated during the Nazi era, and the remaining psychotherapists conformed to the ideological template laid down by the regime.[229] Second, psychotherapists in Weimar operated, in the broadest sense, within a Freudian tradition that Soviet research fundamentally rejected. It is true that both the Freudian perspective and its Pavlovian counterpart emphasized exogenous factors. In this respect, both were antithetical to the doctrine of heredity in psychiatry. Pavlovian research, however, saw itself as decidedly somatic, in contrast to Freudian ideas. Within the conceptual framework centered on higher nervous activity that was established in the Soviet Union, the entire organism was controlled via the uppermost layer of the brain, but this control could be strongly influenced by conditioning.[230]

Ramifications of Pavlovian theory in psychiatric practice

Scientific exchange in psychiatric journals was unquestionably molded by Soviet views. The psychiatric perspective on complaints about "overwork" as found in these publications fits seamlessly into a picture of the 1950s in which workers were to be educated to become good socialists.[231] Yet there was more to this than the adaptation of scientific texts to new circumstances. Effects on practice can be discerned as well. In the clinics and asylums analyzed here, the diagnosis of "psychopathy" appeared ever less often in relation to patient complaints about work. This can be seen both in the issuing of diagnoses consistent with Soviet doctrine, such as "organ neurosis,"[232] and in the description of illness and diagnosis within retirement pension evaluations, in which the question of inability or unwillingness to work was especially pertinent.

Patients who complained of psychological and somatic afflictions due to work were now more often diagnosed with work or organ neurosis, fully in line with psychiatric discourse. At Greifswald especially, but also at Rodewisch and Großschweidnitz, we find descriptions of patients and diagnoses that applied the concept of organ neurosis to the patient exactly as described in the articles published in psychiatric journals. The strikingly comprehensive implementation of socialist diagnostics at Greifswald was probably linked with its director, Hanns Schwarz, who, as mentioned above, was a convinced Pavlovian.[233] One example of the pinpoint implementation of the new doctrine is the following description of the illness afflicting 24-year-old Sina U., who was admitted to Greifswald in 1955 due to persistent hiccups:

> In February of this year, at the end of a political training course, the patient suddenly experienced uncontrollable ructus. The patient did not have a bad taste in her mouth and did not have the feeling that this condition originated in the stomach. It is noteworthy in this context that the patient was intellectually incapable of coping with the course. The ructus subsided through bed rest and appropriate medication, and Miss [U.] resumed her work on May 7. [...]
> Diagnostically, we consider this ructus indicative of organ neurosis.[234]

Both overexertion and underexertion, as well as attempts to compensate for either condition, were considered typical reasons for organ neuroses. They were viewed as signs that the patient had not yet been employed in the ideal position or field of activity. The demand for the ideal job was a double-edged sword. While it was fairly easy to change jobs within GDR companies, this view of illness meant that there was in fact a suitable job for everyone. This had implications for early retirement (and the accompanying pension). Under the rubric of "social therapy," rather than granting individuals' requests for a retirement pension due to illness, attempts were made to find suitable jobs for them.[235] In the retirement pension evaluations compiled at the three psychiatric institutions studied here, "pension neurosis" certainly remained a topic on which physicians commented, for example when tasked with assessing the extent to which the patient "appears to be a retirement pension moocher" (*Rentenkämpfer*).[236] This psychiatric perspective made a snug fit with the GDR's economically driven determination to examine requests for retirement with a critical eye.[237] In the Nazi era, as in East Germany, economic considerations prompted efforts to exploit people's labor power for as long as possible by denying them retirement pensions. But this was implemented quite differently in the GDR, despite ongoing talk of "pension neurosis." It should be noted that the retirement pension evaluations issued at Greifswald, Rodewisch, and Großschweidnitz in the 1950s and early 1960s no longer include diagnoses or descriptions of patients revolving around the terms "psychopathy" and "asocial" so common during the Nazi era.

Typically, physicians in the Nazi era used these terms when they failed to find a condition considered somatic, as in the case of chronic headaches. In the GDR institutions studied here, retirement pension evaluations relating to such complaints were compiled without the old pejorative vocabulary. The expert evaluation of Marie S., who complained of headaches that were preventing her from working, is a good example. In an expert evaluation issued in 1957 at Greifswald, Marie S. was certified as subject to a reduced earning capacity of 50 percent, and diagnosed as suffering from "migraine-like depressive state [*migränöser Verstimmungszustand*] 316 K."[238] The doctors having detected no neurological abnormalities, the patient was described in the evaluation as follows:

> Psychologically, the patient stands out through her primitive description of her complaints, which she expresses with great intensity. Her mood appears slightly depressed.
>
> In diagnostic terms, we believe the patient is experiencing headaches and mood disorders together with a complex of complaints that appears hypochondriacal as a manifestation of migraine equivalents.
>
> From the perspective of our medical specialty, we estimate a reduced earning capacity of 50 percent.[239]

This medical portrayal was still judgmental, when referring, for example, to the "primitive description of her complaints," but it was free of the highly stigmatizing categories of "asocial" and "psychopath" so common during the Nazi era (and earlier). It is not impossible that doctors at other clinics proceeded differently here. However, using the old terminology would have made it clear that the clinic was failing to implement Soviet psychiatric research on the complex of work. It is therefore reasonable to assume that retirement pension evaluations generally adapted to the new linguistic conventions. This is backed up by the fact that contemporary physicians noted the conceptual change in evaluations. A talk on socio-medical assessment at the 15th meeting of the Psychiatric-Neurological Society (Psychiatrisch-Neurologische Gesellschaft) at the Universities of Greifswald and Rostock, for example, highlighted this shift: "The change of form in abnormal reactions from grossly demonstrative forms (hysteria, pseudodementia) to intimate forms (organ neurosis, vegetative dystonia) is particularly evident in the field of social insurance medicine."[240] However, this switch does not necessarily tell us anything about the acceptance of the Soviet approach among the psychiatrists of the GDR. The only thing that seems certain is that they conformed to the prevailing doctrine, at least in official statements. But even if this was a functional adaptation, it constituted a clear break with the Nazi era.[241]

Although the diagnosis of "psychopathy" was rare in the context of work and performance in the 1950s, it did not disappear. In other contexts, it remained an important diagnosis. Above all, "psychopathy" was frequently diagnosed in evaluations of unsoundness of mind in connection with sexual offenses. Nonconforming sexuality, as we have seen, had also been dealt with under the rubric of "psychopathy" during the war, often in conjunction with work, as in the case of women with STDs. While the motif of sexuality continued to play a central role in the psychopathy discourse in East Germany, this did not apply to work and performance. This fits with Sven Korzilius's findings in his study of the criminal prosecution of "asocials" in the GDR. He too notes that in the 1950s, although the regime declared war on "idling" (*Arbeitsbummelei*), criminal prosecution focused on prostitution rather than work.[242]

The thesis that the Pavlov campaign and the Soviet perspective in medical research had no practical impact in the GDR is untenable, at least when it comes to the psychiatric approach to illness in the context of work.[243] Here, a change in practice molded by Pavlov's ideas was already apparent in the 1950s. Doctors asked new questions during committals, but more importantly, they made different diagnoses. While the new diagnoses did not portray the patient in a positive light, in contrast to the past they did not aim to permanently stigmatize people or exclude them from society.

These changes in diagnostic practice did not occur suddenly but at an early stage. Patients who cited overwork and symptoms of fatigue at work were still frequently diagnosed with "psychopathy" at Rodewisch and Greifswald between 1946 and 1949, but hardly ever in the 1950s. If the diagnosis of "psychopathy" was still being made in connection with work in the 1950s, it was in cases where the patient was not working, but it ceased to be ascribed when patients merely complained about their work.

Summary: work and performance in comparative perspective

When it came to decisions at the threshold of the asylum or to how psychiatrists, relatives, and affected persons drew the line between "normality" and "deviancy," work- and performance-related ideas about illness played an important role both in Nazi wartime society and in the two postwar successor states. Continuity and change in these ideas, theories, and practices can be summarized in eight key points.

First, work and performance played a crucial role in wartime committal negotiations. Relatives referred to them not only to legitimize committals, but also to prevent institutionalization. In the latter case, ability to work was put forward as evidence that the patient was a useful member of the "National Community" and that an asylum stay would not be in its best interest. This finding complements researchers' strong emphasis on "inability" and "will" to work as a criterion of exclusion under Nazism.

Second, work-related rationales continued to be important in the committal process in both successor states, but in the FRG they differed from wartime and the GDR in one crucial respect: in West German committals, no connections were made between the individual's performance and the well-being of society as a whole. Here it makes sense to assume that the rationales that made this link in the Nazi period and East Germany represented the (instrumental) appropriation of their regimes' propaganda by both patients and their relatives.

Third, the police and public health authorities in the FRG and the GDR were much less likely to initiate admissions through rationales revolving around the patient's ability and willingness to work. This was bound up with the new modes of committal in both states, which resulted in far fewer committals by police and public health officers. In the GDR, this was due in part to the fact that in the 1950s the focus was on prostitutes and venereal diseases rather than on the exclusion of "asocials." It is quite possible that the links between performance and venereal disease among women shown for the wartime period continued to exist in West and East Germany. But they do not show up in the practice of committal because patients with STDs were no longer admitted to psychiatric institutions solely on the basis of these illnesses.

Fourth, the continuities between the "Third Reich" and the FRG in terms of ideas about the healthy and sick self were significantly greater than in the GDR. This applies both to patients' and physicians' perspectives. While during World War II and in West Germany one's work performance was profoundly important to popular notions of health, and people who were committed to asylums regularly identified "overwork" as the cause of their illness, in the GDR this was true only of a few occupational groups that were able to take advantage of the opportunities for social advancement on offer in the state's early years. Further, medical discourse and practice in the FRG were subject only to minor changes, whereas they underwent significant transformation in the GDR. In the latter, psychopathy discourse, insofar as it related to work behavior,[244] was replaced by a focus on organ and work neurosis. This also had an impact on medical practice. The fact that the medical profession in East Germany maintained a certain distance from the new regime did not mean that it failed to apply the new body of knowledge. This may have been due solely to the fact that expert evaluations of earning capacity entailed departing from the protected space of one's own medical institution. Nevertheless, clear changes can be observed here for patients as well. And even this functionally motivated adaptation reveals the effects of the relationship between science and politics in practice, which in this case were far-reaching.[245]

In the FRG, the classification and evaluation of "overwork" depended heavily on individual physicians and differed even within the same asylum. In the GDR, the differences were smaller. In Greifswald, however, we find a particularly consistent implementation of the Pavlovian approach.

Fifth, the psychiatric evaluation of the working person was based on different paradigms in the East and West. The Soviet concept was undergirded by the model of a flagging "human engine."[246] Articles in the journal *Psychiatrie, Neurologie und medizinische Psychologie* extoled a balanced alternation between activity and rest as a prescription against symptoms of overwork.[247] Some conceptions of "organ neurosis" also worked on the assumption that people may strain themselves beyond their capacities.[248] The West German concept of psychopathy, meanwhile, represents a deterministic variant of what later became known as "human capital."[249] The patient was expected to make considerable efforts to optimize themself in order to meet work demands and ensure their appeal on the labor market. Meanwhile, West German physicians sought the reasons why some patients failed to do so in essentialist notions of class affiliation (the ongoing discourse on "psychopathy" as hereditary) and gender (the female body as placing natural limits on performance—if this took place outside the home). Physicians in the FRG took a positive view of a good attitude toward work and efforts to adapt oneself to its demands, for example in expert evaluations on reduced earning capacity. In such cases, doctors did not perceive the patients as "psychopaths" or "pension neurotics." Whether a patient was a "pension neurotic" remained important in the GDR too. There was a general acceptance that citizens first had to learn the socialist work ethic, yet the "pension moocher" seems to have functioned as an apt trope that was deployed to avoid granting too many retirement pensions.

Sixth, Pavlov's reception in the GDR varied depending on whether it was schizophrenia or work-related deviations that were at issue. The degree of adaptation to the official socialist perspective depended both on the "political" importance of the disease type involved and on whether or not the official dogma strengthened the profession's status as a branch of medicine, as in the case of the new way of diagnosing "work-related complaints" (*Arbeitsbeschwerden*).

Seventh, although the importance of work to a healthy self exhibited gender-specific elements, these were less pronounced than previous research suggests. It is important to note that in the 1940s and 1950s not only men but women too defined the healthy self with reference to work. In the GDR, this self-attribution was in fact more common among women, as it soon lost its relevance to employed patients but persisted with regard to housework, which continued to be considered women's business. The findings on "overwork" relativize this picture somewhat: under the extreme conditions of war, "overwork" was an unsayable reality for men, pointing to a social consensus on a concept of males defined by work and performance. The acceptance of "overwork" in the case of working wives, meanwhile, brings out the differing societal and familial expectations of women. Work in the form of housekeeping or gainful employment exerted a greater influence on women's self-attributions than family and society (as well as the research of the day) expected.

Eighth, the family clearly played a major role in patients' narratives in the early GDR. Even in the case of committals initiated from the workplace, from the perspective of those committed this usually entailed a family problem that merely manifested itself at work. In any case, this finding cannot be described in terms of the dichotomy of gainful employment and leisure time. To what extent people tried to strike a balance between gainful employment and private life, and to what degree these were intertwined, cannot be determined solely in light of the amount of leisure time available and the potential for consumption: the picture in the early GDR was more complex than this. Spheres of life outside of gainful employment were in fact just as important in East Germany as they were in the FRG, at least in connection with mental health and well-being.

Notes

1 LHA Marburg, Patient file sign. 16K10740F, Entry, March 15, 1946, LWV Hesse, 16.
2 Ibid.
3 Arguments related to work were often central in the narratives of patients and their relatives beyond World War II and the postwar period, and they were not limited to Germany. Joost Vijselaar, for example, highlights the great importance of economic circumstances and work within the family in a long-term study of the Netherlands: Vijselaar, "Out and In"; on the aspect of work and the ability to work in the context of both committal practices and everyday practice in asylums around 1900, see Ankele, *Alltag und Aneignung*.
4 On the era-bound production of science, see for instance Sarasin, Philipp et al., "Eine Einleitung," in Philipp Sarasin et al. (eds.), *Bakteriologie und Moderne. Studien zur Biopolitik des Unsichtbaren 1870–1920* (Frankfurt/M., 2007), 14.
5 On the debate about the informative value of patient records and on the problem of the doctor-patient relationship, see for example Condrau, "Alterssicherung"; see also the introduction and conclusion of the present book.
6 Beyond this, it is important to note that even if the consultation was pre-structured by physicians, the information provided by the patients and their relatives was not completely predetermined. In this context, too, processes of appropriation on the part of medical laypersons must be factored in: even if a given question was asked, individuals were not obliged to answer it in detail.
7 The only "socialist" textbook was Giljarowski, *Lehrbuch*.
8 See for example Ewald, Gottfried, *Neurologie und Psychiatrie. Ein Lehrbuch für Studierende und Ärzte* (Munich, 1944), 540.
9 Ibid.
10 While caution is advised here, as it is ultimately unclear what might have been omitted, the questions at least provide a valuable rough guide to how the consultation unfolded.
11 HPA Untergöltzsch, Patient file sign. 6656, Entry, August 8, 1945, SächSta Chemnitz, 32810.
12 On the three dimensions of work in the context of the "Final Solution," namely, extermination through work, rescue through work, and extermination as work, see Sandkühler, Thomas, *"Endlösung" in Galizien. Der Judenmord in Ostpolen und die Rettungsinitiativen von Berthold Beitz 1941–44* (Bonn, 1996), 11–14. On the criterion of inability to work in the process of selecting individuals for murder in the concentration camps, especially toward the end of the war, see the paper by Stefan Hördler at the conference "Arbeit im Nationalsozialismus," in "Tagungsbericht Arbeit im Nationalsozialismus. 13.12.2012–15.12.2012, Berlin," in H-Soz-u-Kult, February 25, 2013, http://hsozkult.geschichte.hu-berlin.de/tagungsberichte/id=4669 (accessed April 7, 2014).

13　Ayaß, "Asoziale," 156 ff.
14　Kranig, Andreas, *Lockerung und Zwang. Zur Arbeitsverfassung im "Dritten Reich"* (Stuttgart, 1983), 142.
15　Though in the Weimar Republic recipients of welfare benefits were already required to perform community service and could be sent to a workhouse if they refused. See Korzilius, "Parasiten," 133.
16　With the onset of the war, the focus on fitness for work, which "preventive medicine" had already sought to ensure, culminated in the shift to occupational health care. The entire field of day-to-day health care was increasingly linked to and oriented toward the workplace. For example, from 1940 onward, only company physicians were allowed to write sick notes in firms important to the war effort. In addition, according to Winfried Süß, "the DAF [German Labor Front] worked systematically to ensure that the sick were cared for in company-owned facilities instead of within the family, in order to enhance their control over them." Süß, "Volkskörper," 261; for a summary of company health care, see Eckart, Wolfgang, *Medizin in der NS-Diktatur. Ideologie, Praxis, Folgen* (Vienna, 2012), 176ff.
17　Hence, at a conference on "Work under National Socialism," Alf Lüdtke and Michael Wildt called for research on the practice of inclusion and exclusion in relation to "work." See "Tagungsbericht Arbeit im Nationalsozialismus."
18　On the need to evaluate health policy inclusion and exclusion, which were not genuinely Nazi in character, differently in the context of Nazi rule, see Thießen, "Medizingeschichte," 562.
19　HPA Untergöltzsch, Patient file sign. 6707, SächSta Chemnitz, 32810.
20　Ibid., Entry, September 2, 1942.
21　Ibid.
22　Ibid., Entry, September 9, 1942.
23　Ibid., Entry, November 28, 1942.
24　Ibid.
25　vBS Bethel, Patient file sign. 2058, HAB, Patient files Mahainam II.
26　HPA Eglfing-Haar, Patient file sign. EH 10389, AB Upper Bavaria, EH.
27　Ibid., Letter, April 12, 1944.
28　Ibid.
29　Ibid.
30　On the topic of war as work from the perspective of soldiers, see Neitzel, Sönke and Welzer, Harald, *Soldaten. Protokolle vom Kämpfen, Töten und Sterben* (Frankfurt/M., 2011), 411ff.
31　See for example HPA Eglfing-Haar, Patient file sign. EH 92, AB Upper Bavaria, EH.
32　On work and exclusion, see also Hörath, Julia, "'Arbeitsscheue Volksgenossen.' Leistungsbereitschaft als Kriterium der Inklusion und Exklusion," URL: http://arbeit-im-nationalsozialismus.oldenbourgverlag.de/open-peer-review/hoerath/ (accessed March 14, 2014).
33　LHA Marburg, Patient file sign. K12962F, Re: Readmission of April 7, 1954, LWV Hesse, 16.
34　For example, vBS Bethel, Patient file sign. 161/2446, Letter, November 10, 1943, HAB, Patient files Mahanaim I. On behavior during bombardments and on discussions about access to bunkers, in which, among other things, it was suggested that working persons ought to take priority over mothers, see also Süß, *Tod*, 347.
35　See Chapter 2, section "Committal practices in a 'society in a state of collapse' (1945–1949)."

36 For the period before the foundation of the two German states, see Kleßmann, *Staatsgründung*.
37 On the renewed engagement with the Christian community in the early FRG, see for example Schildt, *Abendland*.
38 On the new identitarian construct of the housewife as consumer and, as it were, interior decorator of the home, see Schildt, Axel, "Freizeit, Kultur und Häuslichkeit in der 'Wiederaufbau'-Gesellschaft. Zur Modernisierung von Lebensstilen in der Bundesrepublik. Deutschland in den 1950er Jahren," in Hannes Siegrist et al. (eds.), *Europäische Konsumgeschichte. Zur Gesellschafts- und Kulturgeschichte des Konsums (18. bis 20. Jahrhundert)* (Frankfurt/M., 1997), 327–349.
39 LHA Marburg, Patient file sign. 16K14574M, Entry, July 3, 1961, LWV Hesse, 16.
40 Ibid.
41 vBS Bethel, Patient file sign. 39/401, Entry, January 10, 1958, HAB Patient files Mahainam II.
42 LHA Marburg, Patient file sign. 16K13038M, LWV Hesse, 16.
43 Ibid., Entry, August 14, 1956.
44 vBS Bethel, Patient file sign. 4877, Letter [n.d., 1956], HAB, Patient files Gilead III.
45 KA Rodewisch, Patient file sign. 5451, Letter from Dr. K. to patient's father, December 10, 1953, SächSta Chemnitz, 32810.
46 Ibid., Letter from patient's father, October 27, 1953.
47 The rest of the letter is about arranging a visit by the mother to the asylum and related difficulties. Ibid., Letter from the patient's mother [n.d.]. The lack of punctuation reflects the original text.
48 Ibid., Letter from the patient's father, October 27, 1953.
49 KA Rodewisch, Patient file sign. 32681, Entry, May 9, 1950, SächSta, 32810.
50 PsychN Greifswald, Patient file prov. sign. 1949/495, Letter, August 26, 1949, UA Greifswald, PsychN.
51 Ibid., Letter, September 14, 1949.
52 PsychN Greifswald, Patient file prov. sign. 1962/150, Letter, November 21, 1961, UA Greifswald, PsychN (original emphasis).
53 Lindenberger, "Asociality," 222.
54 KA Rodewisch, Patient file sign. 4895, Letters from patient's mother, March 2–September 10, 1953, SächSta Chemnitz, 32810.
55 Ibid., Letter, September 10, 1953.
56 Sabrow, "Sozialismus," 13. On page 18 in the same text, Sabrow explicitly highlights the importance of equality in the semantic world of socialism. In connection with work, equality is also fundamental to the rationale I analyze here.
57 "Overwork" (*Überarbeitung*) is the term used in the sources by medical lay-persons, which is why I place it in quotation marks. Inability to work and unwillingness to work, meanwhile, are terms that encompass a variety of concepts in the sources. While they reflect the evaluations appearing in the sources, they are not necessarily the words used by actors.
58 The only medical record in which a man himself thematized an excessive work-load is that relating to the committal of Walther M. mentioned in Chapter 2, in the section "Between voluntariness and coercion, assistance and long-term residential placement: committals from the perspective of patients in the Nazi era, the GDR, and the FRG." Here it should be noted that the patient was familiar with the asylum and the doctor as a result of numerous previous stays. See LHA Marburg, Patient file sign. K10563M, LWV Hesse, 16.

59 Neuner, *Politik*, 71ff; Lerner, *Men*, 32ff.
60 vBS Bethel, Patient file sign. 27/224, Entry, May 7, 1957, HAB, Patient files Mahanaim II.
61 vBS Bethel, Patient file sign. 27/222, Entry, May 9, 1957, HAB, Patient files Mahanaim II.
62 The frequent and self-evident self-attribution of an excessive workload as a mental problem among women contrasts with Susanne Hoffmann's findings. In her analysis of autobiographical statements, she found this kind of self-attribution exclusively among men, while she identified the self-attribution of physical strain independent of gender. See Hoffmann, *Alltag*, 252. Presumably, these different findings are due to the sources analyzed. Hoffmann's corpus consists of autobiographies, prose narratives written by individuals about their own lives. Though the autobiographies Hoffmann studied were not published, it can be assumed that they were conscious self-representations that could potentially be read, at least by family members. It is possible that the differences are due to the fact that while psychological strain due to work in women was sayable in specific contexts, it did not fit neatly into a self-stylizing auto-biography. The narrative context from which a medical record emerged, on the other hand, was quite different. Of course, these are often conscious self-representations as well, but when a woman made the associated statements, "illness" or "non-normality" had already been ascribed to her. There was now very little prospect of putting forward an exclusively positive story about oneself. Instead, explicit questions were asked about the patient's initial perception of "symptoms of illness" and this in a situation in which many female patients may have hoped to help identify the cause of and improve their condition through the information they provided.
63 HPA Untergöltzsch, Patient file sign. 6976, Entry, April 16, 1948, SächSta Chemnitz, 32810.
64 vBS Bethel, Patient file sign. 3850, HAB, Patient files Gilead III.
65 vBS Bethel, Patient file sign. 161/2443, Entry, January 12, 1943, HAB, Patient files Mahanaim I.
66 On propaganda centered on the strong woman during wartime, see Süß, *Tod*, 74. On how women dealt with demands that they "replace men in industry, the party, the Wehrmacht, and the authorities, and shoulder the extra work arising there and elsewhere as a result of the war," see Kramer, Nicole, *Volksgenossinnen an der "Heimatfront." Mobilisierung, Verhalten, Erinnerung* (Göttingen, 2011), 12. With regard to the period in which this example occurred, Kramer has identified the special importance of the idea of the female comrade who, in addition to efficient household management, also took on other tasks outside the home. She points out that it is in this notion—in contrast to the concept of the mother, which also remained important—that we find the clearest case of the blurring of gender boundaries. See ibid., 344.
67 On the enforcement and widespread embrace of the housewife model in connection with ideas about and the practice of health, see Hoffmann, *Alltag*, 251.
68 Steinbacher, Sybille, "Differenz der Geschlechter? Chancen und Schranken für die 'Volksgenossinnen,'" in Frank Bajohr and Michael Wildt (eds.), *Volksgemeinschaft. Neue Forschungen zur Gesellschaft des Nationalsozialismus* (Frankfurt/M., 2009), 99.
69 vBS Bethel, Patient file sign. 161/2446, Entry, November 10, 1943, HAB, Patient files Mahanaim I. Since anti-aircraft defense was envisaged as a form of citizen-led self-defense on the home front, women in particular were to be recruited to staff it. For women in this field, see Kramer, *Heimatfront*, 103ff. and 111.

70 Franka Maubach shows that the League of German Girls (BDM or Bund Deutscher Mädel) did much to forge women into a community. Expectations were thus linked to real experiences. However, these expectations were also bound up with gender-specific modes of self-interpretation within the "National Community." Nicole Kramer highlights three behavioral models for female national comrades: the mother, the fighter, and the comrade. The prevailing concept of the mother entailed the idea that women must take care of others—as a kind of extended family—and was strongly focused on the community. Maubach, Franka, *Die Stellung halten. Kriegserfahrungen und Lebensgeschichten der Wehrmachthelferinnen* (Göttingen, 2009), 54ff; Kramer, *Heimatfront*, 346ff. On the historical relevance of the dichotomy of expectation and experience, see Koselleck, Reinhart, "'Erfahrungsraum' und 'Erwartungshorizont'—zwei historische Kategorien," in Reinhart Koselleck, *Vergangene Zukunft. Zur Semantik geschichtlicher Zeiten* (Frankfurt/M., 1979), 349–375.

71 In his monograph on these very phenomena, Kury points out that stress is a mass phenomenon in the post-1945 period and argues that the lack of scientific discourse tells us nothing about whether people previously felt stress. Susanne Hoffmann found very similar descriptions of "stress" in her autobiographical sources as early as the beginning of the twentieth century. Kury, *Der Überforderte Mensch*, 267, 11; Hoffmann, *Alltag*, 264.

72 vBS Bethel, Patient file sign. 1875, HAB, Patient files Mahanaim I.

73 Negotiations about illness and health among laypersons took a completely different form when an accepted measuring instrument was involved. See Hess, "Ökonomie," 237 f.

74 LHA Marburg, Patient file sign. 16K14774M, Committal certificate from the Police Administration, March 2, 1962, LWV Hesse, 16.

75 Ibid, Entry, April 9, 1962.

76 Ibid., Entry, April 24, 1962.

77 See for example vBS Bethel, Patient file sign. 2818, Entry, July 26, 1951, HAB, Patient files Morija I.

78 This was not only the case in the medical records. It is striking how many articles on various topics in the psychiatric journal *Der Nervenarzt* contain numerous examples of committals in which the despair felt over the inability to find work was cited as the reason for a suicide attempt. See for example Meinertz, Friedrich, "Was ist inadäquat bei der Schizophrenie?" *Der Nervenarzt* 6 (1955), 232–237, 232.

79 LHA Marburg, Patient file sign. 16K13786M, Entry, January 10, 1959, LWV Hesse, 16.

80 On the overall exceptionally high suicide rate in the GDR and the reasons for it, see Grashoff, *Depression*; Grashoff emphasizes that motives for suicide in East Germany were mostly related to illness, psychoses, and family conflicts. See ibid., 122.

81 On altered frames of reference during the war directly related to the individual sense of failure, see Jeggle, Utz, "Scheitern lernen," in Stefan Zahlmann and Sylka Scholz (eds.), *Scheitern und Biographie. Die andere Seite moderner Lebensgeschichten* (Gießen, 2005), 222.

82 Goeschel, Christian, *Selbstmord im Dritten Reich* (Berlin, 2011), 19.

83 For the same reason, no statements can be made about possible gender-specific differences. In general, however, it has long been undisputed among researchers that unemployment, especially in the first two-thirds of the twentieth century, was addressed as an issue by men far more often than by women. For a summary, see Hoffmann, *Alltag*, 253.

84 See the chapter "Der Leistungsfanatismus des Nationalsozialismus—Ressource für das Wirtschaftswunder?" in Patrick Bahners and Alexander Cammann, (eds.), *Bundesrepublik und DDR. Die Debatte um Hans-Ulrich Wehlers "Deutsche Gesellschaftsgeschichte"* (Munich, 2009), 107–124.

85 The debate was mainly, though not exclusively, focused on the high achievers of the young republic. See ibid.

86 This fits with the findings obtained by Bänzinger on cross-class "busyness" (*Betriebsamkeit*) in the 1950s. See Bänzinger, "Der betriebsame Mensch."

87 Schweig, *Gesundheitsverhalten*, 117. This is the unintended effect of a study that examines only one gender but implicitly makes statements about the other, for example when Schweig identifies capacity for work within the definition of a healthy self as an aspect of specifically male health behavior—on the basis of letters written exclusively by men. Claims, well established in the research, of the class- and occupation-specific internalization of the striving for achievement are in fact being challenged by new research on the cross-class significance of performance and work. See initial findings by Nina Verheyen and Peter-Paul Bänzinger on the cross-class individual significance of work and performance at the turn of the twentieth century, in the Weimar Republic, and in the early FRG: Bänzinger, "Der betriebsame Mensch"; Verheyen, Nina, "Unter Druck. Die Entstehung individuellen Leistungsstrebens um 1900," *Merkur. Zeitschrift für europäisches Denken* 5, 2012, 382–390.

88 New concepts of household management and ideas about how to evaluate it were widely disseminated due to World War I, the house building of the Weimar period, the dissemination of ideas through a bespoke institute, a dedicated journal, the introduction of these ideas into curricula and the support of the women's movement. Borscheid, Peter, "Die 'taylorisierte' Hausfrau. Zu den Auswirkungen der Rationalisierungsbewegung auf den Privathaushalt der 20er Jahre," in Hans-Jürgen Gerhard (ed.), *Struktur und Dimension. Festschrift für Karl Heinrich Kaufhold zum 65. Geburtstag*, vol. 2: *Neunzehntes und Zwanzigstes Jahrhundert* (Stuttgart, 1997), 483.

89 Ibid., 484.

90 Steinbacher, "Differenz," 97.

91 Ibid., 98 f.

92 KA Rodewisch, Patient file sign. 8963, Entry, May 9, 1950, SächSta Chemnitz, 32810.

93 The figures do not reflect the true importance of company physicians, since they often initially committed patients to a hospital from which they were then referred to a sanatorium-nursing home. In the sample, these cases thus appear under the heading "committals by hospitals."

94 Janosch Sch. had a sister living nearby, with whom he had a good relationship, indicating that the reason he was accompanied by a work colleague was not that he had no relatives who might have gone with him. See KA Rodewisch, Patient file sign. 8963, Entry, May 11, 1950, SächSta Chemnitz, 32810.

95 KA Rodewisch, Patient file sign. 5168, Entry, April 29, 1953, SächSta Chemnitz, 32810.

96 On the importance of the company, see for example Kohli, *Arbeitsgesellschaft*, 43.

97 PsychN Greifswald, Patient file prov. sign. 1954/1345, Entry, July 6, 1954, UA Greifswald, PsychN.

98 Ibid.

99 PsychN Greifswald, Patient file prov. sign. 1955/1087, Entry, December 12, 1955, UA Greifswald, PsychN.

100 Bauerkämper, Arnd, "Von der Bodenreform zur Kollektivierung. Zum Wandel der ländlichen Gesellschaft in der Sowjetischen Besatzungszone Deutschlands und in der DDR 1945–1952," in Hartmut Kaelble et al. (eds.), *Sozialgeschichte der DDR* (Stuttgart, 1994), 124ff.
101 Zimmermann, Hartmut, "Überlegungen zur Geschichte der Kader und der Kaderpolitik in der SBZ/DDR," in Hartmut Kaelble et al. (eds.), *Sozialgeschichte der DDR* (Stuttgart, 1994), 335.
102 PsychN Greifswald, Patient file prov. sign. 1955/1087, Entry, December 12, 1955, UA Greifswald, PsychN.
103 Rather than a Foucault-inspired concept of disciplinary power internalized as self-constraint, this interpretation centers on Soviet concepts of the self that may have taken different paths than those proposed by Foucault for the Western world. Hellbeck, Jochen, "Introduction," in Jochen Hellbeck and Klaus Heller (eds.), *Autobiographische Praktiken in Russland. Autobiographical Practices in Russia* (Göttingen, 2004), 11–25.
104 Hellbeck, Jochen, "Russian Autobiographical Practice," in ibid., 279–299.
105 KA Großschweidnitz, Patient file sign. 754, HSta Dresden, 10822.
106 Ibid., Entry, June 5, 1956.
107 See for example Kocka or Hoffmann on the nineteenth century: Kocka, Jürgen, "Mehr Last als Lust. Arbeit und Arbeitsgesellschaft in der europäischen Gesellschaft," JbW 2, 2005, 185–206; Hoffmann, *Alltag*, 249ff. A key psychiatric text was Kraepelin's book *Arbeitskurve* ("The work curve"), which he himself considered his greatest achievement. See Schott and Tölle, *Geschichte der Psychiatrie*, 120.
108 Jureit, "Motive," 167. On the origins of the study of mentality as it informed the *Annales* school, see Durkheim, Emile, *De la division du travail social* (Paris, 1922), 46.
109 On the problem that the invocation of mentalities in the *Annales* tradition may tempt scholars to foreshorten the search for specific causes, see Gilcher-Holthey, Ingrid, "Plädoyer für eine dynamische Mentalitätsgeschichte," GG 3, 1989, 487. According to Gilcher-Holtey, meanwhile, "mentalities are the sum of options for action, whose potency may be intensified and weakened by situational-contextual conditions and intervening variables" (ibid., 496). I am not working here with this dynamic definition of mentality, as it is intended to improve our explanations of actions, whereas my goal is to analyze patterns of thought and their causes in a nuanced way, without touching the level of actions.
110 Schöttler, Peter, "Mentalitäten, Ideologien, Diskurse. Zur sozialgeschichtlichen Thematisierung der 'dritten Ebene,'" in Alf Lüdtke (ed.), *Alltagsgeschichte. Zur Rekonstruktion historischer Erfahrungen und Lebensweisen* (Frankfurt/M., 1989), 85–136.
111 I use the term "world of meaning" (*Sinnwelt*) in line with its usage in everyday history, as in the work of Lüdtke, Lindenberger, and Sabrow. See for example Lüdtke, Alf, (ed.), *Alltagsgeschichte. Zur Rekonstruktion historischer Erfahrungen und Lebensweisen* (Frankfurt/M., 1989), 631; Sabrow, "Sozialismus."
112 See the chapter "Der Leistungsfanatismus des Nationalsozialismus—Ressource für das Wirtschaftswunder?," in Bahners and Cammann, *Bundesrepublik*, 113 f.
113 This is also worth mentioning in light of Malte Thießen's insight that in the postwar period a "community of fate" continued to be invoked at the local political level, as a sort of motivating factor for local reconstruction. At least in personal medical records, there is no equivalent of this local political perpetuation of the appeal to community. It would be interesting to examine whether there was continuity in the "community mythos" in ego-documents of a different

Work and performance 269

provenance. On its local political use, see Thießen, Malte, "Schöne Zeiten? Erinnerungen an die 'Volksgemeinschaft' nach 1945," in Frank Bajohr and Michael Wildt (eds.), *Volksgemeinschaft. Neue Forschungen zur Gesellschaft des Nationalsozialismus* (Frankfurt/M., 2009), 172.

114 On denunciation and "togetherness" during aerial bombardment, see Diewald-Kerkmann, "Denunziantentum und Gestapo"; Süß, *Tod*, 331ff.

115 As early as 1949, the Soviet occupation zone was markedly different from the other zones in this respect: Fulbrook, *Leben*, 50.

116 See for example Kohli, *Arbeitsgesellschaft*, 41.

117 Bänzinger refers to a "busy" (*betriebsam*) self, as he is also concerned with the active organization of leisure time. See Bänzinger, "Der betriebsame Mensch."

118 Kohli, *Arbeitsgesellschaft*, 50.

119 See ibid. and Hübner, *Zukunft*, 181.

120 See Kury, *Der Überforderte Mensch*, 11ff.

121 Kocka, "Last"; Möckel, "Mensch das Recht," 119ff.

122 Sarasin, Philipp, *Reizbare Maschinen. Eine Geschichte des Körpers 1765–1914* (Frankfurt/M., 2001), 321.

123 Ibid.

124 Lerner, "Psychiatry," 14.

125 Nolte, "Gefühl," 195.

126 Karen Nolte assumes that neurasthenia was diagnosed in working women due to prejudices against this group and shows on the basis of medical records from the LHA Marburg that "overwork" was in fact mostly due to financial difficulties. Ibid., 191ff.

127 See Ayaß, *Asoziale*, 13.

128 On the psychiatric discourse surrounding vagabonds in the imperial period, see Althammer, "Pathologische Vagabunden."

129 Kury, *Der Überforderte Mensch*, 49.

130 Ibid., 51.

131 Neuner, *Politik*, 149ff.

132 Donalies, G., "Forensische Psychiatrie und Gutachtertätigkeit," *Der Nervenarzt* 3 (1942), 144.

133 Ibid. The different research views on "psychopathy" and their development can also be traced in Kurt Schneider's book, which was reprinted eight times between 1923 and the end of the Nazi era: Schneider, Kurt, *Die psychopathischen Persönlichkeiten* (Vienna 1923–1943).

134 Bumke, *Lehrbuch*, 159. For a very similar account, see for example Fuhrmann, Manfred and Korbsch, Heinrich, *Lehrbuch der Psychiatrie für Studierende, Ärzte und Juristen* (Leipzig 1937), 87ff.

135 Ibid, 87.

136 On the change in discourse and practice in the Weimar Republic and at the beginning of the Nazi period, especially the supplanting of traumatic neurosis by "pension neurosis," see Neuner, *Politik*.

137 vBS Bethel, Patient file sign. 3850, HAB, Patient files Gilead III.

138 LHA Marburg, Patient file sign. 16K10534M, Entry, January 4, 1945, LWV Hesse, 16.

139 vBS Bethel, Patient file sign. 161/2446, Letter, November 10, 1943, HAB, Patient files Mahanaim I.

140 Of course, the attribution of a "state of nervous exhaustion" did not first appear during World War II. The point is that it was used in a different way during this period in semantic proximity to the discourse of psychopathy.

141 Kury, *Der Überforderte Mensch*, 109ff.

142 Ibid., 114.

143 Ibid., 168.
144 Ibid., 119.
145 Ibid., 123; Roelcke, *Krankheit*, 26.
146 Kury, *Der Überforderte Mensch*, 124.
147 For example, Ewald, *Neurologie und Psychiatrie*, 380. On the far-reaching sig-nificance of Kurt Schneider's "theory of psychopaths" (*Psychopathenlehre*) to American psychiatry and the relevant diagnostic text known as the DSM, see Weber, "Insanity," 22.
148 Ibid, 383.
149 Engstrom, "Question," 392.
150 See the beginning of the chapter "Der Begriff der psychopathischen Persönlichkeit" ("The concept of the psychopathic personality") in the various editions of Schneider, *Persönlichkeiten*. On the shift from the moral norm to the average-based norm in the international context and over the *longue durée*, see Weber, "Insanity," 22.
151 Influential critics were Ernst Kretschmer and Hans Heinze, with whom Schneider dealt, for example, in Schneider, Kurt, "Kritik der klinisch-typologischen Psychopathenbetrachtung," *Der Nervenarzt* 1 (1948), 6–9, 7. Schneider was also an advocate of distinguishing between "psychopath types" and diagnoses; according to him, the term "psychopath" should not in any case appear in diagnoses.
152 Ibid., 9.
153 Ibid.
154 See for example ibid., 7.
155 Hülsmann, Paul, "Die ärztliche Begutachtung von Neurosen für die unterstützende Arbeitslosenhilfe," *Der Nervenarzt* 11 (1953), 461 f.
156 Ibid., 462.
157 Ibid.
158 Von Baeyer, W., "Erschöpfung und Erschöpftsein," *Der Nervenarzt* 5 (1961), 193–199.
159 Ibid., 197.
160 Ibid., 194. One of the few champions of the functional interpretation in German psychiatry was Georg Stertz (1878–1959).
161 This concept has not fundamentally changed to this day. Even the stress concept that became established in Germany in the last quarter of the twentieth century still assumes that the individual worker can deal better with the demands of work in order to avoid "burnout." Patrick Kury, correctly in my view, takes a very negative view of this perspective and calls for stress to be seen once again as a problem for society as a whole, as it was in Sweden in the 1950s and 60 s. See the concluding chapter in Kury, *Der Überforderte Mensch*, 297.
162 On Selye's stress concept and the reasons why it did not gain acceptance in Germany, in contrast to the Anglo-Saxon and Scandinavian countries, see ibid., 109.
163 Von Baeyer, "Erschöpfung und Erschöpftsein," 193.
164 Schultz, J. H., "Diskussionsbeitrag zur Arbeit von W. von Baeyer 'Erschöpfung und Erschöpftsein,'" *Der Nervenarzt* 10 (1961), 467.
165 On Schultz, see Brunner, Jürgen and Steeger, Florian, "*Johannes Heinrich Schultz (1884–1970)—Begründer des Autogenen Trainings*. Ein biographischer Rekonstruktionsversuch im Spannungsfeld von Wissenschaft und Politik," *Bios* 1, 2006, 16–25.
166 This was not an entirely new development but was identified by Stephanie Neuner among the fiercely competing psychiatrists and psychotherapists of the Weimar Republic and with respect to their view of the working person.

For all their other differences, both saw work as curative and the ability to work as the ultimate goal of their treatment. Under Nazism, the remaining psychologists focused chiefly on performance and the will to work as they devoted their efforts to the "New German Psychology" (*Neue Deutsche Seelenkunde*). Schultz, for example, was deputy director of the so-called "Göring Institute," the German Institute for Psychological Research and Psychotherapy (Deutsches Institut für Psychologische Forschung und Psychotherapie), from 1936 to 1945. In an article on Schultz's life, Jürgen Brunner and Florian Steeger make two points that explain this. First, they highlight the fact that the psychotherapists who remained in the Reich had a special interest in "legitimizing and anchoring their work within the tone-setting form of psychiatry, which was geared toward racial hygiene" and were therefore under pressure to achieve results that were in line with Nazi ideology. Second, in connection with this, the main goal of psychotherapy at the Göring Institute was enhancing occupational performance. Hence, the institute was also anchored in the German Labor Front. Schultz's response to Baeyer's article shows that in the early FRG, Schultz defended his position (hard-won during the Nazi period) in mainstream psychiatry against any kind of shift, no matter how small, toward a more moderate view of performance and work expectations. See ibid.

167 The process can be seen in the following case file, among others: vBS Bethel, Patient file sign. 13/186, HAB, Patient files Mahanaim I.

168 Ibid., Entry, September 29, 1953.

169 Ibid.

170 vBS Bethel, Patient file sign. 161/2446, Entry, November 10, 1943, HAB, Patient files Mahanaim I.

171 Kury, *Der Überforderte Mensch*, 223ff.

172 vBS Bethel, Patient file sign. 13/186, Copy of evaluation following observation of September 29, 1953–October 1, 1953 [n.d.], HAB, Patient files Mahanaim I.

173 Ibid.

174 The findings are quite similar for the LHA. Dr. K. at Bethel was selected as an example only because the expert evaluations there were clearly assignable.

175 vBS Bethel, Patient file sign. 141/2051, Evaluation, June 1, 1950, HAB, Patient files Morija I.

176 vBS Bethel, Patient file sign. 52/526, Evaluation, December 21, 1960, HAB, Patient files Morija I.

177 For an evaluation by a physician who regularly used the term "psychopathy" in his evaluations, see for example vBS Bethel, Patient file sign. 193/2818, HAB, Patient files Morija I.

178 vBS Bethel, Patient file sign. 141/2051, Evaluation, June 1, 1950, HAB, Patient files Morija I.

179 vBS Bethel, Patient file sign. 101/1195, HAB, Patient files Mahanaim II.

180 In this chapter, see the section "'Psychopathy' as a Diagnosis in the Nazi Era."

181 See also the chapter "Disease and Diagnostics" on psychiatry's frequent self-description as "expertise" (*Kennerschaft*), which was fed by this constant reference to practice and thus interprets this approach, originally described as deficient, as the result of psychiatrists' difficult-to-acquire "expertise" and "strength of character."

182 Hollmann, Werner, "Soziale Therapie und ärztliche Begutachtung der Arbeitsneurosen," *Psychiatrie, Neurologie und medizinische Psychologie* 8 (1956), 267–275.

183 Ibid., 270.

184 In Rodewisch, the doctor's questions were usually recorded in abbreviated form in brackets in the medical history, as can be seen here.

185 KA Rodewisch, Patient file sign. 8963, Entry, May 11, 1950, SächSta Chemnitz, 32810.
186 In the files from Rodewisch, the question mark in brackets indicates that the doctor looked further into a given issue.
187 Ibid.
188 Keyserlingk, H.v., "Psychopathische Persönlichkeiten, ihre Kriminalität und ihre Stellung vor dem Gesetz," *Psychiatrie, Neurologie und medizinische Psychologie* 6 (1951), 180–207.
189 Bendrat, M., "Zur Frage der Psychopathie," *Psychiatrie, Neurologie und medizinische Psychologie* 1 (1953), 70–77.
190 Ibid., 77.
191 This "bourgeois" standpoint refers to the concept of psychopathy introduced by Kurt Schneider, which was embraced by most psychiatrists in the FRG.
192 This is an allusion to the superficial similarities between the Pavlovian and Freudian approaches. The latter again found a few adherents in the early West Germany, but achieved a broad impact above all in the United States. The common ground is the assumption that it is possible to influence the behavior and character of human beings—in contrast to the hereditary component that was privileged under Nazism.
193 Ibid.
194 According to Pavlov, it is possible to teach people completely new behaviors or to condition them. Aspects of this approach also attracted many adherents in the Western world: "Pavlov was recognized as intellectual progenitor by the founders of behaviorism, behavior therapy, and advertising psychology, John B. Watson (1878–1958) and Burrhus F. Skinner (1904–1990)." See Rüting, *Pavlov*, 123.
195 There was not a single year lacking at least one article on the topic; usually there were several.
196 Werner Hollmann became head physician of the department of internal medicine at Potsdam District Hospital in 1950. In the 1930s, he had been an assistant to Viktor von Weizsäcker in Heidelberg, where he focused on "neurotics."
197 Hollmann, Werner, "Krankheit und soziale Umwelt. Zur sozialen Pathogenese innerer Erkrankungen," *Psychiatrie, Neurologie und medizinische Psychologie* 1 (1951), 15–25.
198 The variant of organ neurosis outlined here is based on the Pavlovian assumption that the organs are infinitely changeable by external influences. See Rüting, *Pavlov*, 123. However, organ neurosis as a diagnosis was not only used in socialist psychiatry. From about 1941 onward, the term organ neurosis was also used for soldiers who had previously been referred to as *Kriegszitterer* or shakers (*Schüttler*). See Quinkert et al., "Einleitung," 20.
199 Hollmann, "Krankheit und soziale Umwelt," 18.
200 Goltermann, *Gesellschaft*, 209.
201 Ibid., 259.
202 In 1940, for example, a series of lectures by him was published in book form: Hollmann, Werner, *Krankheit, Lebenskrise und soziales Schicksal* (Leipzig 1940).
203 Rüting, *Pavlov*, 123.
204 Hollmann, "Krankheit und soziale Umwelt," 18.
205 Ibid., 20.
206 Ibid.
207 Ibid., 23.
208 Ibid., 22 f.
209 Ibid., 23. This was an application of Pavlov's idea that there is a constant interplay between "stimuli" and "inhibitions" and that disturbance of this interplay is the cause of a wide variety of diseases and behaviors.

210 Kury, *Der Überforderte Mensch*, 122.
211 Hoppe, Christa, "Katamnestische Untersuchungen zum Problem der sogenannten 'Managerkrankheit'" *Psychiatrie, Neurologie und medizinische Psychologie* 1 (1961), 23–28, 24.
212 Ibid., 24 f.
213 The finding in this article that psychological consequences of excessive workload occur primarily in the managerial class is consistent with the finding based on the sample for this book that very few people attributed overwork to themselves, but political climbers did so frequently. See the section "Ability to Work and 'Overwork' in the GDR" in this chapter.
214 Ibid., 25.
215 Ibid., 25 f.
216 I believe there are two reasons for this. First, American behavior therapy counted Pavlov among its major influences, and thus parallels can be found in the field of behavioral research at the beginning of the Cold War. Second, the focus on work ability, albeit in a different way and in part for different reasons, was a shared feature of the Western and Eastern blocs, and autogenic training was a cost-effective way to improve it.
217 Roelcke, *Krankheit*, 30.
218 Korzilius, "Parasiten," 40.
219 See, for example, the articles by Werner Hollmann.
220 Through Pavlov's impact, an outdated nineteenth-century concept of unbridled excitation and inhibition was established as, supposedly, empirically proven. See Rüting, *Pavlov*, 153ff.
221 During the Weimar Republic, psychotherapists explained neuroses in relation to work differently than the prevailing doctrine, which attributed them to illicit desires that led to pension neuroses. Psychotherapists, like psychiatrists, did regard sociopolitical reasons as crucial, but in a different way. While the predominant belief system assumed that the welfare state created pension neurotics because it made space for their desires, psychotherapists worked on the assumption that neuroses were triggered by poor social and economic conditions. See Neuner, *Politik*, 149ff.
222 Bendrat, "Zur Frage der Psychopathie."
223 Klimková-Deutschová, E., "Die Doppelbelastung der Frau im Arbeitsprozeß," *Psychiatrie, Neurologie und medizinische Psychologie* 3 (1962), 109–113.
224 Stephan Török, "Das Erlebnis der Arbeit," *Psychiatrie, Neurologie und medizinische Psychologie* 4 (1959), 118–121.
225 As mentioned above, there was no consensus on whether "psychopathy" was a syndrome in the first place.
226 On the efforts of psychiatry to establish itself as a somatic medical specialism, which were virtually foundational to the profession, see Engstrom, *Psychiatry*, 51 and 60 f.
227 On Hanns Schwarz, see the anthology by Fischer and Schmiedebach, *Direktorat*.
228 Some have rightly warned against precipitate use of the so-called "interest model" to explain scientific change and pointed out that ultimately it is often impossible to convincingly demonstrate that interests, as factors not intrinsic to science, have greater explanatory power than the reasoning of physicians. However, in the studies that were reasonably criticized for this, the starting point was fundamentally different. They were focused on the establishment of new interpretations and treatment methods in the absence of a political-ideological rupture of the kind that had occurred in the early GDR. For example, the increase in surgical interventions in the nineteenth century has been interpreted from a professional history perspective as propelled by surgeons' interest in establishing themselves as

an important professional group in their own right. See Schlich, Thomas, "Wissenschaftliche Fakten als Thema der Geschichtsforschung," in Norbert Paul and Thomas Schlich (eds.), *Medizingeschichte. Aufgaben, Probleme, Perspektiven* (Frankfurt/M., 1997), 112 f.

229 On the ideologically conformist New German Psychiatry in connection with ideas about work, see Neuner, *Politik*, 213.

230 For details on the development and establishment of the doctrine of higher nervous activity in Soviet research, see Rüting, *Pavlov*, 109ff.

231 This goal was pursued, among other things, by the establishment of labor brigades in the factories, albeit without much success. See Roesler, *Produktionsbrigaden.*

232 In contrast to the FRG, different clinical pictures were applied in a way that went well beyond avoidance of the term "psychopathy," as recommended by Kurt Schneider. However, the term organ neurosis is not specifically Soviet.

233 Schmiedebach, "Psychoanalyse," 41.

234 PsychN Greifswald, Patient file prov. sign. 1955/582, UA Greifswald, PsychN.

235 Hollmann, "Soziale Therapie," 274.

236 The expression is used, for example, in a statement from Greifswald dated October 17, 1960. In this case, emphasis is placed on the fact that the doctor did not perceive the individual involved as a "pension moocher." See PsychN Greifswald, Patient file prov. sign. 1960/986, UA Greifswald, PsychN.

237 Boldorf, *Rehabilitation*, 467.

238 PsychN Greifswald, Patient file prov. sign. 1957/794, UA Greifswald, PsychN.

239 Ibid., page 5 in the evaluation.

240 "Psychiatrisch-Neurologische Gesellschaft an den Universitäten Greifswald und Rostock. 15. Sitzung am 9. Mai 1956 in Greifswald anläßlich des 50-jährigen Bestehens der Univ.- Nervenklinik Greifswald," *Psychiatrie, Neurologie und medizinische Psychologie* 1 (1957), 29–33, 30.

241 On connections between scientific practice and politics, see Roelcke, "Suche."

242 Korzilius, *Parasiten*, 201ff.

243 See Ernst, *Sozialismus*, 335ff. On the regime's influence on the contents of the journal *Psychiatre, Neurologie und medizinische Psychologie*, see Teitge, Marie and Kumbier, Ekkehardt, "Zur Geschichte der DDR-Fachzeitschrift 'Psychiatrie, Neurologie und medizinische Psychologie,'" *Nervenarzt* 86, 2015, 339–367.

244 This finding tells us nothing about the continuation of psychopathy discourse in other subject areas.

245 On the importance of politics at the various stages of scientific practice, see Roelcke, "Suche."

246 On the model of the fatigable human engine, see Sarasin, *Reizbare Maschinen.*

247 See for example Hoppe, "Katamnestische Untersuchungen," 23–28.

248 As mentioned above, organ neuroses were conceived as a consequence of underexertion but also overexertion.

249 On the rise to prominence of the (non-deterministic) concept of human capital in the Western world during and as a result of the Cold War, see Bernet and Gugerli, "Sputniks Resonanzen."

Conclusion

Patient records as a source: the benefits of a combined hermeneutic and functional approach

Martina R., whose committal to the Marburg Land Sanatorium has run like a thread through this book, was "discharged as healthy and sent home" after four weeks.[1] Her medical record notes: "All the problems in her life were discussed and firm plans were made for the future. She is not to return to her mother-in-law's house but will instead go to other relatives who are willing to take her and her children in."[2] The relevance of the family, then, is emphasized in the course of her discharge, which underscores one of the key findings of this book: committal decisions can only be understood by considering patients' families, patients themselves, and their social milieu.

This finding is based primarily on my analysis of 1,424 patient records. Yet their use as a source is not uncontroversial. In recent years, some scholars have questioned whether medical records tell us anything at all about "substantive" matters.[3] Many studies, meanwhile, seek to provide a functional interpretation of medical records rather than a hermeneutic analysis.[4] This means that our knowledge of the emergence of psychiatric knowledge is, happily, growing continuously. Yet there is far less interest in the way that psychiatry has been embedded in social history and the history of societies, especially when it comes to non-institutional actors. There is general agreement that medical records can be usefully examined to reveal connections between practices of medical documentation and administrative functions, but there is far less consensus over the extent to which they reflect the views of patients.[5] Some authors have insisted that medical records are only a valuable source of information if we wish to analyze "institutional guidelines on the keeping of medical records" and their "materiality and mediality."[6] They are right to point out that these two fields are amenable to analysis and that they provide insights into the relationship between politics and science and, above all, help us reconstruct the institution-bound nature of scientific practice.[7]

In light of this book, however, we can discern certain flaws in the arguments typically made against the hermeneutic analysis of this material.

DOI: 10.4324/9781032716237-7

Doubts about the informative value of medical histories—beyond functional analysis—are based on the assumption that in modern societies illness is associated with disorder, "which must be treated according to scientific precepts and ordered according to rational principles. As a result, the subjective perspective of madness, which has no place within a given order, is omitted from the record and inherently resists (historical) reconstruction. The voices of madness, silenced in the age of reason according to Foucault, are thus characterized as a source of psychiatric history that has often been sought and, just as often, mistakenly believed to have been found."[8]

The present book provides ample reason to doubt the validity of this argument against the hermeneutic interpretation of psychiatric records. The rejectionist perspective regards the attribution of "madness" and the need for institutionalization as givens—ignoring the crucial fact that "non-normality" and "madness" are constructed at the threshold of the asylum. Yet, as we have seen, the threshold of the asylum is not shaped solely by institutional actors—such as physicians and asylum administrators—but also by the role of the asylum for the families of those committed, their social milieu, and sometimes the patients themselves. Epistemologically, medical records shed light on more than just the dichotomous doctor–patient relationship. This book has revealed how much patient records can tell us about the relationship between patients' families on the one hand and medical institutions and physicians on the other. In approaching the patient's social environment, I looked at letters to asylums, but I also scrutinized information in the medical record itself.

The present study leaves us in no doubt that medical records also furnish us with insights into patients' historical positioning. Far from all patients can be aptly described as cases of "disordered madness."[9] Furthermore, the goal of a hermeneutic analysis need not and should not be the reconstruction of "voices of madness." I have explicitly eschewed such an approach. I was even less interested in gaining "insights into the world of madness" or reconstructing authentic "voices of madness."[10] Yet it is quite possible to argue that we can understand some of the patient voices in the case histories. A fundamental distinction must be made here between psychiatric and psychological fragments. The psychiatric anamneses or explorations that I have analyzed do not contain psychological narratives, such as interpretations of dreams[11] or childhood experiences,[12] from which one would have to extract the patients' voices. Moreover, people were admitted to asylums for an array of reasons and at different stages of various illnesses. Many of them were not incapacitated and were not endowed with this status when they entered the asylum. This indicates that not all patients were indiscriminately classified as acting irrationally in every respect. Even in the case of the large number of illnesses whose clinical picture entailed so-called "thought disorders" (*Denkstörungen*), such as schizophrenia and manic-depressive insanity (*manisch-depressives Irresein* or MDI), contemporary psychiatrists assumed that these patients, too, could describe and classify their illness themselves during its onset or certain phases. Doctors on both sides of the Cold War ideological divide took the view, for example, that even "schizophrenics" could describe their illness in its early stages, despite the fact that they were otherwise regarded as the epitome of the "sick" and "other."[13] Both university clinics and asylums had neurological departments, and many of their patients were at no point labeled as suffering from "madness" (*Wahnsinn*). Moreover, within the period studied in this book, individuals with venereal diseases or those classified as "asocials," for example, were identified as requiring an asylum stay. It would hardly make sense to sweepingly deny these two groups the ability to express themselves intelligibly. Ego-documents in the medical records—above all, letters from patients to the asylum—also show quite clearly that many individuals were perfectly capable of rationalizing their illness and their associated concerns. When, for instance, patients put forward generally accepted reasons for a stay in an asylum, such as restoring their ability to work, they were certainly moving within the sphere of rational argumentation proper to a modern industrial society.[14] Like the Scottish medical records examined by Jens Gründler, the ego-documents consulted for the present book were often transcribed verbatim into the records, so patients' statements were not filtered to the point of unusability.[15]

It is in fact understanding the specific conditions under which patient records are created—and in recent years we have come to understand these conditions more clearly—that facilitates a cautious, thoughtful form of content analysis that always remains aware of its limitations. In the course of this volume, then, I reflected on a number of occasions on the origin of medical records, their materiality, their condition, and their purpose. I examined, for example, information in textbooks and psychiatric journals regarding the questions that should be asked when taking a medical history. But I also highlighted the changing conditions under which medical histories were written, which, especially in the period immediately after World War II, reflected material scarcity. Complementing the content analysis of medical records, the circumstances of committal can also be discerned in their genesis and materiality. To take one example, the paper used for Martina R.'s medical records, to which we have returned throughout this book, reflects the asylums' rudimentary resources in the first few postwar years. Martina R.'s medical history was recorded on forms originally from the Haina Land Sanatorium. Since it was apparently impossible to have new forms printed for their own use, in 1946 the staff at the LHA Marburg used these forms from Haina, also located in Hesse. In the immediate postwar period, file covers were reused so often at Marburg that it is sometimes difficult to tell at first glance whose patient history is to be found between them. Information about patients is often recorded on loose, non-standardized sheets. The specific features of the historical context thus shaped medical records in both their materiality and content. Overall, while medical records do not provide comprehensive information on patients' biographies or emotional states, they are a valuable source for studies that connect the history of psychiatry and the history of society: they are artifacts of the interaction of clinic and asylum staff with other institutions as well as with patients and members of their social milieu.

Examining sources in the history of medicine to shed light on the history of everyday life and society would also be a promising means of addressing some themes of relevance to the second half of the twentieth century that the present book has merely touched upon. It would be interesting to analyze periods associated with psychological problems that were conceptualized as gender- and age-specific, such as puberty-related struggles and the "midlife crisis," as well as the gender-specific attribution of somatic diseases or changes. In particular, the assessment of age-specific disease symptoms by laypersons, physicians, and institutions might be informative given the differences in old-age provision in different sociopolitical systems, especially in East–West comparison. The clinical pictures of multiple sclerosis and alcoholism, which are discussed from time to time in this book, should also be considered in this context. In the 1940s and 1950s, multiple sclerosis was still considered a disease that mainly affected men, whereas today it is assumed that the vast majority of sufferers are women. This raises the question of whether this change is linked with gender-specific behavioral patterns within doctor–patient contact and with the self-attribution of illness in the face of different everyday demands and rhythms. Alcoholism was long seen chiefly as a male problem.[16] Here, too, researchers might explore familial and societal role attributions, everyday demands, and class-specific discourses of problematization and the ways in which they changed or remained the same. Questions of this kind, in combination with aspects of the history of science, have proved highly productive in this book. The results of the comparative analysis of committal practices in the "Third Reich," the FRG, and the GDR change our ideas about the relations between state, science, and social practice. In addition, these findings engender a more nuanced picture of the dominant concepts of a healthy self in work-centered states or societies. They also provide insights into the relationship between freedom (and its limits), society, and statehood.

State, science, and social practice

In all three political systems, psychiatry as an institution had little controlling influence over decisions on who was committed and who was not. Certainly, committal practices were shaped by the specific ways that medical institutions were embedded in all three German states and by the ways in which these institutions were oriented toward the sociopolitical system. But what we find in this context are chiefly the indirect and unintended effects of the health care system that impacted on power relations at the threshold of the asylum. In the Nazi period, asylums were obliged to admit people referred from the health office, fostering coalitions between the patient's social milieu and public health officers. The establishment of polyclinics in the GDR as outpatient facilities shifted the power structure even more clearly in favor of the medical laity. Patients now made decisions less often within spaces of medical expertise and more often at home. Social negotiation practices between private and institutional actors were thus embedded in conditions generated by the state. There is, however, no evidence of psychiatry successfully controlling committal decisions.

In line with this, the evidence shows that psychiatric committal practice was relatively independent of all three state systems: it was the decisions made by non-institutional actors that essentially determined access to psychiatric institutions during World War II, in the early FRG, and in the GDR. These non-institutional actors included patients, members of their social milieu—such as neighbors—and, above all, their own families. The institutional actors who were always involved in committals, namely, the asylum and clinic psychiatrists, were largely dependent on the cooperation of families and patients. Furthermore, if they were to admit a patient, they required an initiative from outside their institution and they were subsequently dependent on the information emanating from the doctors who had previously dealt with the patient. The medical attribution of illness was crucial to legitimizing committals. Conversely, such attribution alone did not result in committals. In all three systems, patients were often psychiatrically diagnosed years before their first institutionalization. But they were admitted only when their social environment no longer considered them tolerable or—more rarely, it should be noted—when they themselves sought admission. Medical criteria were necessary for committal, but not sufficient.

In all three systems, the influence of non-institutional actors on medical decisions to admit people to psychiatric facilities is indicative of the role of psychiatry in modern, industrialized, societies in which planning plays a key role. Psychiatric institutions have been described, following Foucault, as indicators and symbols of modernity within the framework of rationalized and planning-based societies. On this view, the "mad," unpredictable, and irrational were locked up on the basis of scientific-medical criteria, as there is no place for them in "reason-based" modernity.[17] But this book shows, first, that access to psychiatric institutions was not primarily determined by scientific actors (physicians) or other actors who had to justify their actions within the framework of state institutions (such as judges). Second, the potential representatives of scientific rationality and objectivity, namely, psychiatrists, described committal decisions and attributions of psychiatric illnesses as an intuitive capacity that they themselves denied scientificity. This self-description correlates with the findings on psychiatric practices in this study: more psychiatric knowledge in the form of increasingly sophisticated medical classifications, for instance, did not lead to more consistent practice. In fact, the obligatory diagnostic categorization carried out in the course of admission depended heavily on local medical traditions, a local embeddedness that is bound up with the powerful position of asylum and clinic directors. At the same time, this local dimension must be understood as the result of path dependencies in practice and as the outcome of local conditions, such as spatial divisions. Especially when it comes to the highly application-oriented science of medicine—but presumably beyond it as well—the results of the present study point to a great diversity of practices at the intermediate institutional level. Without locally imbued tacit knowledge, psychiatric admissions are inconceivable. This book does not provide support for the notion of science as an instrument of the successful centralized control and standardization of interpretations of bodies and behaviors and thus of mechanisms of social inclusion and exclusion.

This is remarkable given that the period under investigation here falls within an era typically characterized by its faith in science and planning euphoria.[18] At least in the committal processes studied here, we find little of this at the level of practice. It is certainly not possible to identify the scientification—in a way that left traces in practice—of social inclusion and exclusion at the threshold of the asylum. Both the self-description of psychiatrists as experts and practitioners as well as the flow of knowledge from families to "experts" reveal the flaws in such a perspective.

Conversely, we can confirm the existence of a compulsion to classify and rationalize that is specific to modern societies. This includes the causal classification of illnesses and exceptional psychological situations in the life of the affected person—by the latter and by members of their social milieu—as well as the medical profession's search for the perfect diagnostic system. The sources reflect optimism and a belief in progress and, in this sense, highlight the influence of scientific concepts on medical laypeople, but they do not show any far-reaching scientification of committal practice. New therapies thus found their way into the rationales put forward by medical "laypersons" in the early FRG and GDR. Women in particular acquired knowledge about treatment options: this book demonstrates a strongly gender-specific form of medical expertise in families from the 1940s to the 1960s. But the transfer of medical expertise to broader population groups was mostly limited to treatment options. Ideas about the causes and course of illness, meanwhile, diverged greatly between families and psychiatrists. The latter attributed misdiagnoses in part to the fact that it was near-impossible to obtain all the information they considered relevant, since patients and members of their social milieu, along with physicians from outside the psychiatric field, generally failed to focus on the issues that the receiving physicians considered crucial. Communication about treatment methods also points to the limits of scientific concepts in practice. Doctors regularly had to explain to their clients that treatments were either not available or had no or very little chance of success.

We can discern in the practice of committals two different orders of justification, shaped, respectively, by scientific and everyday knowledge. Both served to legitimize committals. The psychiatrist, as a self-proclaimed and widely accepted expert, managed these orders at the threshold of the asylum. This made psychiatrists agents of modernity to a special degree, not because they rationalized social practice through scientific knowledge, but because, in their role as "hinge," they coordinated very different orders of knowledge and needs for legitimation, translated them into one another, and made them manageable. The social acceptance of the psychiatrist, as well as the increasing demand for psychiatric places despite meager or moderate success in terms of healing, diagnostic categorization, and the assessment of safety risks, point first and foremost to the great need for regulation and legitimization in all three societies studied in this book. The way psychiatric committals unfolded makes it clear that, if we wish to analyze knowledge societies, we need to pay more attention to the relationship between everyday knowledge and practical knowledge—in conjunction with scientific knowledge. Only in this way can we make statements about the scope of scientific knowledge, while also producing more detailed accounts of practical and everyday knowledge. This should help us finally gain a nuanced sense of how knowledge, of various kinds, did or did not contribute to specific sorts of social change, and why.

In this vein, German psychiatric institutions in the mid-twentieth century tell us something about the (specifically modern?) desire for categorization and plannability. These institutions are not, however, emblematic of far-reaching practical effects of the scientification of the social. They are more representative of societal self-regulation and social control in the private sphere than of institutional or state control and coercion, or of the primacy of science. The centrality of order(-ing) evident in classifications of illness and the sick is in fact symptomatic of the development of psychiatry as a science needed and used by the state. But this focus on order was causal rather than reactive. Psychiatric committals served to reduce complexity and help people deal with everyday existence while maintaining class- and gender-specific norms. The growing demand for asylum and clinic places thus correlated with individuals' increasing difficulties in coping with everyday life, which made it harder, for example, to care for ill family members at home. But this rising demand must also be seen in connection with changes in working conditions. These resulted in greater exhaustion, external monitoring, and psychological pressure. Finally, from the outset, bourgeois families used asylums as a tool of self-thematization and to cement and enforce behavior perceived as befitting their social status. Rather than being driven by growing state control or scientification, the "success" of psychiatric institutions is better understood as a reaction to economic changes and the associated working conditions, along with class or strata formation. At the same time, the master narrative established in both science and society in the 1960s and 1970s of psychiatry's—scientifically rationalized—institutional control over the human being in modernity reflects multiple social and state actors' need for overarching legitimation, for illusions of control, and for ways of alleviating societal tensions.

Work as a category of difference shaped by the sociopolitical system

This book shows that "work" was a core category of difference in all three societies we have looked at. And it is work that throws the specific features and commonalities of the three systems into particularly sharp relief. The category of work was significant at the individual level to the construction of a healthy self, within the social microcosm, at the institutional level from psychiatrists' perspective, and at the state level. Valuations of work, ability to work, and willingness to work are relational and dynamic attributions. They reflected era-specific changes in a special way, since they served to evaluate attitudes, and contemporaries therefore imagined them in less essentialist terms than, for example, gender or "race."

During World War II and in the early FRG, both women and men almost always associated their own illness with a change in their performance, whether in household work or gainful employment. Ability to work thus served as a cross-gender indicator of health. The self-attribution of illness was in fact significantly less gendered than previous research findings have suggested. There is no evidence that men referred more often or more extensively to their ability to work or their performance in the context of illness. In the GDR, the reverse was usually the case. When it came to work outside the home, meanwhile, rationales centered on work, which were omnipresent during World War II and in the FRG, were invoked far less often in the GDR. In the context of household tasks, however, these work-focused rationales remained potent even in the "workers' and peasants' state." Thus, in the 1950s, it was primarily women in the GDR who made connections between the ability to work and health. In cross-gender comparison, work and performance played a smaller role in notions of a healthy self in the early GDR than under Nazism and in the FRG. At the same time, there were more committals from the workplace in East Germany. These, however, were mostly centered on family problems that led to psychological breakdown in the enterprise. The way in which people thematized themselves in the course of committals makes the early GDR look like a society whose members had for the most part withdrawn mentally into the private sphere. In the "workers' and peasants' state," a cross-gender turn to the family is more apparent than in the FRG, at least when it comes to citizens' personal evaluations.

The fact that the criterion of work was mentioned so rarely among employed persons in the GDR suggests that working conditions rooted in the sociopolitical system influenced ideas about the healthy self. We might think here of the lack of opportunities for advancement, which would have brought financial and material advantages. Also significant in this context are the political conditions, which did not allow everyone to have the career they wanted and would have strongly identified with. Important too are the numerous changes that swept through enterprises. These shifts in everyday experience and life chances clearly—and relatively rapidly—shaped people's lives, even extending into basic ideas about their own health. This means that notions of a hard-working and high-performing self are not a constant in the lives of modern people.

The ability and willingness to work were also put forward as markers of normal behavior and belonging. This, however, applied more comprehensively to the two dictatorships than to the West German successor state. In wartime and in the GDR, similar references were made to society as a whole, whereas in the FRG the key benchmark was the immediate social milieu. The enduring importance in the GDR of the criterion of ability and willingness to work in inclusionary and exclusionary arguments suggests that citizens of the "workers' and peasants' state" appropriated its propaganda, while at the same time, everyday working life and career ambitions became less important to many East Germans. For those who aspired to political careers, the changes outlined above did not apply. In contrast to the wartime period, meanwhile, patients' relatives sometimes used references to the diligence and ability to work of the committed to undergird their requests and obtain improvements for their relatives in the asylum. To what extent this had anything to do with the acceptance of socialist ideology or whether it was a matter of purely instrumental appropriation cannot be determined in light of the sources explored in this book. Even in wartime, committals reveal that the promise of the *Volksgemeinschaft* was not just a pledge from above. It is clearer than in the case of the GDR that these were more than instrumentalized propagandistic tropes, that genuine expectations were involved that were sometimes disappointed during the war. For example, a missing "sense of community and comradeship" was addressed in wartime committals. Yet the limits of the community spirit extolled in the "Third Reich" and the GDR were reached in both states when it came to dealing with older citizens. During the war, the elderly were particularly often psychiatrized as disruptive, non-productive "elements" of no relevance to the war. In the GDR, this was perpetuated on the institutional level, albeit without fatal consequences: psychiatric facilities were used to compensate for the lack of old people's homes, and sometimes the two institutions, as in the case of Rodewisch, were simply merged.

Ability to work and performance can help us probe boundary-marking processes in all three systems. Ideas about work and performance thus functioned, to varying degrees, as informal criteria used to determine the formal criteria for entry into an asylum, illness, and threats in everyday life.

Finally, diagnoses of work-related disorders were not unaffected by the political system. The "Third Reich" indisputably saw a narrowing of psychiatric interpretations due to the exclusion and murder of Jewish scholars. This one-sided and backward-looking psychiatric interpretation, in international comparison, also characterized the FRG until the 1960s. Impaired health, which those affected saw as a consequence of an excessive workload, was interpreted by psychiatrists—in a way that targeted certain social groups—as "psychopathy." This interpretation reached its apogee in the persecution of so-called "asocials" under Nazism but persisted without modification in the FRG until the 1960s. This finding is likely relevant to the establishment of later concepts used to convey the results of "work overload" (*Arbeitsüberlastung*) such as stress or burnout. In addition to the history-of-science aspects of the international transfer of the concepts of "managerial disease" and "stress,"[19] one reason for the comparatively late adoption of the stress concept in West Germany may be that an established and accepted alternative already existed in the shape of psychopathy. Only when work overload emerged as a problem of the middle class did the need arise for a new concept to get to grips with it. While the complaints of the "lower class" could be conceptualized as psychopathy, those of the small group of senior personnel in the young state could be portrayed as an understandable, virtually honorable form of overload under the label of "managerial disease." In the GDR, meanwhile, we find changes echoing Soviet interpretations in the field of work-related illnesses, an area that was politically important. The diagnosis of psychopathy lost its significance to the evaluation of ability and will to work, though it remained central to the stigmatization of "moral" and sexual deviation. Psychopathy thus retained its close linkage with the category of gender, encompassing female "prostitution" and male sexual offenses. This reflects the economy of attention typical of the early GDR, which was focused on the field of work: no similarly consequential changes can be discerned in other concepts of illness examined in this study because they were not of immediate ideological interest.

In concentrated form, the prism of "work" reveals continuities and ruptures between the different political systems, as well as shifts in the categories of race, class, and gender, along with the less emphasized category of age. The findings presented in this book suggest that contemporary history as work history—in the sense of an integrative history of society—has much to offer. Work is a relational category in both the past and present. Unlike the categories of race, gender, and age, it has been understood in recent history in a mostly non-essentialist way. This makes the category of work a particularly apt means of analyzing negotiation processes, self-reflection, and intra-societal dynamics.

Freedom (and its limits), society, and statehood

In the context of committal practice, state intervention by health offices, the police or the justice system, and the general population's cooperation with these institutions differed markedly in the three political systems. The way forcible committals unfolded and how often they occurred are particularly revealing of the state's interventionist pretensions and the scope of such intervention—and thus of the relationship between state and society.

The practice of committal during World War II was strongly characterized by collaboration on the part of the family. It was during this era that the degree of state intervention reached its historical apogee but also its highest level of acceptance within society: most forcible committals were initiated or tolerated by the social milieu of those affected. Hospital physicians and health offices worked directly with families, and committals were negotiated between them with no predetermined outcome.

Many forcible committals were explicitly justified with reference to "necessities" arising from the pragmatics and "morality" of war. Some individuals stated, for instance, that their family was unable to reach the air-raid shelter in good time because they were slowed down by a limping grandfather, while women with STDs were interned in asylums to prevent them from infecting soldiers. The affected groups, which had been structurally marginalized in the past but not all of which had been routinely psychiatrized, comprised the elderly, single women, lower-class women with STDs, soldiers afflicted by psychological problems, and so-called "asocials."

Forcible committals during World War II, which took place despite widespread knowledge of the murder of the sick, demonstrate the radicalization of Nazi society. They reflect standards of normality and limits to tolerance in everyday life that were introduced, accepted, and justified as inevitable. How might we explain this? In the "Third Reich," various groups intensified their sense of belonging, which brought them material advantages. They did so by excluding others, in part by expanding on established traditions of marginalization. In addition to the exclusionary criterion of "race," which had been central from the outset, performance and willingness to perform for the "community" were increasingly established and accepted as criteria of belonging. During the war, the state tightened up these criteria, for example, by interning so-called "asocials"[20] and by gearing the state's medical apparatus toward the working population.[21] This book shows that a more ruthless form of boundary marking was simultaneously practiced within and generated by society. Patients' families and members of their social milieu supported the regime and enabled the war to continue by seeking to exclude all those who were unable to contribute, above all for reasons of illness and age. This exclusion was an often painful process, especially within families. But this did not prevent decisions from being made that prioritized the protection of ever smaller groups—such as parts of families—in an attempt to ensure success in war. The practice of committal, then, brings out connections between an inwardly radicalizing and thus increasingly atomized, ultimately disintegrating society and the aspiration to construct, defend, and expand the Nazi "community," together with the faith that this was possible. For the most part, state power and quotidian social practices went hand in hand and, in their interplay, often spawned fatal dynamics of exclusion, especially during the war, which were lived and accepted as normality and justified as inevitable.

Competition and social breakdown affected not only the micro-level, but also the meso- and macro-levels. After the T4 Campaign, the murder of the sick took place on a decentralized basis, catalyzed by relocations initiated from above within the framework of the Brandt Campaign. Thus, at the intermediate level, asylum directors decided whether their patients would live or die. Yet they had little control over access to their asylums. During the war, and especially in 1944 and 1945, hospitals, old people's homes, police, and asylums increasingly competed to avoid dealing with their clientele. In particular, the elderly and women suspected of having venereal diseases were committed by these institutions via the central legitimizing body: the health office. The asylums, which were obliged to admit these "patients," repeatedly tried to prevent this out of self-interest: they pointed out that these were not psychiatric "cases" in order to protect their institutional professionalism. But because the health offices were usually committing people with the support of their families and members of their social milieu, such as neighbors, they rarely succeeded. The practice of committal shows that wartime society as a whole was characterized by a high degree of vertical harmony and steadily decreasing horizontal balance.

In the occupation zones and both successor states of the "Third Reich," the relationship between state and society was far less harmonious when it came to forcible committals than during World War II. Across regimes, postwar society too had an interest in uncomplicated committal to mental asylums that clashed with the protection of individual freedom. Especially in the "society in a state of collapse" (*Zusammenbruchgesellschaft*) but also in the 1950s and 1960s, tensions within the social microcosm were often resolved through committals. This applied, for example, to the situation in camps and in large families living together in cramped conditions, as well as to the integration of "expellees." But the role of the state in forcible committals differed significantly in East and West.

State intervention in the early GDR was the least pronounced among the three systems. In this respect, the two dictatorships differed significantly: there were far fewer formal forcible committals in the GDR than during World War II. The asylums I studied in East Germany, on the other hand, were characterized to a particularly high degree by committal negotiations "outside the state." Committals against the will of the person concerned were usually the result of joint decisions by relatives and physicians, without intervention by health offices, the police, or the legal system. Neither the police nor the health offices filled the legal vacuum, which persisted until 1968, although the transitional provisions still allowed for police intervention in cases of "danger" and for committals certified by a public health officer. Commonly used theoretical models of a *Diktatur der Grenzen* and the concept of a *durchherrschte Gesellschaft*, one in which the tentacles of the state extend into every nook and cranny, are of little use in this context, especially given that the majority of psychiatrists were critical of the new state and cannot be viewed as its agents. A more apt means of explaining this book's findings is the notion of the *sociation* (*Vergesellschaftung*)[22] of one of the state's areas of responsibility. In the psychiatric institutions of the early GDR, decisions about security and freedom, in which modern states otherwise play a leading role, were largely made and implemented in a manner remote from the state.

This sociation appears to have been due to the fact that the SED dictatorship came up against its "limits" in several ways in a field already molded by the social microcosm: while expert evaluations were regularly compiled to determine fitness for work and entitlement to a retirement pension, decisions on forcible committal attracted no state interest at all until the mid-1960s. Clear priorities were set in this regard. Psychiatric expertise was deployed to help establish a "socialist work-oriented society" (*Arbeitsgesellschaft*) from the outset but protecting the freedom of the individual was far from a key goal. Here the limits of state interest had been reached. Psychiatric institutions, moreover, functioned essentially on the basis of great social need. The state provided only rudimentary funding that came nowhere near meeting this need. Finally, the main actors in the context of forcible committals, namely, physicians and families, had no interest in cooperating with state agencies, such as health offices or courts. At least in the 1950s and early 1960s, psychiatry thus symbolized the limits of dictatorship in three ways: the limits of state interest, the limits of state capacities, and the limits of the state's acceptance within society.

Still, the concept of the *Diktatur der Grenzen* falls short here. While this idea is plausible with respect to all those areas in which the state sought to *durchherrschen* society and conveys the extent to which—and why—this could or could not be achieved, this book shows that such *Durchherrschung* was not pursued in every sphere, at least in the early GDR. The possibility that injustice may at times have been due to the state's failure to act, however, takes up little space in discussions of the GDR. Within the Cold War frame of reference, this is hardly surprising, given the strong tendency to think in terms of a dichotomy between liberal capitalist systems and dictatorial socialist ones. Even after 1989, this dichotomy was reproduced without much reflection in theoretical debates on the relationship between the state and society in the GDR. Thus, the sociation of the state and the aspiration to *durchherrschen* society appeared as contradictory rather than complementary characteristics, both underlining the state's dictatorial character.[23] The example of committal practice shows that this conceptual framework is too schematic. The state's disinterest in forcible committal in the early GDR can be explained in light of an interplay between ideological factors and a weak state limited in its capacities. Initially, SED rule shaped everyday life by attempting to thoroughly *durchherrschen* certain fields, while other areas were illegitimately neglected and sociated. In the field of psychiatry, this interplay, which was symptomatic of the early SED regime, presumably had indirect effects on the later phase of real existing socialism: I suspect that the mode of forcible committals by families and asylum physicians, which functioned for two decades, may have laid the ground for the legal regulations introduced in 1968, which largely legitimized existing procedures.

While there were relatively few points of contact between state and society in the practice of committal in the GDR, things were quite different in West Germany. The practice of forcible committal in the western occupation zones

and the FRG was characterized by an antagonism between democratic jur-
idification from above and stubborn resistance to it among the implementing
institutions and the families of those affected. During the occupation,
Bavarian administrative agencies in particular energetically formulated
strategies to avoid implementing American directives aimed at protecting
personal freedom. In the FRG, too, the newly established legal protection
afforded by Article 104 of the Basic Law hardly changed the decision-making
practices surrounding committal. The decisions made by families, family
physicians, and asylum psychiatrists were merely retrospectively legitimized
through the legal system. In the cases analyzed in this book, what we mostly
find is that the patient was first brought to the asylum thanks to a decision
made by a member or members of their family and with the approval of
the family doctor; they were then admitted and subsequently a judge, often
notified by telephone, confirmed the committal.

The Western occupying powers and the FRG placed far greater emphasis
on individual liberties than the GDR, resulting in new legal regulations
intended to protect the individual. These, however, were not specifically
aimed at the field of psychiatry but merely encompassed it, a lack of focus
that is likely to have facilitated the continuation of entrenched practices. The
continuous and inconclusive discussions in the FRG on cost settlement,
which grappled with the character and legitimacy of forcible committals
and who was responsible for them, demonstrate how long the relationship
between freedom and security remained a bone of contention in West
Germany. Both committal practices and discussions of committals there ex-
hibit strong continuities in terms of micro- and meso-level notions of safety,
illness, normality, and everyday tolerance. Precisely because the psychiatric
sector was not a major focus for the state in the FRG, venerable mechanisms
and ideas were widely perpetuated. The differences in the attitude of political
actors in Bavaria and Hesse, however, make it clear that clear statements
and instructions from above could certainly lead to changes.

Analysis of the *practice* of committal directs our attention to processes of
negotiation in the GDR that were remote from the state and sheds light on
the relationship between state and society both in that country and in the
FRG, where it is purposeful actions at the micro- and meso-levels that stand
out. The praxeological approach thus alters our perspective, sparking off
unfamiliar questions that unsettle established interpretations in the field
of contemporary German history. This applies both to the comparison of the
two dictatorships with the FRG and to the classification and evaluation of
psychiatric knowledge and institutions within longer-term developments.
Psychiatric knowledge, that is, became increasingly important as a form of
practical knowledge of great relevance to the state from the final third of the
nineteenth century onward—in the wake of expert evaluations, warfare, and
intelligence testing. It served the state in its pursuit of regulation, control,
planning, and prophylaxis. This expertise was provided in part by in-patient
evaluations. This, however, applied only to a small proportion of committals:

more than three-quarters of all committals in the mid-twentieth century were initiated to varying degrees from within society. Much of what went on in asylums was important to the state chiefly as a cost factor, and the increasing number of committals soon became a major problem. At the same time, internally the asylums were subject to differentiation: a distinction was made between calm (*ruhig*) and restless (*unruhig*) patients, between cases of treatment and care, between dangerous and non-dangerous residents, between patients who were capable of work and those who were not, and between the affluent and those dependent on welfare. When it comes to the further course of the twentieth century, the establishment of child and adolescent psychiatry as a specialty in its own right also fits this picture of differentiation. This effort to achieve finer degrees of classification within the asylum contrasts with a practice of committal marked by its flexibility and adaptation to social conditions as well as by the diverse pathways and actors involved. The striking breadth of asylum use is not fully reflected in public debates on psychiatry. In addition to the much-discussed forcible committals, there were also those in which patients sought admission, for example, out of fear of themselves, but also in the hope of receiving help and of being able to cope with family or working life after an inpatient stay. The tension between coercion and voluntariness that opens up here can be understood particularly well at the level of practice, though it cannot be resolved analytically. Attempts to categorize within the asylum can only be understood against the background of the asylum's flexible threshold. Their extremely heterogeneous "pathological material" (that is, the patients) gave the asylums the opportunity to subdivide people in multiple ways on the basis of differing criteria. The asylums themselves thus seem to mirror a highly differentiated society, one in which classification by experts plays a significant role. On the other hand, the diverse practice of committal suggests that the desired order was possible only within the enclosed space of the asylum and that it was ultimately the fairly open form of access to the asylum that was the prerequisite for its differentiated interior. Hence, the symbolism of the ordering of "lunatics" inside the asylum always highlights the failure to assign psychiatry an unambiguous functional role within society. Various actors repeatedly demanded that it be assigned as clear a role as possible, but this was never to be achieved. In their ambivalence, psychiatric institutions are in fact symptomatic of high modernity.[24] They are both a symbol of concentrated scientific and governmental attempts to order and regulate the "social" and also places that exist and expand because these efforts fail. In this sense, psychiatric institutions are chiefly an instrument of social self-regulation from below and thus a symptom of the adaptation of social microcosms to modern processes of rationalization.

Notes

1 LHA Marburg, Patient file sign. 16K10740F, Entry, April 18, 1946.

2 Ibid., Entry, April 14, 1946.
3 One of the authors who strongly oppose this view is Ledebur, Sophie, *Das Wissen der Anstaltspsychiatrie in der Moderne. Zur Geschichte der Heil- und Pflegeanstalten Am Steinhof Wien* (Vienna, 2011), 144 f. For Roy Porter's demand, preceding this criticism, to include the patient's view in studies in the history of medicine, see the much-cited article: Porter, Roy, "The Patient's View. Doing Medical History from Below," *Theory and Society* 14, 1985, 175–198. On the rare implementation of this demand, see Meier et al., *Psychiatrie*, 41.
4 These studies are primarily concerned with the emergence of psychiatric knowledge. The present volume builds on many of their results without, however, taking a primarily history-of-knowledge approach. Particularly important to this book are four anthologies, two of them on medical case histories, plus monographs on the clinical pictures of schizophrenia and multiple sclerosis, which I have frequently drawn on: Behrens, Rudolf and Carsten Zelle (eds.), *Der ärztliche Fallbericht. Epistemische Grundlagen und textuelle Strukturen dargestellter Beobachtung* (Wiesbaden, 2012), esp. Behrens, Rudolf and Carsten Zelle, "Vorwort," in ibid., vii–xii; Brändli, Sybille et al. (eds.), *Zum Fall machen, zum Fall werden. Wissensproduktion und Patientenerfahrung in Medizin und Psychiatrie des 19. und 20. Jahrhunderts* (Frankfurt/M., 2009); Wernli, Martina (ed.), *Wissen und Nicht-Wissen in der Klinik. Dynamiken der Psychiatrie um 1900* (Bielefeld, 2012); Hess and Schmiedebach, *Am Rande des Wahnsinns*; Bernet, *Schizophrenie*; Murray, *Multiple Sclerosis*. As a representative of others, I would also mention Hess, Volker, "Formalisierte Beobachtung. Die Genese der modernen Krankengeschichte am Beispiel der Berliner und Pariser Medizin (1725–1830)," *Medizinhistorisches Journal* 45, 2010, 293–340; Ledebur, *Anstaltspsychiatrie*.
5 On this range of opinions, see Conference Report, *Psychiatrische Krankenakten als Material der Wissenschaftsgeschichte. Methodisches Vorgehen am Einzelfall.* May 17–May 19, 2007, Berlin, in H-Soz-u-Kult, June 10, 2007, http://hsozkult.geschichte.hu-berlin.de/tagungsberichte/id=1602 (accessed June 21, 2014).
6 Sophie Ledebur justifies her decision to analyze the psychiatric records of the Viennese Am Steinhof asylum in a purely functional way with the argument that a fundamental distinction must be made between a functional and a hermeneutic approach, with the latter unsuccessfully attempting to reconstruct something that the source simply does not provide, namely, "the experiential worlds and the horizons of the meaning of those affected." Ledebur, *Anstaltspsychiatrie*, 144 f.
7 Ibid., 145. See also Bernet, "Eintragen," 64; Sammet, Kai, "Paratext und Text. Über das Abheften und die Verwendung psychiatrischer Krankenakten. Beispiele aus den Jahren 1900 bis 1930," *Schriftenreihe der Deutschen Gesellschaft zur Geschichte der Nervenheilkunde* 12, 2006, 339–367.
8 Meier et al., *Psychiatrie*, 41; also paraphrased in Ledebur, *Anstaltspsychiatrie*, 145.
9 Many patients were not so ill that they could no longer reflect on their situation, or their illnesses were episodic, so that there were sometimes extremely clear and barely comprehensible statements or letters from the same person.
10 On the criticism that a hermeneutic approach aims to reconstruct "experiential worlds" and the "silenced voices of madness," see Ledebur, *Anstaltspsychiatrie*, 144.
11 In dream interpretation, for example, it is scarcely possible to separate the patient's voice from the doctor's interpretation. See Behrens and Zelle, "Vorwort," xi.
12 Psychiatry and psychology largely went their separate ways between the 1940s and 1960s. Especially in state asylums, psychiatry, which saw itself to a very large extent as a somatic discipline, undoubtedly enjoyed supremacy. On the separate path of psychology, see Roelcke, "Psychotherapy," 486 f.

13 For example, an April 1955 article in *Psychiatrie, Neurologie und medizinische Psychologie* on schizophrenia states: "As long as the disease process is still in its early stages, the sick can describe the subjective picture of their illness." Tscholakow, "Zur pathophysiologischen Analyse," 97.

14 Of course, this does not apply to all patients. There are ego-documents in the sample taken for this book whose meaning is not immediately obvious.

15 Gründler, *Armut und Wahnsinn*, 115.

16 On the Weimar Republic and the Nazi period, see Hauschildt, *Trinkerfürsorge*.

17 Foucault, *Psychology*, 132.

18 On processes of scientification and the knowledge society in this period, see Szöllösi-Janze, "Wissensgesellschaft."

19 See Kury, *Der Überforderte Mensch*.

20 See Ayaß, "Asoziale."

21 Süß, "Volkskörper," 263ff.

22 On sociation in the GDR, see Jessen, "Gesellschaft," 106 f.

23 Jessen's concept of a complementary process of growing state control over society and the sociation of the state increasingly faded into the background amid a boom in research on *Durchherrschung* and its scope. In reviews of the state of research, the concept is mentioned only cursorily, if at all. See, for example, the summary of the state of research in Kocka, Jürgen, "Wissenschaft und Politik in der DDR," in Kocka, Jürgen and Renate Mayntz (eds.), *Wissenschaft und Wiedervereinigung: Disziplinen im Umbruch* (Berlin, 1998), 435–459. Interpretive constructs such as *Fürsorgediktatur* ("welfare dictatorship"), *Versorgungsdiktatur* ("provisioning dictatorship"), and *Erziehungsdiktatur* ("educational dictatorship"), which seek to resolve the contradiction of emancipatory elements and dictatorial practice, also assume an all-pervasive aspiration to total domination of society. On these concepts, see Jarausch, Konrad, "Fürsorgediktatur, Version: 1.0," *Docupedia-Zeitgeschichte*, February 11, 2010, URL: http://docupedia.de/zg/F.C3. BCrsorgediktatur?oldid=106417 (accessed April 11, 2014).

24 On the concept of high modernity, see Herbert, "Liberalisierung."

Appendix

Abbreviations

AB Oberbayern	Archiv des Bezirks Oberbayern (Archive of the District of Upper Bavaria)
ALR	Allgemeines Landrecht (General State Law; in Prussia, the basis for the commitment of mentally ill individuals until the founding of the Empire was the General State Law of 1794)
BA	Bundesarchiv (Federal Archive)
BRD	Bundesrepublik Deutschland (Federal Republic of Germany)
DAF	Deutsche Arbeitsfront (German Labor Front)
DDR	Deutsche Demokratische Republik (German Democratic Republic)
DSM	Diagnostic and Statistical Manual of Mental Disorders (US diagnostic handbook, first published in 1952)
DZVG	Deutsche Zentralverwaltung für das Gesundheitswesen (German Central Administration for Healthcare in the Soviet occupation zone)
EH	Eglfing-Haar
FRG	Federal Republic of Germany
GDR	German Democratic Republic
GG	Grundgesetz (Basic Law, the constitution of the FRG)
GgGSB	Gesetz gegen gefährliche Gewohnheitsverbrecher und über die Maßregeln der Sicherung und Besserung" ("Law against Dangerous Recidivists and on Protection and Rehabilitation Measures" of November 24, 1933)
GzVeN	Gesetz zur Verhütung erbkranken Nachwuchses" ("Law for the Prevention of Hereditarily Diseased Offspring" of July 14, 1933)
HAB	Hauptarchiv der von Bodelschwinghschen Stiftungen Bethel (Main Archive of the von Bodelschwingh Foundations Bethel)

HPA	Heil- und Pflegeanstalt (sanatorium-nursing home)
HSta	Hauptstaatsarchiv (Main State Archive)
ICD	International Statistical Classification of Diseases and Related Health Problems
KA	Krankenanstalten (hospitals)
LA	Landesanstalt (Land asylum)
LHA	Landesheilanstalt (Land sanatorium)
LK	Landeskrankenhaus (Land hospital)
LWV	Landeswohlfahrtsverband (Land welfare association)
MDI	manisch-depressives Irresein (manic-depressive insanity)
MfG	Ministerium für Gesundheitswesen (Ministry of Health, GDR)
MS	Multiple Sklerose (multiple sclerosis)
NS	Nationalsozialismus (National Socialism, Nazism)
PVG	Polizeiverwaltungsgesetz (Police Administration Law of June 1, 1931)
SächSta	Sächsisches Staatsarchiv (Saxony State Archive)
SBZ	Sowjetische Besatzungszone (Soviet occupation zone)
PsychN	Psychiatrische und Nervenklinik (Psychiatric and neurological clinic)
SMI	Staatsministerium des Inneren (State Ministry of the Interior)
StdA	Stadtarchiv (City Archive)
PStGB	Polizeistrafgesetzbuch (Police Criminal Code; in this book, always the Police Criminal Code for Bavaria of December 26, 1871)
StGB	Strafgesetzbuch (Criminal Code)
StPO	Strafprozessordnung (Code of Criminal Procedure)
T	Table
vBS	von Bodelschwinghsche Stiftungen (von Bodelschwingh Foundations)
ČSR	Tschechoslowakische Republik (Czechoslovak Republic [1945–1960])
ČSSR	Tschechoslowakische Sozialistische Republik (Czechoslovak Socialist Republic [1960–1990])
WHO	World Health Organization
ZPO	Zivilprozessordnung (Code of Civil Procedure)

1. Statistical analysis of the committal pathway

Explanations of the statistical analysis:

- "Unavailable" indicates that no information was recorded in the medical records.
- The category "indeterminate," meanwhile, was used when information was present in the medical records but could not be deciphered definitively

because, for example, abbreviations could not be confidently decoded or different pieces of information were recorded but it was unclear which was correct.

• Compulsory committals are divided into three subcategories. A distinction is made between judicial committals and those initiated by the police and public health office. The latter two cases were committals "on grounds of danger," and they were legitimized by the same legal regulations (PVG, in Bavaria Article 80/II PStGB). The difference between them is that the committals referred to here as "by the police" were initially carried out without a medical certificate, whereas the category "health office" (*Gesundheitsamt*) entailed the issuance of a certificate by a public health officer.

• Committals for "Evaluation § 51" were expert assessments of unsoundness of mind.

• "Nazi labor camps" in the tables means camps where foreign forced laborers were held during the Nazi era, while "foreigner camps post-WWII" refers to those that continued to exist for a time after the war until the forced laborers were able to return to their home countries.

Tables: Committal pathway from 1941 to end of war

Permanent residence prior to committal (tables 1–5)

T1 Greifswald University Psychiatric Clinic

		Frequency	Percent	Valid Percent	Cumulative Percent
Valid	Indeterminate	3	4.1	4.1	4.1
	At home	65	89	89	93.2
	Refugee camp	4	5.5	5.5	98.6
	Military use	1	1.4	1.4	100
	Total	73	100	100	

T2 Untergöltzsch Sanatorium-Nursing Home (Rodewisch from 1947)

		Frequency	Percent	Valid Percent	Cumulative Percent
Valid	Indeterminate	7	8.3	8.3	8.3
	At home	49	58.3	58.3	66.7
	Psychiatric institution or department	6	7.1	7.1	73.8
	Prison	3	3.6	3.6	77.4
	Old people's home	5	6	6	83.3

(Continued)

T2 (Continued)

	Frequency	Percent	Valid Percent	Cumulative Percent
Refugee camp	1	1.2	1.2	84.5
Military use	5	6	6	90.5
Nursing home	6	7.1	7.1	97.6
Refugee	1	1.2	1.2	98.8
Staying with relatives	1	1.2	1.2	100
Total	84	100	100	

T3 Eglfing-Haar Sanatorium-Nursing Home

		Frequency	Percent	Valid Percent	Cumulative Percent
Valid	Indeterminate	13	16.7	16.7	16.7
	Street	1	1.3	1.3	17.9
	Reserve hospital	4	5.1	5.1	23.1
	At home	43	55.1	55.1	78.2
	Psychiatric institution or department	4	5.1	5.1	83.3
	Prison	2	2.6	2.6	85.9
	Old people's home	1	1.3	1.3	87.2
	Home for the blind	1	1.3	1.3	88.5
	Nazi labor camp	1	1.3	1.3	89.7
	Foreigners' camp post-WWII	3	3.8	3.8	93.6
	Sanatorium	2	2.6	2.6	96.2
	Educational institution	1	1.3	1.3	97.4
	Refugee camp	1	1.3	1.3	98.7
	Children's home	1	1.3	1.3	100
	Total	78	100	100	

T4 Marburg Land Sanatorium

		Frequency	Percent	Valid Percent	Cumulative Percent
Valid	Indeterminate	12	13.2	13.2	13.2
	At home	54	59.3	59.3	72.5
	Psychiatric institution or department	2	2.2	2.2	74.7
	Prison	1	1.1	1.1	75.8
	Old people's home	4	4.4	4.4	80.2
	Nazi labor camp	2	2.2	2.2	82.4
	Educational institution	4	4.4	4.4	86.8
	Military use	4	4.4	4.4	91.2
	Hospital	2	2.2	2.2	93.4
	War captivity/forced laborer	6	6.6	6.6	100
	Total	91	100	100	

T5 Von Bodelschwingh Asylums Bethel

		Frequency	Percent	Valid Percent	Cumulative Percent
Valid	Indeterminate	7	17.9	17.9	17.9
	At home	27	69.2	69.2	87.2
	Psychiatric institution or department	3	7.7	7.7	94.9
	Military use	1	2.6	2.6	97.4
	War captivity	1	2.6	2.6	100
	Total	39	100	100	

Place of residence immediately prior to committal (tables 6–10)

T6 Greifswald University Psychiatric Clinic

		Frequency	Percent	Valid Percent	Cumulative Percent
Valid	Indeterminate	10	13.7	13.7	13.7
	At home	50	68.5	68.5	82.2
	Non-psych. hospital	8	11	11	93.2
	From prison	1	1.4	1.4	94.5
	Refugee/resettler camp	3	4.1	4.1	98.6
	Workplace	1	1.4	1.4	100
	Total	73	100	100	

T7 Untergöltzsch Sanatorium-Nursing Home (Rodewisch from 1947)

		Frequency	Percent	Valid Percent	Cumulative Percent
Valid	Indeterminate	9	10.7	10.7	10.7
	At home	28	33.3	33.3	44
	Another psych. hospital	11	13.1	13.1	57.1
	Non-psych. hospital	12	14.3	14.3	71.4
	Prison	1	1.2	1.2	72.6
	Old people's home	9	10.7	10.7	83.3
	Of no fixed abode	1	1.2	1.2	84.5
	Military use	4	4.8	4.8	89.3
	By relatives	1	1.2	1.2	90.5
	Nursing home	6	7.1	7.1	97.6
	Refugee/resettler camp	2	2.4	2.4	100
	Total	84	100	100	

T8 Eglfing-Haar Sanatorium-Nursing Home

		Frequency	*Percent*	*Valid Percent*	*Cumulative Percent*
Valid	Indeterminate	9	11.5	11.5	11.5
	At home	14	17.9	17.9	29.5
	Another psych. hospital	34	43.6	43.6	73.1
	Non-psych. hospital	17	21.8	21.8	94.9
	Prison	2	2.6	2.6	97.4
	Via psychiatric counseling center	2	2.6	2.6	100
	Total	78	100	100	

T9 Marburg Land Sanatorium

		Frequency	*Percent*	*Valid Percent*	*Cumulative Percent*
Valid	Indeterminate	18	19.8	19.8	19.8
	At home	25	27.5	27.5	47.3
	Another psych. hospital	11	12.1	12.1	59.3
	Non-psych. hospital	21	23.1	23.1	82.4
	Prison	5	5.5	5.5	87.9
	Youth welfare office	1	1.1	1.1	89
	Old people's home	2	2.2	2.2	91.2
	Of no fixed abode	1	1.1	1.1	92.3
	Military use	1	1.1	1.1	93.4
	Educational institution	4	4.4	4.4	97.8
	Labor camp	2	2.2	2.2	100
	Total	91	100	100	

T10 Von Bodelschwingh Foundations Bethel

		Frequency	*Percent*	*Valid Percent*	*Cumulative Percent*
Valid	Indeterminate	9	23.1	23.1	23.1
	At home	18	46.2	46.2	69.2
	Another psych. hospital	3	7.7	7.7	76.9
	Non-psych. hospital	7	17.9	17.9	94.9
	Apprehended on the street	1	2.6	2.6	97.4
	Military use	1	2.6	2.6	100
	Total	39	100	100	

Committing institution (tables 11–15)

T11 Greifswald University Psychiatric Clinic

		Frequency	Percent	Valid Percent	Cumulative Percent
Valid	Indeterminate	12	16.4	16.4	16.4
	By the police	2	2.7	2.7	19.2
	Health Office	2	2.7	2.7	21.9
	Hospital	8	11	11	32.9
	Psychiatric department/clinic	2	2.7	2.7	35.6
	Medical practice	25	34.2	34.2	69.9
	From home without referral by a doctor	1	1.4	1.4	71.2
	External psychiatric care; outpatient examination by the receiving clinic's doctors leads to committal	5	6.8	6.8	78.1
	Evaluation (ability to work, invalidity, result of work-related accident)	4	5.5	5.5	83.6
	Evaluation § 51	2	2.7	2.7	86.3
	Evaluation hereditary health court	9	12.3	12.3	98.6
	Health insurance fund	1	1.4	1.4	100
	Total	73	100	100	

T12 Untergöltzsch Sanatorium-Nursing Home (Rodewisch from 1947)

		Frequency	Percent	Valid Percent	Cumulative Percent
Valid	Indeterminate	14	16.7	16.7	16.7
	By the police	2	2.4	2.4	19
	Judicial	1	1.2	1.2	20.2
	Health Office	21	25	25	45.2
	Hospital	12	14.3	14.3	59.5
	Psychiatric department/clinic	14	16.7	16.7	76.2
	Medical practice	15	17.9	17.9	94
	From home without referral by a doctor	4	4.8	4.8	98.8
	Evaluation of hereditary health court	1	1.2	1.2	100
	Total	84	100	100	

T13 Eglfing-Haar Sanatorium-Nursing Home

		Frequency	*Percent*	*Valid Percent*	*Cumulative Percent*
Valid	Indeterminate	11	14.1	14.1	14.1
	By the police	31	5.1	5.1	19.2
	Judicial	3	3.8	3.8	23
	Health Office	4	39.7	39.7	62.8
	Hospital	12	15.4	15.4	78.2
	Psychiatric department/ clinic	11	14.1	14.1	92.3
	Medical practice	3	3.8	3.8	96.2
	From home without referral by a doctor	3	3.8	3.8	100
	Total	78	100	100	

T14 Marburg Land Sanatorium

		Frequency	*Percent*	*Valid Percent*	*Cumulative Percent*
Valid	Indeterminate	10	11	11	11
	By the police	2	2.2	2.2	13.2
	Judicial	2	2.2	2.2	15.4
	Health Office	4	4.4	4.4	19.8
	Hospital	17	18.7	18.7	38.5
	Psychiatric department/ clinic	14	15.4	15.4	53.8
	Medical practice	22	24.2	24.2	78
	From home without referral by a doctor	1	1.1	1.1	79.1
	Evaluation (ability to work, invalidity, result of work-related accident)	1	1.1	1.1	80.2
	Evaluation § 51	14	15.4	15.4	95.6
	For evaluation by hereditary health court	3	3.3	3.3	98.9
	For evaluation (incapacitation)	1	1.1	1.1	100
	Total	91	100	100	

T15 Von Bodelschwingh Foundations Bethel

		Frequency	Percent	Valid Percent	Cumulative Percent
Valid	Indeterminate	12	30.8	30.8	30.8
	By the police	2	5.1	5.1	35.9
	Hospital	8	20.5	20.5	56.4
	Psychiatric department/clinic	1	2.6	2.6	59
	Medical practice	6	15.4	15.4	74.4
	From home without referral by a doctor	1	2.6	2.6	76.9
	Through informal inquiry	8	20.5	20.5	97.4
	Evaluation (ability to work, invalidity, result of work-related accident)	1	2.6	2.6	100
	Total	39	100	100	

Tables: Committal pathway from end of war to 1949 inclusive

Permanent residence prior to committal (tables 16–20)

T16 Greifswald University Psychiatric Clinic

		Frequency	Percent	Valid Percent	Cumulative Percent
Valid	Indeterminate	7	7.4	7.5	7.5
	Wanderhof NS	2	2.1	2.2	9.7
	Military detention	1	1.1	1.1	10.8
	Street	1	1.1	1.1	11.8
	At home	70	74.5	75.3	87.1
	Refugee camp	10	10.6	10.8	97.8
	Military use	1	1.1	1.1	98.9
	War captivity	1	1.1	1.1	100
	Total	93	98.9	100	
Unavailable	System	1	1.1		
	Total	94	100		

T17 Untergöltzsch Sanatorium-Nursing Home (Rodewisch from 1947)

		Frequency	Percent	Valid Percent	Cumulative Percent
Valid	Indeterminate	3	3.8	5.1	5.1
	At home	37	46.8	62.7	67.8
	Psychiatric institution or department	4	5.1	6.8	74.6
	Old people's home	11	13.9	18.6	93.2

(*Continued*)

T17 (Continued)

		Frequency	Percent	Valid Percent	Cumulative Percent
	Refugee camp	1	1.3	1.7	94.9
	Nursing home	2	2.5	3.4	98.3
	Salvation Army men's shelter	1	1.3	1.7	100
	Total	59	74.7	100	
	System	20	25.3		
Unavailable	Total	79	100		
	Total	94	100		

T18 Eglfing-Haar Sanatorium-Nursing Home

		Frequency	Percent	Valid Percent	Cumulative Percent
Valid	Indeterminate	8	11.4	11.4	11.4
	Street	3	4.3	4.3	15.7
	At home	41	58.6	58.6	74.3
	Prison	1	1.4	1.4	75.7
	Foster family	1	1.4	1.4	77.1
	Old people's home	5	7.1	7.1	84.3
	Foreigners' camp post-WWII	6	8.6	8.6	92.9
	Refugee camp	4	5.7	5.7	98.6
	Children's home	1	1.4	1.4	100
	Total	70	100	100	

T19 Marburg Land Sanatorium

		Frequency	Percent	Valid Percent	Cumulative Percent
Valid	Indeterminate	12	12.8	12.8	12.8
	Street	1	1.1	1.1	13.8
	At home	65	69.1	69.1	83
	Psychiatric institution or department	3	3.2	3.2	86.2
	Prison	1	1.1	1.1	87.2
	Refugee camp	9	9.6	9.6	96.8
	Hospital	1	1.1	1.1	97.9
	War captivity	2	2.1	2.1	100
	Total	94	100	100	

T20 Von Bodelschwingh Foundations Bethel

		Frequency	Percent	Valid Percent	Cumulative Percent
Valid	Indeterminate	4	12.1	12.1	12.1
	At home	25	75.8	75.8	87.9
	Prison	1	3	3	90.9
	Refugee camp	2	6.1	6.1	97
	War captivity	1	3	3	100
	Total	33	100	100	

Place of residence immediately prior to committal (tables 21–25)

T21 Greifswald University Psychiatric Clinic

		Frequency	Percent	Valid Percent	Cumulative Percent
Valid	Unspecified	20	21.3	21.7	21.7
	From home	53	56.4	57.6	79.3
	Non-psych. hospital	14	14.9	15.2	94.6
	Prison	1	1.1	1.1	95.7
	Refugee/resettler camp	4	4.3	4.3	100
	Total	92	97.9	100	
Unavailable	System	2	2.1		
	Total	94	100		

T22 Untergöltzsch Sanatorium-Nursing Home (Rodewisch from 1947)

		Frequency	Percent	Valid Percent	Cumulative Percent
Valid	Unspecified	4	5.1	6.8	6.8
	From home	23	29.1	39	45.8
	From another psych. Hospital	4	5.1	6.8	52.5
	From non-psych. hospital	8	10.1	13.6	66.1
	From prison	1	1.3	1.7	67.8
	Old people's home	13	16.5	22	89.8
	Apprehended on the street	1	1.3	1.7	91.5
	By relatives	2	2.5	3.4	94.9
	Nursing home	1	1.3	1.7	96.6
	Salvation Army men's shelter	1	1.3	1.7	98.3
	Refugee/resettler camp	1	1.3	1.7	100
	Total	59	74.7	100	
Unavailable	System	20	25.3		
	Total	79	100		

T23 Eglfing-Haar Sanatorium-Nursing Home

		Frequency	Percent	Valid Percent	Cumulative Percent
Valid	Indeterminate	4	5.7	5.7	5.7
	From home	21	30	30	35.7
	From another psych. hospital	23	32.9	32.9	68.6
	Non-psych. hospital	18	25.7	25.7	94.3
	Prison	1	1.4	1.4	95.7
	Old people's home	1	1.4	1.4	97.1
	Apprehended on the street	1	1.4	1.4	98.6
	Of no fixed abode	1	1.4	1.4	100
	Total	70	100	100	

T24 Marburg Land Sanatorium

		Frequency	Percent	Valid Percent	Cumulative Percent
Valid	Indeterminate	13	13.8	13.8	13.8
	At home	40	42.6	42.6	56.4
	From another psych. hospital	18	19.1	19.1	75.5
	From non-psych. hospital	17	18.1	18.1	93.6
	From prison	2	2.1	2.1	95.7
	Old people's home	2	2.1	2.1	97.9
	Apprehended on the street	1	1.1	1.1	98.9
	From educational institution	1	1.1	1.1	100
	Total	94	100	100	

T25 Von Bodelschwingh Foundations Bethel

		Frequency	Percent	Valid Percent	Cumulative Percent
Valid	Indeterminate	5	15.2	15.2	15.2
	At home	24	72.7	72.7	87.9
	Non-psych. hospital	2	6.1	6.1	93.9
	Prison	1	3	3	97
	Apprehended on the street	1	3	3	100
	Total	33	100	100	

Committing institution (tables 26–30)

T26 Greifswald University Psychiatric Clinic

		Frequency	Percent	Valid Percent	Cumulative Percent
Valid	Indeterminate	19	20.2	20.4	20.4
	By the police	3	3.2	3.2	23.7
	Hospital	14	14.9	15.1	38.7
	Medical practice/rural outpatient clinic/polyclinic	40	42.6	43	81.7
	From home without referral by a doctor	2	2.1	2.2	83.9
	External psychiatric care; outpatient examination by the receiving clinic's doctors leads to committal	3	3.2	3.2	87.1
	Summoned for evaluation (ability to work, invalidity, result of work-related accident)	7	7.4	7.5	94.6
	Evaluation § 51	4	4.3	4.3	98.9
	Evaluation (care)	1	1.1	1.1	100
	Total	93	98.9	100	
Unavailable	System	1	1.1		
	Total	94	100		

T27 Untergöltzsch Sanatorium-Nursing Home (Rodewisch from 1947)

		Frequency	Percent	Valid Percent	Cumulative Percent
Valid	Indeterminate	16	20.3	27.1	27.1
	By the police	2	2.5	3.4	30.5
	Health Office	5	6.3	8.5	39
	Hospital	8	10.1	13.6	52.5
	Psychiatric department/clinic	5	6.3	8.5	61
	Medical practice/rural outpatient clinic/polyclinic	22	27.8	37.3	98.3
	From home without referral by a doctor	1	1.3	1.7	100
	Total	59	74.7	100	
Unavailable	System	20	25.3		
	Total	79	100		

T28 Eglfing-Haar Sanatorium-Nursing Home

		Frequency	Percent	Valid Percent	Cumulative Percent
Valid	Indeterminate	7	10	10.1	10.1
	By the police	4	5.7	5.8	15.9
	Health Office	2	2.9	2.9	18.8
	Hospital	15	21.4	21.7	40.6
	Psychiatric department/clinic	23	32.9	33.3	73.9
	Medical practice	13	18.6	18.8	92.8
	From home without referral by a doctor	5	7.1	7.2	100
	Total	69	98.6	100	
Unavailable	System	1	1.4		
	Total	70	100		

T29 Marburg Land Sanatorium

		Frequency	Percent	Valid Percent	Cumulative Percent
Valid	Indeterminate	9	9.6	9.6	9.6
	By the police	1	1.1	1.1	10.6
	Judicial	4	4.3	4.3	14.9
	Health Office	2	2.1	2.1	17
	Hospital	12	12.8	12.8	29.8
	Psychiatric department/clinic	19	20.2	20.2	50
	Medical practice	39	41.5	41.5	91.5
	From home without referral by a doctor	2	2.1	2.1	93.6
	Evaluation § 51	4	4.3	4.3	97.9
	Evaluation (incapacitation)	1	1.1	1.1	98.9
	Evaluation (divorce)	1	1.1	1.1	100
	Total	94	100	100	

T30 Von Bodelschwingh Foundations Bethel

		Frequency	Percent	Valid Percent	Cumulative Percent
Valid	Indeterminate	12	36.4	36.4	36.4
	By the police	1	3	3	39.4
	Health Office	5	15.2	15.2	54.5
	Hospital	2	6.1	6.1	60.6
	Medical practice	10	30.3	30.3	90.9
	From home without referral by a doctor	2	6.1	6.1	97
	Through unofficial request	1	3	3	100
	Total	33	100	100	

Tables: Committal pathway, 1950–1955

Permanent residence prior to committal (tables 31–34)

T31 Greifswald University Psychiatric Clinic

		Frequency	Percent	Valid Percent	Cumulative Percent
Valid	Indeterminate	3	3.8	3.9	3.9
	Reserve hospital	1	1.3	1.3	5.2
	At home	72	91.1	93.5	98.7
	Prison	1	1.3	1.3	100
	Total	77	97.5	100	
Unavailable	System	2	2.5		
	Total	79	100		

T32 Untergöltzsch Sanatorium-Nursing Home (Rodewisch from 1947)

		Frequency	Percent	Valid Percent	Cumulative Percent
Valid	Indeterminate	2	2.8	3.1	3.1
	At home	55	76.4	85.9	89.1
	Prison	2	2.8	3.1	92.2
	Old people's home	2	2.8	3.1	95.3
	Home for the blind	1	1.4	1.6	96.9
	Hospital	1	1.4	1.6	98.4
	Staying with relatives	1	1.4	1.6	100
	Total	64	88.9	100	
Unavailable	System	8	11.1		
	Total	72	100		

T33 Marburg Land Sanatorium

		Frequency	Percent	Valid Percent	Cumulative Percent
Valid	Indeterminate	12	12.8	12.9	12.9
	At home	65	69.1	69.9	82.8
	Psychiatric institution or department	11	11.7	11.8	94.6
	Old people's home	4	4.3	4.3	98.9
	Refugee camp	1	1.1	1.1	100
	Total	93	98.9	100	
Unavailable	System	1	1.1		
	Total	94	100		

T34 Von Bodelschwingh Foundations Bethel

		Frequency	Percent	Valid Percent	Cumulative Percent
Valid	Indeterminate	1	1.6	1.6	1.6
	At home	60	93.8	93.8	95.3
	Old people's home	1	1.6	1.6	96.9
	Refugee camp	2	3.1	3.1	100
	Total	64	100	100	

Place of residence immediately prior to committal (tables 35–38)

T35 Greifswald University Psychiatric Clinic

		Frequency	Percent	Valid Percent	Cumulative Percent
Valid	Indeterminate	7	8.9	9.1	9.1
	From home	56	70.9	72.7	81.8
	Another psych. hospital	1	1.3	1.3	83.1
	From non-psych. hospital	11	13.9	14.3	97.4
	From prison	2	2.5	2.6	100
	Total	77	97.5	100	
Unavailable	System	2	2.5		
	Total	79	100		

T36 Untergöltzsch Sanatorium-Nursing Home (Rodewisch from 1947)

		Frequency	Percent	Valid Percent	Cumulative Percent
Valid	Indeterminate	12	16.7	18.8	18.8
	From home	24	33.3	37.5	56.3
	Another psych. hospital	4	5.6	6.3	62.5
	Non-psych. hospital	17	23.6	26.6	89.1
	Prison	2	2.8	3.1	92.2
	Old people's home	2	2.8	3.1	95.3
	Apprehended on the street	1	1.4	1.6	96.9
	Police	1	1.4	1.6	98.4
	Workplace	1	1.4	1.6	100
	Total	64	88.9	100	
Unavailable	System	8	11.1		
	Total	72	100		

T37 Marburg Land Sanatorium

		Frequency	Percent	Valid Percent	Cumulative Percent
Valid	Indeterminate	10	10.6	10.8	10.8
	At home	37	39.4	39.8	50.5
	Another psych. hospital	20	21.3	21.5	72
	Non-psych. hospital	20	21.3	21.5	93.5
	Prison	2	2.1	2.2	95.7
	Old people's home	4	4.3	4.3	100
	Total	93	98.9	100	
Unavailable	System	1	1.1		
	Total	94	100		

T38 Von Bodelschwingh Foundations Bethel

		Frequency	Percent	Valid Percent	Cumulative Percent
Valid	Indeterminate	2	3.1	3.1	3.1
	At home	57	89.1	89.1	92.2
	Non-psych. hospital	4	6.3	6.3	98.4
	Old people's home	1	1.6	1.6	100
	Total	64	100	100	

Committing institution (tables 39–42)

T39 Greifswald University Psychiatric Clinic

		Frequency	Percent	Valid Percent	Cumulative Percent
Valid	Indeterminate	10	12.7	13	13
	By the police	1	1.3	1.3	14.3
	Hospital	12	15.2	15.6	29.9
	Medical practice/rural outpatient clinic/polyclinic	22	27.8	28.6	58.4
	External psychiatric care; outpatient examination by the receiving clinic's doctors leads to committal	8	10.1	10.4	68.8
	Evaluation (ability to work, invalidity, result of work-related accident)	17	21.5	22.1	90.9
	Evaluation § 51	1	1.3	1.3	92.2
	Evaluation (Care)	1	1.3	1.3	93.5
	By company doctor	3	3.8	3.9	97.4
	Interruption evaluation	1	1.3	1.3	98.7
	Evaluation asylum placement	1	1.3	1.3	100
	Total	77	97.5	100	
Unavailable	System	2	2.5		
	Total	79	100		

T40 Untergöltzsch Sanatorium-Nursing Home (Rodewisch from 1947)

		Frequency	Percent	Valid Percent	Cumulative Percent
Valid	Indeterminate	11	15.3	17.2	17.2
	By the police	3	4.2	4.7	21.9
	Judicial	1	1.4	1.6	23.4
	Health Office	4	5.6	6.3	29.7
	Hospital	18	25	28.1	57.8
	Psychiatric department/ clinic	3	4.2	4.7	62.5
	Medical practice/rural outpatient clinic/ polyclinic	20	27.8	31.3	93.8
	Evaluation (ability to work, invalidity, result of work-related accident)	1	1.4	1.6	95.3
	Evaluation § 51	3	4.2	4.7	100
	Total	64	88.9	100	
Unavailable	System	8	11.1		
	Total	72	100		

T41 Marburg Land Sanatorium

		Frequency	Percent	Valid Percent	Cumulative Percent
Valid	Indeterminate	7	7.4	7.5	7.5
	By the police	3	3.2	3.2	10.8
	Judicial	6	6.4	6.5	17.2
	Health Office	5	5.3	5.4	22.6
	Hospital	17	18.1	18.3	40.9
	Psychiatric department/ clinic	20	21.3	21.5	62.4
	Medical practice	27	28.7	29	91.4
	From home without referral by a doctor	3	3.2	3.2	94.6
	Evaluation § 51	5	5.3	5.4	100
	Total	93	98.9	100	
Unavailable	System	1	1.1		
	Total	94	100		

T42 Von Bodelschwingh Foundations Bethel

		Frequency	Percent	Valid Percent	Cumulative Percent
Valid	Indeterminate	6	9.4	9.4	9.4
	By the police	1	1.6	1.6	10.9
	Hospital	6	9.4	9.4	20.3
	Psychiatric department/clinic	1	1.6	1.6	21.9
	Medical practice	33	51.6	51.6	73.4
	From home without referral by a doctor	4	6.3	6.3	79.7
	External psychiatric care; outpatient examination by the receiving clinic's doctors leads to committal	1	1.6	1.6	81.3
	Evaluation (ability to work, invalidity, result of work-related accident)	12	18.8	18.8	100
	Total	64	100	100	

Tables: Committal pathway, 1956–1963

Permanent residence prior to committal (tables 43–46)

T43 Greifswald University Psychiatric Clinic

		Frequency	Percent	Valid Percent	Cumulative Percent
Valid	Indeterminate	3	5.9	5.9	5.9
	At home	45	88.2	88.2	94.1
	Psychiatric institution or department	2	3.9	3.9	98
	Old people's home	1	2	2	100
	Total	51	100	100	

T44 Großschweidnitz Land Sanatorium

		Frequency	Percent	Valid Percent	Cumulative Percent
Valid	Indeterminate	5	7.5	7.5	7.5
	Wanderhof	1	1.5	1.5	9
	At home	50	74.6	74.6	83.6
	Psychiatric institution or department	2	3	3	86.6
	Prison	4	6	6	92.5
	Old people's home	2	3	3	95.5
	Refugee camp	1	1.5	1.5	97
	Nursing home	2	3	3	100
	Total	67	100	100	

T45 Marburg Land Sanatorium

		Frequency	Percent	Valid Percent	Cumulative Percent
Valid	Indeterminate	7	7.8	7.9	7.9
	Wanderhof	2	2.2	2.2	10.1
	At home	67	74.4	75.3	85.4
	Psychiatric institution or department	7	7.8	7.9	93.3
	Prison	1	1.1	1.1	94.4
	Old people's home	1	1.1	1.1	95.5
	Educational institution	2	2.2	2.2	97.8
	Hospital	1	1.1	1.1	98.9
	Bundeswehr	1	1.1	1.1	100
	Total	89	98.9	100	
Unavailable	System	1	1.1		
	Total	90	100		

T46 von Bodelschwingh Foundations Bethel

		Frequency	Percent	Valid Percent	Cumulative Percent
Valid	Indeterminate	1	1.8	1.8	1.8
	At home	51	89.5	89.5	91.2
	Psychiatric institution or department	3	5.3	5.3	96.5
	Old people's home	1	1.8	1.8	98.2
	Refugee camp	1	1.8	1.8	100
	Total	57	100	100	

Place of residence immediately prior to committal (tables 47–50)

T47 Greifswald University Psychiatric Clinic

		Frequency	Percent	Valid Percent	Cumulative Percent
Valid	Indeterminate	4	7.8	7.8	7.8
	At home	37	72.5	72.5	80.4
	Another psych. hospital	2	3.9	3.9	84.3
	Non-psych. hospital	6	11.8	11.8	96.1
	Prison	1	2	2	98
	Old people's home	1	2	2	100
	Total	51	100	100	

T48 Großschweidnitz Land Sanatorium

		Frequency	Percent	Valid Percent	Cumulative Percent
Valid	Indeterminate	4	6	6	6
	At home	37	55.2	55.2	61.2
	Another psych. hospital	2	3	3	64.2
	Non-psych. hospital	12	17.9	17.9	82.1
	Prison	6	9	9	91
	Old people's home	2	3	3	94
	Nursing home	2	3	3	97
	Police	1	1.5	1.5	98.5
	Refugee/resettler camp	1	1.5	1.5	100
	Total	67	100	100	

T49 Marburg Land Sanatorium

		Frequency	Percent	Valid Percent	Cumulative Percent
Valid	Indeterminate	11	12.2	12.4	12.4
	At home	46	51.1	51.7	64
	Another psych. hospital	15	16.7	16.9	80.9
	Non-psych. hospital	8	8.9	9	89.9
	Prison	3	3.3	3.4	93.3
	Youth welfare office	1	1.1	1.1	94.4
	Old people's home	1	1.1	1.1	95.5
	Apprehended on the street	1	1.1	1.1	96.6
	Educational institution	2	2.2	2.2	98.9
	Bundeswehr	1	1.1	1.1	100
	Total	89	98.9	100	
Unavailable	System	1	1.1		
	Total	90	100		

T50 Von Bodelschwingh Foundations Bethel

		Frequency	Percent	Valid Percent	Cumulative Percent
Valid	Indeterminate	2	3.5	3.5	3.5
	At home	51	89.5	89.5	93
	Another psych. hospital	2	3.5	3.5	96.5
	Old people's home	1	1.8	1.8	98.2
	Police	1	1.8	1.8	100
	Total	57	100	100	

Committing institution (tables 51–54)

T51 Greifswald University Psychiatric Clinic

		Frequency	Percent	Valid Percent	Cumulative Percent
Valid	Indeterminate	3	5.9	6	6
	Hospital	6	11.8	12	18
	Psychiatric department/clinic	1	2	2	20
	Medical practice/Rural outpatient clinic/polyclinic	18	35.3	36	56
	From home without referral by a doctor	1	2	2	58
	External psychiatric care; outpatient examination by the receiving clinic's doctors leads to committal	5	9.8	10	68
	Evaluation (ability to work, invalidity, result of work-related accident)	9	17.6	18	86
	Evaluation § 51	4	7.8	8	94
	Evaluation (incapacitation)	1	2	2	96
	By company doctor	2	3.9	4	100
	Total	50	98	100	
Unavailable	System	1	2		
	Total	51	100		

T52 Großschweidnitz Land Sanatorium

		Frequency	Percent	Valid Percent	Cumulative Percent
Valid	Indeterminate	7	10.4	10.4	10.4
	By the police	3	4.5	4.5	14.9
	Judicial	2	3	3	17.9
	Health Office	1	1.5	1.5	19.4
	Hospital	12	17.9	17.9	37.3
	Psychiatric department/clinic	2	3	3	40.3
	Medical practice/Rural outpatient clinic/polyclinic	27	40.3	40.3	80.6
	External psychiatric care; outpatient examination by the receiving clinic's doctors leads to committal	4	6	6	86.6
	Evaluation (ability to work, invalidity, result of work-related accident)	1	1.5	1.5	88.1
	Evaluation § 51	6	9	9	97
	By company doctor	1	1.5	1.5	98.5
	Health insurance fund	1	1.5	1.5	100
	Total	67	100	100	

T53 Marburg Land Sanatorium

		Frequency	Percent	Valid Percent	Cumulative Percent
Valid	Indeterminate	12	13.3	13.5	13.5
	By the police	6	6.7	6.7	20.2
	Judicial	9	10	10.1	30.3
	Hospital	8	8.9	9	39.3
	Psychiatric department/clinic	11	12.2	12.4	51.7
	Medical practice	32	35.6	36	87.6
	From home without referral by a doctor	4	4.4	4.5	92.1
	Evaluation (ability to work, invalidity, result of work-related accident)	2	2.2	2.2	94.4
	Evaluation § 51	4	4.4	4.5	98.9
	Evaluation (Care)	1	1.1	1.1	100
	Total	89	98.9	100	
Unavailable	System	1	1.1		
	Total	90	100		

T54 Von Bodelschwingh Foundations Bethel

		Frequency	Percent	Valid Percent	Cumulative Percent
Valid	Indeterminate	4	7	7	7
	Judicial	1	1.8	1.8	8.8
	Hospital	2	3.5	3.5	12.3
	Medical practice	37	64.9	64.9	77.2
	From home without referral by a doctor	3	5.3	5.3	82.5
	Evaluation (Ability to work, invalidity, result of work-related accident)	10	17.5	17.5	100
	Total	57	100	100	

2. Further statistical analyses

T55 Termination of stay at Greifswald University Psychiatric Clinic, 1950

		Frequency	Percent	Valid Percent	Cumulative Percent
Valid	Discharged from clinic	114	89.1	89.8	89.8
	Died at clinic	5	3.9	3.9	93.7
	Transferred to another psychiatric or nursing establishment	4	3.1	3.1	96.9
	Absconded	1	0.8	0.8	97.6
	Transferred to a surgical clinic or another non-psych. and non-neurol. ward	3	2.3	2.4	100
	Total	127	99.2	100	
Unavailable	System	1	0.8		
	Total	128	100		

T56 HPA Untergöltzsch 1941 to end of war, gender distribution in compulsory committals

		Frequency	Percent	Valid Percent	Cumulative Percent
Valid	Male	7	33.3	33.3	33.3
	Female	14	66.7	66.7	100
	Total	21	100	100	

Sources and bibliography

Sources

Unprinted sources

Archive of the District of Upper Bavaria

Yearbooks Eglfing-Haar 1941–1959
Patient files 1941–1949: 180 randomly selected case files

Archive of the Hesse Land Welfare Association

Patient files 1941–1963: 370 randomly selected case files

Bavarian Main State Archive Munich

Files of the State Ministry of the Interior
No. 80911 Care of the mentally ill 1947–1955
No. 80914 Care of the mentally ill 1961

Federal Archive Koblenz

B106/36773 Deprivation of liberty and restrictions for the mentally ill, 1951–1963
B142/1017 Isolation of infected persons and commitment of the mentally ill. Implementation of Article 104 of the Basic Law, 1949–1955
B189/9106 International agreements on the exchange of information with respect to asylum committals, discharges, and death of the mentally ill—general, 1955–1969

Federal Archive Lichterfelde

DQ1 Ministry of Health
22109 Ministry of Health, Dept. of Health Protection Organization, Psychiatry
21228 Ministry of Health, Dept. of Health Protection. Sector General Health Protection/Psychiatry, Submissions from the general public, S–Z 1963
21230 Ministry of Health, Submissions from the general public 1959–62 Multiple sclerosis
3902, Department of Health, Submissions Psychiatry 1952–54
6691, Department of Health, 1955–67, Sector special medical care, Psychiatry

21600 Ministry of Health, State institutions, including Großschweidnitz and Rodewisch, Stralsund and Ueckermünde

Main Archive of the von Bodelschwingh Foundations Bethel

Patient files 1941–1963: 220 case files on the basis of the GORT system from the following holdings:
Mahanaim1
Mahanaim2
Morija1
Morija2
Gilead III

Hesse Main State Archive Marburg

Collection 180, No. 3589 Supervision and commitment of the mentally ill 1901–1947
Collection 401.13. No. 34: Disease control 1945–1953
Collection 401.15, No. 83: Health services
Collection 401.17, No. 219: Hessian agent at the Furth im Wald Border Crossing Point: Reports on the Admission of Displaced Persons into the Federal Territory and into the State of Hesse, 1950–1951

Greifswald Land Archive

Rep 200 9.1. Health and Social Services,
Sign. 14 District Assembly and Council of the District of Rostock, Dept. of Health; Situation reports on the care of psychiatric and neurological patients, 1957
Sign. 56 Council of the District of Rostock. Dept. of Health; specialized organs of the local councils, health care, Rostock district, work, reports

Schwerin Main Land Archive

5.12–7/1 Ministry of Medical Affairs. 10054 Terms of admission. vol. 2.

Saxony Main State Archive Dresden

Collection 10822, Großschweidnitz Land Asylum, Medical records 1956–63: 66 case files on the basis of the GORT system

Saxony State Archive Chemnitz

Collection 32810 Saxony Hospital for Psychiatry and Neurology Rodewisch (Land hospital), Medical records 1941–1955: 248 randomly selected case files

State Archive Munich

Collection: Police Headquarters. No. 7979 collective file: Haar Sanatorium-Nursing Home, 1941

318 *Sources and bibliography*

Collection District Administrative Office Munich,
No. 59141 Sanatorium-nursing home 1941–44
No. 20261 Mentally ill, crippled, deaf and dumb, blind 1851–1943

Munich City Archive

Collection health care, No. 117 Health Office, Marriage Counseling Center

Greifswald University Archive

Patient files 1941–1963: 400 case files on the basis of the GORT system

Printed sources

Psychiatric journals

Psychiatrie, Neurologie und medizinische Psychologie, 1949–1963
Der Nervenarzt, 1941–1963

Psychiatric textbooks and monographs

Bumke, Oswald, *Lehrbuch der Geisteskrankheiten* (Munich, 1936).
Ewald, Gottfried, *Neurologie und Psychiatrie. Ein Lehrbuch für Studierende und Ärzte* (Munich, 1944).
Ewald, Gottfried, *Neurologie und Psychiatrie. Ein Lehrbuch für Studierende und Ärzte* (Munich, 1948).
Ewald, Gottfried, *Neurologie und Psychiatrie. Ein Lehrbuch für Studierende und Ärzte* (Munich, 1954).
Ewald, Gottfried, *Neurologie und Psychiatrie. Ein Lehrbuch für Studierende und Ärzte* (Munich, 1959).
Fuhrmann, Manfred and Heinrich Korbsch, *Lehrbuch der Psychiatrie für Studierende, Ärzte und Juristen* (Leipzig, 1937).
Giljarowski, W. A., *Lehrbuch der Psychiatrie* (Berlin, 1960).
Hollmann, Werner, *Krankheit, Lebenskrise und soziales Schicksal* (Leipzig, 1940).
Kolle, Kurt, *Psychiatrie. Ein Lehrbuch für Studierende und Ärzte* (Berlin, 1943).
Kolle, Kurt, *Psychiatrie. Ein Lehrbuch für Studierende und Ärzte* (Berlin, 1949).
Kolle, Kurt, *Psychiatrie. Ein Lehrbuch für Studierende und Ärzte* (Stuttgart, 1961).
Lange, Johannes, *Kurz gefasstes Lehrbuch der Psychiatrie* (Leipzig, 1936).
Schneider, Kurt, *Die psychopathischen Persönlichkeiten* (Vienna, 1923–1943, first to eighth editions).

Bibliography

Althammer, Beate, "Pathologische Vagabunden. Psychiatrische Grenzziehungen um 1900," *GG*, vol. 3, 2013, 306–337.
Aly, Götz (ed.), *Aktion T4. 1939–1945. Die "Euthanasie"-Zentrale in der Tiergartenstrasse 4* (Berlin, 1989).
Aly, Götz, *Die Belasteten. "Euthanasie" 1939–1945. Eine Gesellschaftsgeschichte* (Frankfurt/M., 2013).

Andrews, Jonathan and Anne Digby, "Introduction. Gender and Class in the Historiography of British and Irish Psychiatry," in Andrews, Jonathan and Anne Digby (eds.), *Sex and Seclusion, Class and Custody. Perspectives on Gender and Class in the History of British and Irish Psychiatry* (Amsterdam, 2004), 7–44.

Ankele, Monika, *Alltag und Aneignung in Psychiatrien um 1900. Selbstzeugnisse von Frauen aus der Sammlung Prinzhorn* (Vienna, 2009).

Arenz, Dirk, *Eine kleine Geschichte der Schizophrenie* (Bonn, 2008).

Arndt, Agnes et al. (eds.), *Vergleichen, verflechten, verwirren? Europäische Geschichtsschreibung zwischen Theorie und Praxis* (Göttingen, 2011).

Ash, Mitchell G., "Kurt Gottschaldt and Psychological Research in Nazi and Socialist Germany," in Kristie Macrakis and Dieter Hoffmann (eds.), *Science under Socialism. East Germany in Comparative Perspective* (Cambridge, 1999), 286–301.

Ayaß, Wolfgang, *"Asoziale" im Nationalsozialismus* (Stuttgart, 1995).

Ayaß, Wolfgang, *"Gemeinschaftsfremde." Quellen zur Verfolgung von "Asozialen" 1933–1945* (Koblenz, 1998).

Bahners, Patrick and Alexander Cammann (eds.), *Bundesrepublik und DDR. Die Debatte um Hans-Ulrich Wehlers 'Deutsche Gesellschaftsgeschichte'* (Munich, 2009).

Bajohr, Frank and Michael Wildt, "Einleitung," in Frank Bajohr and Michael Wildt (eds.), *Volksgemeinschaft. Neue Forschungen zur Gesellschaft des Nationalsozialismus* (Frankfurt/M., 2009), 7–24.

Balz, Viola, *Zwischen Wirkung und Erfahrung—eine Geschichte der Psychopharmaka. Neuroleptika in der Bundesrepublik Deutschland, 1950–1980* (Bielefeld, 2010).

Bauerkämper, Arnd, "Von der Bodenreform zur Kollektivierung. Zum Wandel der ländlichen Gesellschaft in der Sowjetischen Besatzungszone Deutschlands und in der DDR 1945–1952," in Hartmut Kaelble et al. (eds.), *Sozialgeschichte der DDR* (Stuttgart, 1994), 119–143.

Bauerkämper, Arnd, *Ländliche Gesellschaft in der kommunistischen Diktatur. Zwangsmodernisierung und Tradition in Brandenburg 1945–1963* (Cologne, 2002).

Baumann, Jürgen, *Unterbringungsrecht und systematischer und synoptischer Kommentar zu den Unterbringungsgesetzen der Länder* (Tübingen, 1966).

Bänzinger, Peter-Paul, "Der betriebsame Mensch: ein Bericht (nicht nur) aus der Werkstatt," *Österreichische Zeitschrift für Geschichtswissenschaften*, vol. 2, 2012, 222–236.

Behnke, Klaus and Jürgen Fuchs (eds.), *Zersetzung der Seele: Psychologie und Psychiatrie im Dienste der Stasi* (Hamburg, 1995).

Behrens, Rudolf and Carsten Zelle (eds.), *Der ärztliche Fallbericht. Epistemische Grundlagen und textuelle Strukturen dargestellter Beobachtung* (Wiesbaden, 2012).

Behrens, Rudolf and Carsten Zelle, "Vorwort," in ibid., vii-xii.

Benzenhöfer, Udo and Wolfgang Eckart, *Medizin im Spielfilm des Nationalsozialismus* (Tecklenburg, 1999).

Berger, Georg, *Die Beratenden Psychiater des deutschen Heeres während des Zweiten Weltkrieges* (Freiburg, 1997).

Bernet, Brigitta, "'Eintragen' und Ausfüllen': Der Fall des psychiatrischen Formulars," in Sibylle Brändli et al. (eds.), *Zum Fall machen, zum Fall werden* (Frankfurt/M. 2009), 62–91.

Bernet, Brigitta, *Schizophrenie. Entstehung und Entwicklung eines psychiatrischen Krankheitsbildes um 1900* (Zürich, 2013).

Bernet, Brigitta and David Gugerli, "Sputniks Resonanzen. Der Aufstieg der Humankapiteltheorie im Kalten Krieg—eine Argumentationsskizze," *Historische Anthropologie*, vol. 3, 2011, 433–446.

Beyer, Christoph, *Von der Kreisirrenanstalt zum Pfalzklinikum. Eine Geschichte der Psychiatrie in Klingenmünster* (Kaiserslautern, 2009).

Bischof, Hans Ludwig, "Heil- und Pflegeanstalt Gabersee," in Michael von Cranach and Hans-Ludwig Siemen (eds.), *Psychiatrie im Nationalsozialismus. Die Bayerischen Heil- und Pflegeanstalten zwischen 1933 und 1945* (Munich, 1999), 363–379.

Blasius, Dirk, *"Einfache Seelenstörung." Geschichte der deutschen Psychiatrie 1800–1945* (Frankfurt/M., 1994).

Boldorf, Marcel, "Rehabilitation und Hilfen für Behinderte," in *1949–1961 Deutsche Demokratische Republik. Im Zeichen des Aufbaus des Sozialismus (Geschichte der Sozialpolitik in Deutschland seit 1945, vol. 8)* (Berlin, 2004), 455–494.

Borggräfe, Henning, *Schützenvereine im Nationalsozialismus. Pflege der "Volksgemeinschaft" und Vorbereitung auf den Krieg (1933–1945)* (Münster, 2011).

Borscheid, Peter, "Die 'taylorisierte' Hausfrau. Zu den Auswirkungen der Rationalisierungsbewegung auf den Privathaushalt der 20er Jahre," in Hans-Jürgen Gerhard (ed.), *Struktur und Dimension. Festschrift für Karl Heinrich Kaufhold zum 65. Geburtstag 2: Neunzehntes und Zwanzigstes Jahrhundert* (Stuttgart, 1997), 477–484.

Bourdieu, Pierre, *Die feinen Unterschiede. Kritik der gesellschaftlichen Urteilskraft* (Frankfurt/M., 1982).

Bourdieu, Pierre, *Sozialer Sinn. Kritik der theoretischen Vernunft* (Frankfurt/M., 1987).

Brändli, Sybille et al. (eds.), *Zum Fall machen, zum Fall werden. Wissensproduktion und Patientenerfahrung in Medizin und Psychiatrie des 19. und 20. Jahrhunderts* (Frankfurt/M., 2009).

Bretschneider, Falk et al. (eds.), *Personal und Insassen von "Totalen Institutionen"— zwischen Konfrontation und Verflechtung* (Leipzig, 2011).

Brink, Cornelia, *Grenzen der Anstalt. Psychiatrie und Gesellschaft in Deutschland 1860–1980* (Göttingen, 2010).

Brunner, Jürgen and Florian Steeger, "Johannes Heinrich Schultz (1884–1970)— Begründer des Autogenen Trainings. Ein biographischer Rekonstruktionsversuch im Spannungsfeld von Wissenschaft und Politik," *Bios*, vol. 1, 2006, 16–25.

Bruns, Florian, *Medizinethik im Nationalsozialismus. Entwicklungen und Protagonisten in Berlin (1939–1945)* (Stuttgart, 2009).

Burleigh, Michael, *Tod und Erlösung. Euthanasie in Deutschland 1900–1945* (Zürich, 2002).

Castel, Robert, "Vom Widerspruch der Psychiatrie," in Franco Basaglia and Franca Basaglia-Ongaro (eds.), *Befriedungsverbrechen. Über die Dienstbarkeit des Intellektuellen* (Frankfurt/M., 1980), 81–96.

Christians, Annemone, *Amtsgewalt und Volksgesundheit. Das öffentliche Gesundheitswesen im nationalsozialistischen München* (Göttingen, 2013).

Cocks, Geoffrey, *Psychotherapy in the Third Reich. The Göring Institute* (New York, 1985).

Collins, Harry M., "Tacit Knowledge, Trust and the Q of Sapphire," *Social Studies of Science*, vol. 3, 2001, 71–85.

Conci, Marco, *Sullivan neu entdecken. Leben und Werk Harry Stack Sullivans und seine Bedeutung für Psychiatrie, Psychotherapie und Psychoanalyse* (Gießen, 2005).

Conrad, Christoph, "Alterssicherung," in Hans Günter Hockerts (ed.), *Drei Wege deutscher Sozialstaatlichkeit. NS-Diktatur, Bundesrepublik und DDR im Vergleich* (Munich, 1998), 101–116.

Conze, Eckart, "Sicherheit als Kultur. Überlegungen zu einer 'modernen' Politikgeschichte' der Bundesrepublik Deutschland," *VfZ*, vol. 3, 2005, 357–380.

Cranach, Michael von and Hans-Ludwig Siemen (eds.), *Psychiatrie im Nationalsozialismus. Die Bayerischen Heil- und Pflegeanstalten zwischen 1933 und 1945* (Munich, 1999).

Condrau, Flurin, "The Patient's View Meets the Clinical Gaze," *Social History of Medicine*, vol. 3, 2007, 525–540.

Daston, Lorraine, "On Scientific Observation," *Isis*, vol. 1, 2008, 97–110.

Daston, Lorraine and Peter Galison, *Objectivity* (New York, 2010).

Degen, Barbara, *Bethel in der NS-Zeit. Die verschwiegene Geschichte* (Bad Homburg v. d. Höhe, 2014).

Diewald-Kerkmann, Gisela, "Denunziantentum und Gestapo. Die freiwilligen 'Helfer' aus der Bevölkerung," in Gerhard Paul and Klaus-Michael Mallmann (eds.), *Die Gestapo. Mythos und Realität* (Darmstadt, 1995), 288–305.

Dipper, Christof, "Moderne, Version: 1.0," *Docupedia-Zeitgeschichte*, URL: http://docupedia.de/zg/Moderne?oldid=84639 (accessed April 9, 2014).

Durkheim, Emile, *De la division du travail social* (Paris, 1922).

Ebbinghaus, Angelika and Klaus Dörner (eds.), *Vernichten und Heilen. Der Nürnberger Ärzteprozeß und seine Folgen* (Berlin, 2002).

Eberle, Annette, "Sozial–Asozial. Ausgrenzung und Verfolgung in der bayerischen Fürsorgepraxis 1934–1945," in *München und der Nationalsozialismus. Menschen, Orte, Strukturen* (Berlin, 2008), 207–226.

Eckart, Wolfgang, *Medizin in der NS-Diktatur. Ideologie, Praxis, Folgen* (Vienna, 2012).

Eckart, Wolfgang and Robert Jütte, *Medizingeschichte. Eine Einführung* (Cologne, 2007).

Eghigian, Greg, "The Psychologization of the Socialist Self. East German Forensic Psychology and its Deviants, 1945–1975," *German History*, vol. 2, 2004, 181–205.

Ehlerding, Mark, *Sind Klassifikationen sinnvoll? Zur Anwendbarkeit des Person-In-Environment System in der Klinischen Sozialarbeit* (Munich, 2002).

Ehmer, Joseph and Edith Sauer, "Arbeit," in Friedrich Jaeger (ed.), *Enzyklopädie der Neuzeit*, vol. 1 (Stuttgart, 2005), 507–533.

Eirund, Wolfgang, "Auswirkungen biologischer Krankheitsmodelle auf die psychiatrische Behandlung—eine medizin-historische Studie am Beispiel von Krankenakten aus zwei Jahrhunderten," in Christina Vanja et al. (eds.), *Wissen und irren. Psychiatriegeschichte aus zwei Jahrhunderten—Eberbach und Eichberg* (Kassel, 1999), 94–107.

Elkeles, Barbara, "Die schweigsame Welt von Arzt und Patient. Einwilligung und Aufklärung in der Arzt-Patient-Beziehung des 19. und frühen 20. Jahrhunderts," *Medizin, Gesellschaft und Geschichte*, vol. 8, 1989, 63–91.

Ellerbrock, Dagmar, *"Healing Democracy"—Demokratie als Heilmittel. Gesundheit, Krankheit und Politik in der amerikanischen Besatzungszone, 1945–1949* (Bonn, 2004).

Engstrom, Eric J., *Clinical Psychiatry in Imperial Germany. A History of Psychiatric Practice* (Ithaca, 2003).

Engstrom, Eric J., "Beyond Dogma and Discipline. New Directions in the History of Psychiatry," *Current Opinion in Psychiatry*, vol. 19, 2006, 595–599.

Engstrom, Eric J., "'On the Question of Degeneration' by Emil Kraepelin (1908)," *History of Psychiatry*, vol. 3, 2007, 389–398.

Engstrom, Eric J. et al., "Preface," in Eric J. Engstrom et al. (eds.), *Knowledge and Power. Perspectives in the History of Psychiatry* (Berlin, 1999), 9–10.

Engstrom, Eric J. and Matthias M. Weber, "Introduction to Special Issue: Making Kraepelin History. A Great Idea?", *History of Psychiatry*, vol. 3, 2007, 267–273.

Ernst, Anne Sabine, *"Die beste Prophylaxe ist der Sozialismus." Ärzte und medizinische Hochschullehrer in der SBZ/DDR 1945–1961* (Münster, 1997).

Fabisch, Hans et al., "Schizophrenie. Zur Geschichte der Schizophrenie Diagnostik," *Psychopraxis. Zeitschrift für Psychiatrie und Neurologie*, vol. 1, 2000, 26–32.

Faulstich, Heinz, *Hungersterben in der Psychiatrie* (Freiburg, 1993).

Faulstich, Heinz, *Von der Irrenfürsorge zur Euthanasie* (Freiburg, 1993).

Finnane, Mark, *Insanity and the Insane in Post-Famine Ireland* (London, 1981).

Fischer, Wolfgang and Hans-Peter Schmiedebach (eds.), Die Greifswalder *Universitäts- und Nervenklinik unter dem Direktorat von Hanns Schwarz 1946 bis 1965* (Greifswald, 1999).

Foucault, Michel, *Psychologie und Geisteskrankheit* (Frankfurt/M., 1968).

Foucault, Michel, *Wahnsinn und Gesellschaft* (Frankfurt/M., 1969).

Foucault, Michel, "Andere Räume," in Karlheinz Barck (ed.), *Aisthesis. Wahrnehmungen heute oder Perspektiven einer anderen Ästhetik. Essais* (Leipzig, 1991), 34–46.

Foucault, Michel, *Sicherheit, Territorium, Bevölkerung. Geschichte der Gouvernementalität I. Vorlesungen am Collège de France (1977–1978)* (Frankfurt/M., 2004).

Foucault, Michel, *Die Geburt der Biopolitik. Geschichte der Gouvernementalität II. Vorlesungen am Collège de France (1978–79)* (Frankfurt/M., 2004).

Foucault, Michel, *Die Ordnung des Diskurses* (Frankfurt/M., 2007).

Frevert, Ute, "Vertrauen—eine historische Spurensuche," in Ute Frevert (ed.), *Vertrauen–Historische Annäherungen* (Göttingen, 2003), 7–66.

Frevert, Ute, "Does Trust Have a History? Max Weber Lecture No. 2009/01, 2," URL: http://cadmus.eui.eu/bitstream/handle/1814/11258/MWP_LS_2009_01.pdf;jsessionid=43C3D99861F422AC1B3ED3BF0897FE25?sequence=1 (accessed July 2, 2014).

Friedländer, Henry, *Der Weg zum NS-Genozid. Von der Euthanasie zur Endlösung* (Berlin, 1997).

Fritzsche, Peter, *Life and Death in the Third Reich* (Harvard, 2008).

Fuchs, Petra et al. (eds.), *"Das Vergessen ist Teil der Vernichtung selbst." Lebensgeschichten von Opfern der nationalsozialistischen "Euthanasie"* (Göttingen, 2007).

Fulbrook, Mary, *Ein ganz normales Leben. Alltag und Gesellschaft in der DDR* (Darmstadt, 2008).

Fulbrook, Mary, *Dissonant lives. Generations and Violence through German dictatorships* (Oxford, 2011).

Gerhard, Uta, "Editorial," *L'Homme. Europäische Zeitschrift für feministische Geschichtswissenschaft*, vol. 19, 2008, 7–14.

Gilcher-Holthey, Ingrid, "Plädoyer für eine dynamische Mentalitätsgeschichte," *GG*, vol. 3, 1989, 476–497.

Gilman, Sander L., "Constructing Schizophrenia as a Category of Mental Illness," in Edwin R. Wallace and John Gach (eds.), *History of Psychiatry and Medical Psychology. With an Epilogue on Psychiatry and the Mind-Body Relation* (New York, 2008), 461–483.

Gitter, Wolfgang, "Soziale Sicherung bei Unfall und Berufskrankheit," in *1949–1961 Deutsche Demokratische Republik. Im Zeichen des Aufbaus des Sozialismus (Geschichte der Sozialpolitik in Deutschland seit 1945, vol. 8)* (Berlin, 2004), 437–452.

Goeschel, Christian, *Selbstmord im Dritten Reich* (Berlin, 2011).

Goffman, Erving, *Asyle. Über die soziale Situation von Patienten und anderer Insassen* (Berlin, 1973).

Goldberg, Ann, "Conventions of Madness. Bürgerlichkeit and the Asylum in the Vormärz," *Central European History*, vol. 2, 2000, 173–193.

Goldstein, Jan, *Console and Classify. The French Psychiatric Profession in the Nineteenth Century* (Chicago, 1992).

Goldstein, Jan, "Bringing the Psyche into Scientific Focus," in Theodore M. Porter and Dorothy Ross (eds.), *The Cambridge History of Science 7: The Modern Social Sciences* (Cambridge, 2003), 131–153.

Golinski, Jan, *Making Natural Knowledge. Constructivism and the History of Science* (Chicago, 2005).

Goltermann, Svenja, *Die Gesellschaft der Überlebenden. Deutsche Kriegsheimkehrer und ihre Gewalterfahrungen im Zweiten Weltkrieg* (Munich, 2009).

Gotto, Bernhard, *Nationalsozialistische Kommunalpolitik. Administrative Normalität und Systemstabilisierung durch die Augsburger Stadtverwaltung 1933–1945* (Munich, 2009).

Grashoff, Udo, *"In einem Anfall von Depression ..." Selbsttötung in der DDR* (Berlin, 2006).

Greyerz, Kaspar von et al., "Einführung. Schauplätze wissensgeschichtlicher Forschung," in Kaspar von Greyerz et al. (eds.), *Wissenschaftsgeschichte und Geschichte des Wissens im Dialog—Connecting Science and Knowledge* (Göttingen, 2013), 9–34.

Grundmann, Kornelia, "Vom Kaiserreich über die Weimarer Zeit bis zum Nationalsozialismus: Die Landesheilanstalt zur Zeit von Prof. Dr. Jahrmärker (1914–1937)," in Peter Sandner et al. (eds.), *Heilbar und nützlich. Ziele und Wege der Psychiatrie in Marburg an der Lahn* (Marburg, 2001), 247–275.

Gründler, Jens, *Armut und Wahnsinn. "Arme Irre" und ihre Familien im Spannungsfeld von Psychiatrie und Armenfürsorge in Glasgow 1875–1921* (Munich, 2013).

Grüsser, Otto-Joachim, "Richard Jung (1911–1986)," *Neuropsychologia*, vol. 4, 1987, 739–741.

Hachtmann, Rüdiger, "Arbeitsverfassung," in Hans Günter Hockerts (ed.), *Drei Wege deutscher Sozialstaatlichkeit. NS-Diktatur, Bundesrepublik und DDR im Vergleich* (Munich, 1998), 27–55.

Hahn, Susanne, "Pflegebedürftige alte Menschen im Nationalsozialismus," in Christoph Kopke (ed.), *Medizin und Verbrechen. Festschrift zum 60. Geburtstag von Walter Wuttke* (Ulm, 2001), 131–142.

Hanrath, Sabine, *Zwischen Euthanasie und Psychiatriereform. Anstaltspsychiatrie in Westfalen und Brandenburg: Ein deutsch-deutscher Vergleich (1945–1964)* (Paderborn, 2004).

Hauschildt, Elke, *"Auf den richtigen Weg zwingen … ." Trinkerfürsorge 1922–1945* (Freiburg, 1995).

Hähner-Rombach, Sylvelyn, *Gesundheit und Krankheit im Spiegel von Petitionen an den Landtag von Baden-Württemberg 1946 bis 1980* (Stuttgart, 2011).

Hellbeck, Jochen, "Introduction," in Jochen Hellbeck and Klaus Heller (eds.), *Autobiographische Praktiken in Russland. Autobiographical Practices in Russia* (Göttingen, 2004), 11–25.

Hellbeck, Jochen, "Russian Autobiographical Practice," in ibid., 279–299.

Helwig, Gisela and Barbara Hille, "Familie-, Jugend- und Altenpolitik," in *1949–1961 Deutsche Demokratische Republik. Im Zeichen des Aufbaus des Sozialismus (Geschichte der Sozialpolitik in Deutschland seit 1945, vol. 8)* (Berlin, 2004), 495–553.

Herbert, Ulrich, *Fremdarbeiter. Politik und Praxis des "Ausländer-Einsatzes" in der Kriegswirtschaft des "Dritten Reiches"* (Berlin, 1985).

Herbert, Ulrich, "Traditionen des Rassismus," in Ulrich Herbert (ed.), *Arbeit, Volkstum, Weltanschauung. Über Fremde und deutsche im 20. Jahrhundert* (Frankfurt/M., 1995), 11–29.

Herbert, Ulrich, *Best. Biographische Studien über Radikalismus, Weltanschauung und Vernunft 1903–1989* (Bonn, 1996).

Herbert, Ulrich, "Liberalisierung als Lernprozeß. Die Bundesrepublik in der deutschen Geschichte–eine Skizze," in Ulrich Herbert (ed.), *Wandlungsprozesse in Westdeutschland. Belastung, Integration, Liberalisierung 1945–1980* (Göttingen, 2002), 7–49.

Hess, Volker, "Die moralische Ökonomie der Normalisierung. Das Beispiel Fiebermessen," in Werner Sohn and Herbert Mehrtens (eds.), *Normalität und Abweichung. Studien zur Theorie und Geschichte der Normalisierungsgesellschaft* (Opladen, 1999), 222–243.

Hess, Volker, "Formalisierte Beobachtung. Die Genese der modernen Krankengeschichte am Beispiel der Berliner und Pariser Medizin (1725–1830)," *Medizinhistorisches Journal*, vol. 45, 2010, 293–340.

Hess, Volker and Benoit Majerus, "Writing the History of Psychiatry in the 20th Century," *History of Psychiatry*, vol. 22, 2011, 139–145.

Hess, Volker and Heinz-Peter Schmiedebach (eds.), *Am Rande des Wahnsinns. Schwellenräume einer urbanen Moderne* (Vienna, 2012).

Hockerts, Hans Günter, *Sozialpolitische Entscheidungen im Nachkriegsdeutschland. Alliierte und deutsche Sozialversicherungspolitik* (Stuttgart, 1980).

Hockerts, Hans Günter, "Einführung," in Hans Günter Hockerts (ed.), *Drei Wege Deutscher Sozialstaatlichkeit. NS-Diktatur, Bundesrepublik und DDR im Vergleich* (Munich, 1998), 7–27.

Hoffmann, Dierk, "Sicherung bei Alter, Invalidität und für Hinterbliebene, Sonderversorgungssysteme," in *1949–1961 Deutsche Demokratische Republik. Im Zeichen des Aufbaus des Sozialismus (Geschichte der Sozialpolitik in Deutschland seit 1945, vol. 8)* (Berlin, 2004), 347–387.

Hoffmann, Dierk and Michael Schwartz, "Politische Rahmenbedingungen," in *1949–1961 Deutsche Demokratische Republik. Im Zeichen des Aufbaus des Sozialismus (Geschichte der Sozialpolitik in Deutschland seit 1945, vol. 8)* (Berlin, 2004), 1–73.

Hoffmann, Dierk and Michael Schwartz, "Gesellschaftliche Strukturen und sozialpolitische Handlungsfelder," in ibid., 75–158.

Hoffmann, Susanne, *Gesunder Alltag im 20. Jahrhundert? Geschlechterspezifische Diskurse und gesundheitsrelevante Verhaltensstile in deutschsprachigen Ländern* (Stuttgart, 2010).

Hörath, Julia, "'Arbeitsscheue Volksgenossen.' Leistungsbereitschaft als Kriterium der Inklusion und Exklusion," URL: http://arbeit-im-nationalsozialismus. oldenbourg-verlag.de/open-peer-review/hoerath/ (accessed March 14, 2014).

Huppmann, Gernot, "Milieuschäden intramural untergebrachter Geisteskranker: eine historiographisch-medizinpsychologische Studie zum 'Anstaltssyndrom,'" in Gernot Huppmann (ed.), *Prolegomena einer medizinischen Psychologie der Hoffnung* (Würzburg, 2006), 455–502.

Hübner, Peter, "Die Zukunft war gestern. Soziale und mentale Trends in der DDR-Industriearbeiterschaft," in Hartmut Kaelble et al. (eds.), *Sozialgeschichte der DDR* (Stuttgart, 1994), 171–187.

Hübner, Peter, *Arbeiter in der SBZ-DDR* (Essen, 1999).

Hübner, Peter, "Betriebe als Träger der Sozialpolitik, betriebliche Sozialpolitik," in *1949–1961 Deutsche Demokratische Republik. Im Zeichen des Aufbaus des Sozialismus (Geschichte der Sozialpolitik in Deutschland seit 1945, vol. 8)* (Berlin, 2004), 727–774.

Hübner, Peter, *Arbeit, Arbeiter und Technik in der DDR 1971 bis 1989. Zwischen Fordismus und digitaler Revolution* (Bonn, 2014).

Hürtgen, Renate, *Ausreise per Antrag: der lange Weg nach drüben. Eine Studie über Herrschaft und Alltag in der DDR-Provinz* (Göttingen, 2014).

Imbusch, Peter, "Macht und Herrschaft in der wissenschaftlichen Kontroverse," in Peter Imbusch (ed.), *Macht und Herrschaft. Sozialwissenschaftliche Theorien und Konzeptionen* (Wiesbaden, 2013), 9–35.

Jarausch, Konrad, "Fürsorgediktatur, Version: 1.0," *Docupedia-Zeitgeschichte*, February 11, 2010, URL: http://docupedia.de/zg/F.C3.BCrsorgediktatur?oldid= 106417 (accessed April 11, 2014).

Jeggle, Utz, "Scheitern lernen," in Stefan Zahlmann and Sylka Scholz (eds.), *Scheitern und Biographie. Die andere Seite moderner Lebensgeschichten* (Gießen, 2005), 221–236.

Jessen, Ralph, "Polizei und Gesellschaft. Zum Paradigmenwechsel in der Polizeigeschichtsforschung," in Gerhard Paul and Klaus-Michael Mallmann (eds.), *Die Gestapo. Mythos und Realität* (Darmstadt, 1995), 19–46.

Jessen, Ralph, "Die Gesellschaft im Staatssozialismus. Probleme einer Sozialgeschichte der DDR," *GG*, vol. 1, 1995, 96–110.

Jessen, Ralph, *Akademische Elite und kommunistische Diktatur. Die ostdeutsche Hochschullehrerschaft in der Ulbricht-Ära* (Göttingen, 1999).

Jureit, Ulrike, "Motive-Mentalitäten-Handlungsspielräume. Theoretische Anmerkungen zu Handlungsoptionen von Soldaten," in Christian Hartmann et al. (eds.), *Verbrechen der Wehrmacht. Bilanz einer Debatte* (Munich, 2005), 163–170.

Jütte, Robert, *Medizin im Nationalsozialismus. Bilanz und Perspektiven der Forschung* (Göttingen, 2011).

Kaelble, Hartmut, "Die Debatte über Vergleich und Transfer und was jetzt?," *H-Soz-u-Kult*, February 8, 2005, URL: http://hsozkult.geschichte.hu-berlin.de/forum/id= 574&type=artikel (accessed June 7, 2014).

Kaufmann, Doris, *Aufklärung, bürgerliche Selbsterfahrung und die "Erfindung" der Psychiatrie in Deutschland, 1770–1850* (Göttingen, 1995).

Kaufmann, Doris, "Nervenschwäche, Neurasthenie und 'sexuelle Frage' im deutschen Kaiserreich," in Christine Wolters et al. (ed.), *Abweichung und Normalität. Psychiatrie in Deutschland vom Kaiserreich bis zur Deutschen Einheit* (Bielefeld, 2013), 197–209.

Kaufmann, Franz-Xaver, "Sicherheit. Das Leitbild beherrschbarer Komplexität," in Stephan Lessenich (ed.), *Wohlfahrtstaatliche Grundbegriffe. Historische und aktuelle Diskurse* (Frankfurt/M., 2003), 73–104.

Klee, Ernst, *"Euthanasie" im NS-Staat. Die Vernichtung lebensunwerten Lebens* (Frankfurt/M., 1983).

Klee, Ernst, *Das Personenlexikon zum "Dritten Reich." Wer war was vor und nach 1945* (Frankfurt/M., 2005).

Kleßmann, Christoph, *Die doppelte Staatsgründung: Deutsche Geschichte 1945–1955* (Bonn, 1991).

Kleßmann, Christoph, *Arbeiter im "Arbeiterstaat" DDR. Deutsche Traditionen, sowjetisches Modell, westdeutsches Magnetfeld (1945–1971)* (Bonn, 2007).

Klöppel, Ulrike, "1954. Brigade Propaphenin arbeitet an der Ablösung des Megaphen. Der prekäre Beginn der Psychopharmakaproduktion der DDR," in Nicholas Eschenbuch et al. (eds.), *Arzneimittel des 20. Jahrhunderts. Historische Skizzen von Lebertran bis Contergan* (Bielefeld, 2009), 199–223.

Kocka, Jürgen, "Eine durchherrschte Gesellschaft," in Hartmut Kaelble et al. (eds.), *Sozialgeschichte der DDR* (Stuttgart, 1994), 547–553.

Kocka, Jürgen, "Wissenschaft und Politik in der DDR," in Jürgen Kocka and Renate Mayntz (eds.), *Wissenschaft und Wiedervereinigung: Disziplinen im Umbruch* (Berlin, 1998), 435–459.

Kocka, Jürgen, "Mehr Last als Lust. Arbeit und Arbeitsgesellschaft in der europäischen Gesellschaft," *JbW*, vol. 2, 2005, 185–206.

Kohli, Martin, "Die DDR als Arbeitsgesellschaft? Arbeit, Lebenslauf und soziale Differenzierung," in Hartmut Kaelble et al. (eds.), *Sozialgeschichte der DDR* (Stuttgart, 1994), 31–61.

Kollmeier, Kathrin, *Ordnung und Ausgrenzung. Die Disziplinarpolitik der Hitler-Jugend* (Göttingen, 2007).

Korzilius, Sven, *"Asoziale" und "Parasiten" im Recht der SBZ/DDR* (Cologne, 2005).

Koselleck, Reinhart, "'Erfahrungsraum' und 'Erwartungshorizont'—zwei historische Kategorien," in Reinhart Koselleck (ed.), *Vergangene Zukunft. Zur Semantik geschichtlicher Zeiten* (Frankfurt/M., 1979), 349–375.

Kossert, Andreas, *Kalte Heimat. Die Geschichte der deutschen Vertriebenen nach 1945* (Bonn, 2008).

Kramer, Nicole, *Volksgenossinnen an der "Heimatfront." Mobilisierung, Verhalten, Erinnerung* (Göttingen, 2011).

Kranig, Andreas, *Lockerung und Zwang. Zur Arbeitsverfassung im "Dritten Reich"* (Stuttgart, 1983).

Krumpolt, Holm, "Die Landesanstalt Großschweidnitz als 'T4' Zwischenanstalt und als Tötungsansanstalt (1939–1945)," in Stiftung Sächsische Gedenkstätten (ed.), *Nationalsozialistische Euthanasieverbrechen. Beiträge zur Aufarbeitung ihrer Geschichte in Sachsen* (Dresden, 2004), 137–147.

Kundrus, Birthe, "Regime der Differenz. Volkstumspolitische Inklusion und Exklusion im Warthegau und im Generalgouverment, 1939–1945," in Frank Bajohr and Michael Wildt (eds.), *Volksgemeinschaft. Neue Forschungen zur Gesellschaft des Nationalsozialismus* (Frankfurt/M., 2009), 105–123.

Kundrus, Birthe, "Der Holocaust. Die 'Volksgemeinschaft' als Verbrechensgemeinschaft?," in Hans-Ulrich Thamer and Simone Erpel (eds.), *Hitler und die Deutschen. Volksgemeinschaft und Verbrechen* (Berlin, 2010), 130–136.

Kundrus, Birthe and Sybille Steinbacher, "Einleitung," in Birthe Kundrus (ed.), *Kontinuitäten und Diskontinuitäten. Der Nationalsozialismus in der Geschichte des 20. Jahrhunderts* (Göttingen, 2013), 9–29.

Kupke, Christian, "Was ist so unverständlich am Wahn? Philosophisch-kritische Darstellung des Jaspers'schen Unverständlichkeitstheorems," *Journal für Philosophie & Psychiatrie*, vol. 1, 2008, 1–12.

Kury, Patrick, *Der Überforderte Mensch. Eine Wissensgeschichte vom Stress zum Burnout* (Frankfurt/M., 2012).

Labisch, Alfons and Reinhard Spree, "Neuere Entwicklungen und aktuelle Trends in der Sozialgeschichte der Medizin in Deutschland—Rückschau und Ausblick," *VSWG*, vol. 3, 1997, 305–321.

Lachmund, Jens and Gunnar Stollberg, *Patientenwelten. Krankheit und Medizin vom späten 18. Bis zum frühen 20. Jahrhundert im Spiegel von Autobiographien* (Opladen, 1995).

Landwehr, Achim, "Diskurs und Diskursgeschichte," *Docupedia-Zeitgeschichte*, February 11, 2010, URL: http://docupedia.de/zg/Diskurs_und_Diskursgeschichte?oldid=84596, 6 (accessed July 22, 2014).

Ledebur, Sophie, *Das Wissen der Anstaltspsychiatrie in der Moderne. Zur Geschichte der Heil- und Pflegeanstalten Am Steinhof Wien* (Vienna, 2011).

Lengwiler, Martin, "Auf dem Weg zur Sozialtechnologie. Die Bedeutung der frühen Militärpsychiatrie für die Professionalisierung der Psychiatrie in Deutschland," in Eric. J. Engstrom and Volker Roelcke (eds.), *Psychiatrie im 19. Jahrhundert. Forschungen zur Geschichte von psychiatrischen Institutionen, Debatten und Praktiken im deutschen Sprachraum* (Mainz, 2003), 245–263.

Lerner, Paul, "Psychiatry and Casualties of War in Germany, 1914–18," *Journal of Contemporary History*, vol. 1, 2000, 13–28.

Lerner, Paul, *Hysterical Men. War, Psychiatry, and the Politics of Trauma in Germany, 1890–1930* (Ithaca, 2003).

Leuenberger, Christine, "Socialist Psychotherapy and its Dissidents," *Journal of the History of the Behavioral Sciences*, vol. 37, 2001, 261–273.

Lindenberger, Thomas, "Die Diktatur der Grenzen. Zur Einleitung," in Thomas Lindenberger (ed.), *Herrschaft und Eigen-Sinn in der Diktatur. Studien zur Gesellschaftsgeschichte der DDR* (Cologne, 1999), 13–44.

Lindenberger, Thomas, "Herrschaft und Eigen-Sinn in der Diktatur. Das Alltagsleben in der DDR und sein Platz in der Erinnerungskultur des vereinten Deutschlands," *Aus Politik und Zeitgeschichte*, vol. 40, 2000, URL: http://www.bpb.de/apuz/25409/herrschaft-und-eigen-sinn-in-der-diktatur?p=all (accessed April 11, 2014).

Lindenberger, Thomas, "In den Grenzen der Diktatur. Die DDR als Gegenstand von 'Gesellschaftsgeschichte,'" in Rainer Eppelmann et al. (eds.), *Bilanz und Perspektiven der DDR-Forschung* (Paderborn, 2003), 239–245.

Lindenberger, Thomas, "'Asociality' and Modernity. The GDR as a Welfare Dictatorship," in Katherine Pence and Paul Betts (eds.), *Socialist Modern. East German Everyday Culture and Politics* (Ann Arbor, 2011), 211–233.

Lindner, Ulrike, "Unterschiedliche Traditionen und Konzepte. Frauen und Geschlechtskrankheiten als Problem der Gesundheitspolitik in Großbritannien und Deutschland," in Ulrike Lindner and Merith Niehuss (eds.), *Ärztinnen–Patientinnen. Frauen im deutschen und britischen Gesundheitswesen des 20. Jahrhunderts* (Cologne, 2002), 215–242.

Lindner, Ulrike, *Gesundheitspolitik in der Nachkriegszeit. Großbritannien und die Bundesregierung Deutschland im Vergleich* (Munich, 2004).

Longerich, Peter, *"Davon haben wir nichts gewusst!" Die Deutschen und die Judenverfolgung 1933–1945* (Bonn, 2006).

Lutz, Petra, "Herz und Vernunft. Angehörige von 'Euthanasie'-Opfern im Schriftwechsel mit den Anstalten," in Heiner Fangerau and Karen Nolte (eds.), *"Moderne" Anstaltspsychiatrie im 19. Und 20. Jahrhundert–Legitimation und Kritik* (Stuttgart, 2006), 143–168.

Lutz, Petra et al., "NS-Gesellschaft und 'Euthanasie'. Die Reaktionen der Eltern ermordeter Kinder," in Christoph Mundt et al. (eds.), *Psychiatrische Forschung und NS-"Euthanasie." Beiträge zu einer Gedenkveranstaltung an der Psychiatrischen Universitätsklinik Heidelberg* (Heidelberg, 2001), 97–113.

Lüdtke, Alf, "Einleitung. Herrschaft als soziale Praxis," in Alf Lüdtke (ed.), *Herrschaft als soziale Praxis. Historische und sozialanthropologische Studien* (Göttingen, 1991), 9–63.

Lüdtke, Alf, *"Sicherheit" und "Wohlfahrt." Polizei, Gesellschaft und Herrschaft im 19. Und 20. Jahrhundert* (Frankfurt/M., 1992).

Lüdtke, Alf, *Eigen-Sinn. Fabrikalltag, Arbeitererfahrungen und Politik vom Kaiserreich bis in den Faschismus* (Hamburg, 1993).

Lüdtke, Alf, "'Helden der Arbeit'-Mühen beim Arbeiten," in Hartmut Kaelble et al. (eds.), *Sozialgeschichte der DDR* (Stuttgart, 1994), 189–213.

Lüdtke, Alf, "People Working. Everyday Life and German Fascism," *History Workshop Journal*, vol. 50, 2000, 76–92.

Lüdtke, Alf, "'Fehlgreifen in der Wahl der Mittel.' Optionen im Alltag militärischen Handelns," *Mittelweg 36*, vol. 12, 2003, issue 1, 61–75.

Lüdtke, Alf, "The World of Men's Work, East and West," in Katherine Pence and Paul Betts (eds.), *Socialist Modern. East German Everyday Culture and Politics* (Ann Arbor, 2011), 234–249.

Mallmann, Klaus-Michael, "Die V-Leute der Gestapo. Umrisse einer kollektiven Biographie," in Gerhard Paul and Klaus-Michael Mallmann (eds.), *Die Gestapo. Mythos und Realität* (Darmstadt, 1995), 268–288.

Mallmann, Klaus-Michael and Gerhard Paul, "Die Gestapo. Weltanschauungsexekutive mit gesellschaftlichem Rückhalt," in Klaus-Michael Mallmann and Gerhard Paul (eds.), *Die Gestapo im Zweiten Weltkrieg. "Heimatfront" und besetztes Europa* (Darmstadt, 2000), 599–650.

Mallmann, Klaus-Michael and Gerhard Paul, *Karrieren der Gewalt. Nationalsozialistische Täterbiographien* (Darmstadt, 2004).

Mallmann, Klaus-Michael and Andrej Angrick (eds.), *Die Gestapo nach 1945. Konflikte, Karrieren, Konstruktionen* (Darmstadt, 2009).

Maubach, Franka, *Die Stellung halten. Kriegserfahrungen und Lebensgeschichten der Wehrmachthelferinnen* (Göttingen, 2009).

Meier, Marietta et al., *Zwang zur Ordnung. Psychiatrie im Kanton Zürich, 1870–1970* (Zürich, 2007).

Meuschel, Sigrid, "Überlegungen zu einer Herrschafts- und Gesellschaftsgeschichte der DDR," *GG*, vol. 1, 1993, 5–14.

Meyer, Beate, "Erfühlte und erdachte 'Volksgemeinschaft.' Erfahrungen 'jüdischer Mischlinge' zwischen Integration und Ausgrenzung," in Frank Bajohr and Michael Wildt (eds.), *Volksgemeinschaft. Neue Forschungen zur Gesellschaft des Nationalsozialismus* (Frankfurt/M., 2009), 144–164.

Moeller, Robert, *War Stories. The Search for a Usable Past in the Federal Republic of Germany* (Berkeley, 2001).

Moldzio, Andrea, *Schizophrenie—eine philosophische Erkrankung?* (Würzburg, 2004).

Möckel, Benjamin, "'Mit 70 Jahren hat kein Mensch das Recht, sich alt zu fühlen.'—Altersdiskurse und Bilder des Alters in der NS-Sozialpolitik," *Österreichische Zeitschrift für Geschichtswissenschaften*, vol. 22, 2013, 112–134.

Murray, T. Jock, *Multiple Sclerosis. The History of a Disease* (New York, 2005).

Müller, Roland, "Militärpsychiatrie im Zweiten Weltkrieg. Die Reservelazarette III und IV in der Landesheilanstalt," in Peter Sandner et al. (eds.), *Heilbar und nützlich. Ziele und Wege der Psychiatrie in Marburg an der Lahn* (Marburg, 2001), 305–314.

Neitzel, Sönke and Harald Welzer, *Soldaten. Protokolle vom Kämpfen, Töten und Sterben* (Frankfurt/M., 2011).

Nellen, Stefan and Robert Suter, "Unfälle, Vorfälle, Fälle: Eine Archäologie des polizeilichen Blicks," in Sybille Brändli et al. (eds.), *Zum Fall machen, zum Fall werden. Wissensproduktion und Patientenerfahrung in Medizin und Psychiatrie des 19. Und 20. Jahrhunderts* (Frankfurt/M., 2009), 159–181.

Neubert, Ehrhart, *Geschichte der Opposition in der DDR 1949–1989* (Berlin, 2000).

Neuner, Stephanie, *Politik und Psychiatrie. Die staatliche Versorgung psychisch Kriegsbeschädigter in Deutschland 1920–1939* (Göttingen, 2011).

Nolte, Karen, "'So ein Gefühl, als wenn sich jeder Nerv im Kopf zusammenziehe.' Die 'moderne' Diagnose Nervosität—Zum Konzept der Marburger Anstalt am Beispiel der Behandlung 'nervöser' Patientinnen (1876–1918)," in Peter Sandner et al. (eds.), *Heilbar und nützlich. Ziele und Wege der Psychiatrie in Marburg an der Lahn* (Marburg, 2001), 184–200.

Paul, Gerhard and Klaus-Michael Mallmann (eds.), *Die Gestapo. Mythos und Realität* (Darmstadt, 1995).

Paul, Gerhard and Klaus-Michael Mallmann, *Die Gestapo im Zweiten Weltkrieg. "Heimatfront" und besetztes Europa* (Darmstadt, 2000).

Peukert, Detlef, *Volksgenossen und Gemeinschaftsfremde. Anpassung, Ausmerze und Aufbegehren unter dem Nationalsozialismus* (Cologne, 1982).

Pfister, Ulrich, "Unterschicht," in Friedrich Jaeger (ed.), *Enzyklopädie der Neuzeit* 13 (Stuttgart, 2011), 1089–1092.

Pohl, Dieter, *Verfolgung und Massenmord in der NS-Zeit 1933–1945* (Darmstadt, 2003).

Polanyi, Michael, *Personal Knowledge. Towards a Post-Critical Philosophy* (Chicago, 1958).

Port, Andrew I., *Die rätselhafte Stabilität der DDR. Arbeit und Alltag im sozialistischen Deutschland* (Berlin, 2010).

Porter, Roy, "Introduction," in Roy Porter (ed.), *Patients and Practitioners. Lay Perceptions of Medicine in Pre-Industrial Society* (Cambridge, 1985), 1–22.

Porter, Roy, "The Patient's View. Doing Medical History from Below," *Theory and Society*, vol. 14, 1985, 175–198.

Putz, Christa, "Narrative Heterogenität und dominante Darstellungsweise. Zur Produktion von Fallnarrativen in der deutschsprachigen Sexualmedizin und Psychoanalyse, 1890 bis 1930," in Sibylle Brändli et al. (eds.), *Zum Fall machen, zum Fall werden* (Frankfurt/M., 2009), 92–120.

Quinkert, Babette et al., "Einleitung," in Babette Quinkert et al. (eds.), *Krieg und Psychiatrie 1914–1950* (Göttingen, 2010), 9–28.

Raffnsøe, Sverre et al., *Foucault. Studienhandbuch* (Munich, 2011).

Reemtsma, Jan Philipp, "Über den Begriff 'Handlungsspielräume,'" *Mittelweg 36*, vol. 3, 2004, 5–23.

Reichel, Peter, *Erfundene Erinnerung. Weltkrieg und Judenmord in Film und Theater* (Vienna, 2004).

Reichhardt, Sven, "Praxeologische Geschichtswissenschaft. Eine Diskussionsanregung," *Sozial. Geschichte*, vol. 3, 2007, 43–65.

Rieß, Volker, "Zentrale und dezentrale Radikalisierung. Die Tötungen 'unwerten Lebens' in den annektierten west- und nordpolnischen Gebieten 1939–1941," in Klaus-Michael Mallmann and Bogdan Musial (eds.), *Genesis des Genozids—Polen 1939–1941* (Darmstadt, 2004), 127–145.

Roelcke, Volker, *Krankheit und Kulturkritik. Psychiatrische Gesellschaftsdeutungen im bürgerlichen Zeitalter (1790–1914)* (Frankfurt/M., 1999).

Roelcke, Volker, "Psychotherapy between Medicine, Psychoanalysis, and Politics. Concepts, Practices, and Institutions in Germany, c. 1945–1992," *Medical History*, vol. 4, 2004, 473–492.

Roelcke, Volker, "Auf der Suche nach der Politik in der Wissensproduktion. Plädoyer für eine historisch-politische Epistemologie," *Berichte zur Wissenschaftsgeschichte*, vol. 33, 2010, 176–192.

Roelcke, Volker, "Die Etablierung der psychiatrischen Genetik, ca. 1900–1960. Wechselbeziehungen zwischen Psychiatrie, Eugenik und Humangenetik," in Christine Wolters et al. (eds.), *Abweichung und Normalität. Psychiatrie in Deutschland vom Kaiserreich bis zur Deutschen Einheit* (Bielefeld, 2013), 111–135.

Roesler, Jörg, "Die Produktionsbrigaden in der Industrie der DDR. Zentrum der Arbeitswelt?" in Hartmut Kaelble et al. (eds.), *Sozialgeschichte der DDR* (Stuttgart, 1994), 144–170.

Rosa, Hartmut et al., *Soziologische Theorien* (Konstanz, 2013).

Rose, Wolfgang, *Anstaltspsychiatrie in der DDR. Die brandenburgischen Kliniken zwischen 1945 und 1990* (Berlin, 2005).

Roth, Karl Heinz, "'Ich klage an'—Aus der Entstehungsgeschichte eines Propaganda-Films," in Götz Aly (ed.), *Aktion T4. 1939–1945. Die "Euthanasie"-Zentrale in der Tiergartenstrasse* (Berlin, 1989), 93–116.

Rüting, Torsten, *Pavlov und der Neue Mensch. Diskurse und Disziplinierung in Sowjetrussland* (Munich, 2002).

Rupieper, Hermann-J. et al. (eds.), *Die mitteldeutsche Chemieindustrie und ihre Arbeiter im 20. Jahrhundert* (Halle, 2005).

Sabrow, Martin, "Sozialismus als Sinnwelt. Diktatorische Herrschaft in kulturhistorischer Perspektive," *Potsdamer Bulletin für Zeithistorische Studien*, vol. 40/41, 2007, 9–23.

Sachse, Carola, *Der Hausarbeitstag. Gerechtigkeit und Gleichberechtigung in Ost und West 1939–1994* (Göttingen, 2002).

Sammet, Kai, "Paratext und Text. Über das Abheften und die Verwendung psychiatrischer Krankenakten. Beispiele aus den Jahren 1900 bis 1930," *Schriftenreihe der Deutschen Gesellschaft zur Geschichte der Nervenheilkunde*, vol. 12, 2006, 339–367.

Sandkühler, Thomas, *"Endlösung" in Galizien. Der Judenmord in Ostpolen und die Rettungsinitiativen von Berthold Beitz 1941–44* (Bonn, 1996).

Sandner, Peter et al. (ed.), *Heilbar und nützlich. Ziele und Wege der Psychiatrie in Marburg an der Lahn* (Marburg, 2001).

Sandner, Peter et al., "Einleitung," in ibid., 14–20.

Sarasin, Philipp, *Reizbare Maschinen. Eine Geschichte des Körpers 1765–1914* (Frankfurt/M., 2001).

Sarasin, Philipp et al., "Eine Einleitung," in Philipp Sarasin et al. (eds.), *Bakteriologie und Moderne. Studien zur Biopolitik des Unsichtbaren 1870–1920* (Frankfurt/M., 2007), 8–43.

Schagen, Udo and Sabine Schleiermacher, "Gesundheitswesen und Sicherung bei Krankheit," in *1949–1961 Deutsche Demokratische Republik. Im Zeichen des Aufbaus des Sozialismus (Geschichte der Sozialpolitik in Deutschland seit 1945, vol. 8)* (Berlin, 2004), 390–435.

Schewe, Jörg, "Die Geschichte der Sicherungsverwahrung. Entstehung, Entwicklung und Reform" (Dissertation, Kiel, 1999).

Schikorra, Christa, *Kontinuitäten der Ausgrenzung. "Asoziale" Häftlinge im Frauen-Konzentrationslager Ravensbrück* (Berlin, 2001).

Schildt, Axel, "Freizeit, Kultur und Häuslichkeit in der 'Wiederaufbau'-Gesellschaft. Zur Modernisierung von Lebensstilen in der Bundesrepublik. Deutschland in den 1950er Jahren," in Hannes Siegrist et al. (eds.), *Europäische Konsumgeschichte. Zur Gesellschafts- und Kulturgeschichte des Konsums (18. bis 20. Jahrhundert)* (Frankfurt/M., 1997), 327–349.

Schildt, Axel, *Zwischen Abendland und Amerika. Studien zur westdeutschen Ideenlandschaft der 50er Jahre* (Munich, 1999).

Schlich, Thomas, "How Gods and Saints Became Transplant Surgeons. The Scientific Article as a Model for the Writing of History," *History of Science*, vol. 33, 1995, 311–331.

Schlich, Thomas, "Wissenschaftliche Fakten als Thema der Geschichtsforschung," in Norbert Paul and Thomas Schlich (eds.), *Medizingeschichte. Aufgaben, Probleme, Perspektiven* (Frankfurt/M., 1997), 107–129.

Schmidt, Gerhardt, *Selektion in der Heilanstalt 1939–1945* (Stuttgart, 1965).

Schmiedebach, Heinz-Peter, "Psychoanalyse, Psychotherapie und die Lehre von Pawlow im Werk von Hanns Schwarz," in Wolfgang Fischer and Heinz-Peter Schmiedebach (eds.), *Die Greifswalder Universitäts- und Nervenklinik unter dem Direktorat von Hanns Schwarz 1946 bis 1965* (Greifswald, 1999), 30–47.

Schmuhl, Hans-Walter, "Die Patientenmorde," in Angelika Ebbinghaus and Klaus Dörner (eds.), *Vernichten und Heilen. Der Nürnberger Ärzteprozeß und seine Folge* (Berlin, 2001), 295–331.

Schott, Heinz and Rainer Tölle, *Geschichte der Psychiatrie. Krankheitslehren, Irrwege, Behandlungsformen* (Munich, 2006).

Schöttler, Peter, "Mentalitäten, Ideologien, Diskurse. Zur sozialgeschichtlichen Thematisierung der 'dritten Ebene,'" in Alf Lüdtke (ed.), *Alltagsgeschichte. Zur Rekonstruktion historischer Erfahrungen und Lebensweisen* (Frankfurt/M., 1989), 85–136.

Schulz, Günther, "Soziale Sicherung von Frauen und Familien," in Hans Günter Hockerts (ed.), *Drei Wege deutscher Sozialstaatlichkeit. NS-Diktatur, Bundesrepublik und DDR im Vergleich* (Munich, 1998), 117–150.

Schulz, Jörg, "Die Rodewischer Thesen von 1963. Ein Versuch zur Reform der DDR-Psychiatrie," in Franz-Werner Kersting (ed.), *Psychiatriereform als Gesellschaftsreform. Die Hypothek des Nationalsozialismus und der Aufbruch der sechziger Jahre* (Paderborn, 2003), 87–100.

Schwegel, Andreas, *Der Polizeibegriff im NS-Staat* (Tübingen, 2005).

Schwartz, Michael and Constantin Goschler, "Ausgleich von Kriegs- und Diktaturfolgen, soziales Entschädigungsrecht," in *1949–1961 Deutsche Demokratische Republik. Im Zeichen des Aufbaus des Sozialismus (Geschichte der Sozialpolitik in Deutschland seit 1945, vol. 8)* (Berlin, 2004), 589–654.

Schweig, Nicole, *Gesundheitsverhalten von Männern. Gesundheit und Krankheit in Briefen 1800–1950* (Stuttgart, 2008).

Schwoch, Rebecka, "'... leider muss ich feststellen, dass man mich hier abgestellt hat.' Alte Menschen in den Wittenauer Heilstätten 1945 und 1946," in Thomas Beddies and Andrea Dörris (eds.), *Die Patienten der Wittenauer Heilstätten in Berlin 1919–1960* (Husum, 1999), 462–498.

Scull, Andrew, *Social Order-Mental Disorder. Anglo-American Psychiatry in Historical Perspective* (London, 1989).

Seegers, Lu, "Being Fatherless. Memories of War Children in Germany, England and Poland," *The International Journal of Evacuee and War Child Studies*, vol. 4, 2006, 87–90.

Selye, Hans, *The Story of the Adaption Syndrome* (Montreal, 1952).

Showalter, Elaine, *The Female Malady. Women, Madness and English Culture 1830–1980* (New York, 1985).

Siebenborn, Eva, "Darstellungsprobleme im medizinischen Fallbericht am Beispiel einer Hystérie Pulmonaire (1888)," in Rudolf Behrens and Carsten Zelle (eds.), *Der ärztliche Fallbericht. Epistemische Grundlagen und textuelle Strukturen darges-tellter Beobachtung* (Wiesbaden, 2012), 107–135.

Siemen, Hans-Ludwig, "Die bayerischen Heil- und Pflegeanstalten während des Nationalsozialismus," in Michael von Cranach and Hans-Ludwig Siemen (eds.), *Psychiatrie im Nationalsozialismus. Die Bayerischen Heil- und Pflegeanstalten zwi-schen 1933 und 1945* (Munich, 1999), 417–475.

Spary, Emma C., "Kennerschaft versus chemische Expertise," in Kaspar von Greyerz et al. (eds.), *Wissenschaftsgeschichte und Geschichte des Wissens im Dialog—Connecting Science and knowledge* (Göttingen, 2013), 35–60.

Steinbacher, Sybille, "Differenz der Geschlechter? Chancen und Schranken für die 'Volksgenossinnen,'" in Frank Bajohr and Michael Wildt (eds.), *Volksgemeinschaft. Neue Forschungen zur Gesellschaft des Nationalsozialismus* (Frankfurt/M., 2009), 94–104.

Steinbacher, Sybille, *Wie der Sex nach Deutschland kam. Der Kampf um Sittlichkeit und Anstand in der frühen Bundesrepublik* (Munich, 2011).

Stengel, Erwin, "Classification of Mental Disorders," *Bulletin of the World Health Organization*, vol. 21, 1959, 601–663.

Steuwer, Janosch, "Was meint und nützt das Sprechen von der 'Volksgemeinschaft'? Neue Literatur zur Gesellschaftsgeschichte des Nationalsozialismus," *AfS*, vol. 53, 2013, 487–534.

Stockdreher, Petra, "Heil- und Pflegeanstalt Eglfing-Haar," in Michael von Cranach and Hans-Ludwig Siemen (eds.), *Psychiatrie im Nationalsozialismus. Die Bayerischen Heil- und Pflegeanstalten zwischen 1933 und 1945* (Munich, 1999), 327–363.

Suzuki, Akituito, *Madness at Home. The Psychiatrists, the Patient, and the Family in England 1820–1860* (Berkeley, 2006).

Süß, Dietmar, *Tod aus der Luft. Kriegsgesellschaft und Luftkrieg in Deutschland und England* (Munich, 2011).

Süß, Sonja, *Politisch mißbraucht? Psychiatrie und Staatssicherheit in der DDR* (Berlin, 1999).

Süß, Winfried, *Der "Volkskörper" im Krieg. Gesundheitspolitik, Gesundheitsverhältnisse und Krankenmord im nationalsozialistischen Deutschland, 1939–1945* (Munich, 2003).

Süß, Winfried, "Medizin im Krieg," in Robert Jütte (ed.), *Medizin im Nationalsozialismus. Bilanz und Perspektiven der Forschung* (Göttingen, 2011), 190–200.

Szasz, Thomas, *The Myth of Mental Illness. Foundations of a Theory of Personal Conduct* (New York, 1961).

Szöllösi-Janze, Margit, "Wissensgesellschaft—ein neues Konzept zur Erschließung der deutsch-deutschen Zeitgeschichte?" in Hans Günter Hockerts (ed.), *Koordinaten deutscher Geschichte in der Epoche des Ost-West-Konflikts* (Munich, 2004), 277–307.

Szöllösi-Janze, Margit, "Wissensgesellschaft in Deutschland: Überlegungen zur Neubestimmung der deutschen Zeitgeschichte über Verwissenschaftlichungsprozesse," *GG*, vol. 30, 2004, 275–311.

Teitge, Marie and Kumbier, Ekkehardt, "Zur Geschichte der DDR-Fachzeitschrift 'Psychiatrie, Neurologie und medizinische Psychologie,'" *Der Nervenarzt*, vol. 86, 2015, 339–367.

Thiekötter, Andrea, *Pflegeausbildung in der Deutschen Demokratischen Republik* (Frankfurt/M., 2006).

Thieler, Kerstin, "Volksgenossen unter Vorbehalt. Die Herrschaftspraxis der NSDAP-Kreisleitungen und die Zugehörigkeit zur 'Volksgemeinschaft,'" in Detlef Schmiechen-Ackermann (ed.), *"Volksgemeinschaft." Mythos, wirkungsmächtige soziale Verheißung oder soziale Realität im "Dritten Reich"? Propaganda und Selbstmobilisierung im NS-Staat* (Paderborn, 2011), 211–225.

Thießen, Malte, "Schöne Zeiten? Erinnerungen an die 'Volksgemeinschaft' nach 1945," in Frank Bajohr and Michael Wildt (eds.), *Volksgemeinschaft. Neue Forschungen zur Gesellschaft des Nationalsozialismus* (Frankfurt/M., 2009), 165–188.

Thießen, Malte, "Medizingeschichte in der Erweiterung. Perspektiven für eine Sozial- und Kulturgeschichte der Moderne," *AfS*, vol. 53, 2013, 535–599.

Tönsmeyer, Tatjana and Annette Vowinckel, "Sicherheit und Sicherheitsempfinden als Thema der Zeitgeschichte: Eine Einleitung," *Zeithistorische Forschungen/ Studies in Contemporary History*, Online-Ausgabe 2, 2010, URL: http://www. zeithistorische-forschungen.de/16126041-Inhalt-2-2010 (accessed April 1, 2014).

Verheyen, Nina, "Unter Druck. Die Entstehung individuellen Leistungsstrebens um 1900," *Merkur. Zeitschrift für europäisches Denken*, vol. 5, 2012, 382–390.

Vijselaar, Joost, "Out and In. The Family and the Asylum. Patterns of Admission and Discharge in Three Dutch Psychiatric Hospitals 1890–1950," in Marijke Gijswijt-Hofstra (ed.), *Psychiatric Cultures Compared. Psychiatry and Mental Health Care in the Twentieth Century. Comparisons and Approaches* (Amsterdam, 2005), 277–294.

Voßkuhle, Andreas, "Der Gefahrenbegriff im Polizei- und Ordnungsrecht," *Juristische Schulung*, vol. 10, 2007, 908–910.

Wagner, Christina, *Psychiatrie und Nationalsozialismus in der Sächsischen Landesheil- und Pflegeanstalt Untergöltzsch* (Dresden, 2002).

Wagner, Leonie, *Nationalsozialistische Frauenansichten. Weiblichkeitskonzeptionen und Politikverständnis führender Frauen im Nationalsozialismus* (Berlin, 2010).

Wagner, Patrick, *Hitlers Kriminalisten. Die deutsche Kriminalpolizei und der Nationalsozialismus* (Munich, 2002).

Wagner-Kyora, Georg, *Vom "nationalen" zum "sozialistischen" Selbst. Zur Erfahrungsgeschichte deutscher Chemiker und Ingenieure im 20. Jahrhundert* (Stuttgart, 2009).

Walter, Bernd, "Fürsorgepflicht und Heilungsanspruch. Die Überforderung der Anstalt (1870–1930)," in Franz-Werner Kersting et al. (eds.), *Nach Hadamar. Zum Verhältnis von Psychiatrie und Gesellschaft im 20. Jahrhundert* (Paderborn, 1993), 66–97.

Walton, John L., "Lunacy in the Industrial Revolution. A Study of Asylum Admissions in Lancashire, 1845–50," *Journal of Social History*, vol. 13, 1979, 1–21.

Watzka, Carlos, "Zur Interdependenz von Personal und Insassen in 'Totalen Institutionen.' Probleme und Potentiale von Erving Goffmans 'Asyle,'" in Falk Bretschneider et al. (eds.), *Personal und Insassen von "Totalen Institutionen"—zwischen Konfrontation und Verflechtung* (Leipzig, 2011), 25–56.

Weber, Joachim, "Von der 'moral insanity' über die Psychopathie zur Persönlichkeitsstörung. Ein psychiatriegeschichtlicher Rückblick," in Reinhard Steinberg (eds.), *Persönlichkeitsstörungen. 22. Psychiatrie-Symposium* (Regensburg, 2002), 13–28.

Weber, Max, "Die protestantische Ethik und der Geist des Kapitalismus," in Max Weber (ed.), *Gesammelte Aufsätze zur Religionssoziologie I* (Tübingen, 1988), 17–206.

Weber, Max, *Wirtschaft und Gesellschaft. Grundriss der verstehenden Soziologie* (Tübingen, 2013).

Wehler, Hans-Ulrich, *Deutsche Gesellschaftsgeschichte, vol. 5: Bundesrepublik und DDR 1949–1990* (Munich, 2008).

Wentker, Hermann, "Forschungsperspektiven und -desiderate der DDR-Geschichte," in Daniel Hechler et al. (eds.), *Promovieren zur deutsch-deutschen Zeitgeschichte. Handbuch* (Berlin, 2009), 25–40.

Weinberger, Friedrich, "Schizophrenie ohne Symptome? Zum systematischen Mißbrauch der Psychiatrie in der DDR," *Zeitschrift des Forschungsverbundes SED-Staat*, vol. 25, 2009, 120–132.

Welskopp, Thomas, "Stolpersteine auf dem Königsweg. Methodische Anmerkungen zum internationalen Vergleich in der Gesellschaftsgeschichte," *AfS*, vol. 35, 1995, 339–367.

Werner, Michael and Bénédicte Zimmermann, "Vergleich, Transfer, Verflechtung," *GG*, vol. 4, 2002, 607–636.

Wernli, Martina (ed.), *Wissen und Nicht-Wissen in der Klinik. Dynamiken der Psychiatrie um 1900* (Bielefeld, 2012).

Wierling, Dorothee, *Geboren im Jahr Eins. Der Geburtsjahrgang 1949—Versuch einer Kollektivbiographie* (Berlin, 2002).

Wildt, Michael, "'Volksgemeinschaft'. Eine Antwort auf Ian Kershaw," *Zeithistorische Forschungen*, vol. 8, 2011, 102–109.

Wright, David, "Getting Out of the Asylum. Understanding the Confinement of the Insane in the Nineteenth Century," *Social History of Medicine*, vol. 10, 1997, 137–155.

Zeller, Uwe, *Psychotherapie in der Weimarer Zeit. Die Gründung der Allgemeinen Ärztlichen Gesellschaft für Psychotherapie (AÄGP)* (Tübingen, 2001).

Zimmermann, Hartmut, "Überlegungen zur Geschichte der Kader und der Kaderpolitik in der SBZ/DDR," in Hartmut Kaelble et al. (eds.), *Sozialgeschichte der DDR* (Stuttgart, 1994), 322–356.

Index

Note: Page numbers in blood refer to tables. Page numbers followed by "n" refer to notes.

prostitution 117, 119, 240, 243, 259, 284
provincial associations
(*Provinzialverbände*) 47
Prussia: General State Law (*Allgemeines Landrecht*, ALR) 38; Prussian Police Administration Law (*Polizeiverwaltungsgesetz*, PVG) 38, 39
pseudodementia 258
psychiatric committals *see* committals
psychiatric discourse 14, 32n127, 238–240, 243, 253, 254, 257
psychiatric illness 7, 14, 36, 43, 153, 165, 173, 203n69, 279
psychiatric institutions, role of 36–40
psychiatric knowledge 8, 15, 19, 35, 37, 163, 170, 183, 184, 214, 275, 279, 288, 290n4; as foil for interpretation of social problems 42–44; as war-related knowledge 40–42
Psychiatric Polyclinic of Karl Marx University: changes in committal pathways 73
psychiatrische und Nervenkliniken (psychiatric and neurological clinics) 34
psychiatrists: among themselves 177–182; differing diagnoses by 182–184; as expert 155–170; as providers of expert evaluations 40; role of 153–154; self-placement 154
psychiatry: national 171; regional 171; as supplier of knowledge 40–42
Psychiatry Inquiry of 1975 2
psycho-cognitive (*seelisch-geistig*) disturbances 251
psychopathic personalities 156
psychopaths (*Psychopathin*) 81, 156, 179, 224, 238–239, 258; asocial female 115–121; as community aliens (*Gemeinschaftsfremde*) 240; "inferiority" of 251; unstable (*haltlos*) 240, 244; weak-willed 244
psychopathy 44, 117, 118, 164–165, 169, 179, 242–249, 283; as diagnosis in Nazi era 239–242
psycho-physical experiments 204n84
psychotherapy 168–170, 200, 205n114, 206n122, 271n166
public health officers (*Amtsärzte*) 182
public safety 79; "danger to public safety" (*Gefahr für die öffentliche*

Sicherheit) 106, 113; "threat to public safety" (*Gefährdung der öffentlichen Sicherheit*) 12, 105–122
purposefulness (*Eigensinn*) 4
psychological stress 42, 169, 235, 242

"quartering institutions" (*Verwahranstalten*) 36–38, 84

racism, internal 8, 16, 215
"raving madness" (*tobender Wahnsinn*) 37, 40
raw food therapy 197
reactive depression 128, 151, 188, 189
recovery 36–38
Reich Penal Code (*Reichstrafgesetzbuch*, RStGB): § 42b 45, 50n81, 104; § 51 45
Reich's Insurance Office 40
relatives, initiation of committals by 58–64
restlessness (*innere Unruhe*) 229, 233
Rodewisch Sanatorium-Nursing Home *see* Untergöltzsch/Rodewisch Sanatorium-Nursing Home
Roelcke, Volker 43
Rosenkötter, Lutz 169
Rüdin, Ernst 44, 51n88
Rümke, Henricus Cornelius 204n72
Rüting, Torsten 175

"safeguarding cases" (*Bewahrungsfälle*) 78
safety 1, 11, 35, 36, 39, 40, 45, 46, 77, 79–81, 87, 131, 133, 135, 152, 281; "danger to public safety" (*Gefahr für die öffentliche Sicherheit*) 106, 113; "danger to the safety" (*Gefahr für die Sicherheit*) 103; definition of 135; risk 12; "threat to public safety" (*Gefährdung der öffentlichen Sicherheit*) 12, 51n83, 105–122
salary 249–250
sanatorium-nursing homes 7, 9, 33–36, 39, 41, 43, 46, 56, 57, 61, 62, 65, 68–70, 79, 80, 94n66, 95n77, 103–105, 107–111, 114, 116, 118, 119, 130, 143n33, 144n53, 144n71, 158, 185, 190, 267n93
Saxony Land Sanatorium-Nursing Home for the Mentally Ill (Sächsische

For Product Safety Concerns and Information please contact our EU
representative GPSR@taylorandfrancis.com
Taylor & Francis Verlag GmbH, Kaufingerstraße 24, 80331 München, Germany

www.ingramcontent.com/pod-product-compliance
Lightning Source LLC
Chambersburg PA
CBHW052118230326
41598CB00080B/3837

*9 7 8 1 0 3 2 7 1 6 2 2 0 *